GULF WAR and HEALTH

VOLUME 5

INFECTIOUS DISEASES

Abigail E. Mitchell, Laura B. Sivitz, Robert E. Black, *Editors*

Committee on Gulf War and Health: Infectious Diseases

Board on Population Health and Public Health Practice

INSTITUTE OF MEDICINE
OF THE NATIONAL ACADEMIES

THE NATIONAL ACADEMIES PRESS
Washington, D.C.
www.nap.edu

THE NATIONAL ACADEMIES PRESS 500 Fifth Street, NW Washington, DC 20001

NOTICE: The project that is the subject of this report was approved by the Governing Board of the National Research Council, whose members are drawn from the councils of the National Academy of Sciences, the National Academy of Engineering, and the Institute of Medicine. The members of the committee responsible for the report were chosen for their special competences and with regard for appropriate balance.

This study was supported by Contract V101(93)P-2155 between the National Academy of Sciences and the Department of Veterans Affairs. Any opinions, findings, conclusions, or recommendations expressed in this publication are those of the author(s) and do not necessarily reflect the view of the organizations or agencies that provided support for this project.

International Standard Book Number-10: 0-309-10106-9 (Book)
International Standard Book Number-13: 978-0-309-10106-6 (Book)
International Standard Book Number-10: 0-309-65706-7 (PDF)
International Standard Book Number-13: 978-0-309-65706-8 (PDF)

Library of Congress Control Number: 2006934962

Additional copies of this report are available from the National Academies Press, 500 Fifth Street, NW, Lockbox 285, Washington, DC 20055; (800) 624-6242 or (202) 334-3313 (in the Washington metropolitan area); Internet, http://www.nap.edu.

For more information about the Institute of Medicine, visit the IOM home page at **www.iom.edu.**

Printed in the United States of America.

The serpent has been a symbol of long life, healing, and knowledge among almost all cultures and religions since the beginning of recorded history. The serpent adopted as a logotype by the Institute of Medicine is a relief carving from ancient Greece, now held by the Staatliche Museen in Berlin.

"Knowing is not enough; we must apply.
Willing is not enough; we must do."

—Goethe

INSTITUTE OF MEDICINE

OF THE NATIONAL ACADEMIES

Advising the Nation. Improving Health.

COMMITTEE ON GULF WAR AND HEALTH: INFECTIOUS DISEASES

ROBERT E. BLACK, MD, MPH, Edgar Berman Professor and Chair, Department of International Health, Johns Hopkins University, Bloomberg School of Public Health, Baltimore, MD

MARTIN J. BLASER, MD, Frederick H. King Professor of Internal Medicine, Chair of the Department of Medicine, and Professor of Microbiology, New York University School of Medicine, New York

RICHARD D. CLOVER, MD, Dean and Professor, School of Public Health and Information Sciences, University of Louisville, KY

MYRON S. COHEN, MD, J. Herbert Bate Distinguished Professor of Medicine and Microbiology, Immunology and Public Health, University of North Carolina School of Medicine, Chapel Hill

JERROLD J. ELLNER, MD, Professor and Chair of the New Jersey Medical School at the University of Medicine and Dentistry of New Jersey, Newark

JEANNE MARRAZZO, MD, MPH, Associate Professor, Department of Medicine, University of Washington School of Medicine, Seattle

MEGAN MURRAY, MD, ScD, MPH, Assistant Professor of Epidemiology, Harvard University, School of Public Health, Boston, MA

EDWARD C. OLDFIELD III, MD, Director, Division of Infectious Diseases, Eastern Virginia Medical School, Norfolk

RANDALL R. REVES, MD, MSc, Professor, Division of Infectious Diseases, University of Colorado Health Sciences Center, Denver

EDWARD T. RYAN, MD, Director, Tropical and Geographic Medicine Center, Massachusetts General Hospital, and Associate Professor of Medicine, Harvard Medical School, Boston, MA

STEN H. VERMUND, MD, PhD, Amos Christie Chair and Director, Vanderbilt University Institute for Global Health, and Professor of Pediatrics, Medicine, Preventive Medicine, and Obstetrics and Gynecology, Vanderbilt University School of Medicine, Nashville, TN

DAWN M. WESSON, PhD, Associate Professor, Tulane School of Public Health and Tropical Medicine, New Orleans, LA

STAFF

ABIGAIL E. MITCHELL, PhD, Senior Program Officer
LAURA B. SIVITZ, MSJ, Senior Program Associate
DEEPALI M. PATEL, Senior Program Associate
MICHAEL J. SCHNEIDER, MPH, Senior Program Associate
PETER JAMES, Research Associate
DAMIKA WEBB, Research Assistant
DAVID J. TOLLERUD, Program Assistant
RENEE WLODARCZYK, Program Assistant
NORMAN GROSSBLATT, Senior Editor
ROSE MARIE MARTINEZ, ScD, Director, Board on Population Health and Public Health Practice

REVIEWERS

This report has been reviewed in draft form by persons chosen for their diverse perspectives and technical expertise in accordance with procedures approved by the National Research Council's Report Review Committee. The purpose of this independent review is to provide candid and critical comments that will assist the institution in making its published report as sound as possible and to ensure that the report meets institutional standards of objectivity, evidence, and responsiveness to the study charge. The review comments and draft manuscript remain confidential to protect the integrity of the deliberative process. We wish to thank the following for their review of this report:

Lawrence R. Ash, Professor Emeritus, Department of Epidemiology, University of California, Los Angeles School of Public Health
Michele Barry, Tropical Medicine and International Health Programs, Yale University School of Medicine
Herbert DuPont, School of Public Health, University of Texas Health Science Center at Houston and St. Luke's Episcopal Hospital
Robert Edelman, Travelers' Health Clinic, University of Maryland
David Hill, National Travel Health Network and Centre, Hospital for Tropical Diseases, London
Richard T. Johnson, Department of Neurology, The Johns Hopkins Hospital
Arthur Reingold, Division of Epidemiology, University of California, Berkeley
Philip K. Russell, Professor Emeritus, Johns Hopkins School of Public Health
Mark Wallace, Independent Infectious Diseases Consultant and United States Navy, Retired

Although the reviewers listed above have provided many constructive comments and suggestions, they were not asked to endorse the conclusions or recommendations nor did they see the final draft of the report before its release. The review of this report was overseen by **George Rutherford,** Institute of Global Health, University of California, San Francisco, and **Elaine L. Larson,** School of Nursing, Columbia University. Appointed by the National Research Council, they were responsible for making certain that an independent examination of this report was carried out in accordance with institutional procedures and that all review comments were carefully considered. Responsibility for the final content of this report rests entirely with the authoring committee and the institution.

PREFACE

Infectious diseases have been a problem for military personnel throughout history. The consequences in previous conflicts have ranged from frequent illnesses disrupting daily activities and readiness to widespread deaths. Preventive measures, early diagnosis, and treatment greatly limit the exposures and acute illnesses of troops today in comparison with those in armies of the past, but infections and consequent acute illnesses still occur. In addition, long-term adverse health outcomes of some pathogens are increasingly recognized.

The deployment of about 700,000 US troops to the Persian Gulf region in the Gulf War of 1991 potentially exposed them to pathogens that they had not encountered at home. After returning from that short campaign, some veterans reported symptoms and expressed the concern that they may have been exposed to biologic, chemical, or physical agents during their service in the Persian Gulf. In response to those concerns, the US Department of Veterans Affairs (VA) commissioned the Institute of Medicine (IOM) to review the scientific evidence on possible long-term adverse health outcomes of exposure to specific biologic, chemical, and physical agents and to draw conclusions on the strength of that evidence with regard to delayed and chronic illnesses of the veterans.

The authorizing legislation for the work of IOM included several infectious diseases endemic in the Persian Gulf region. In the charge to our committee, VA asked that we not limit consideration to those diseases but rather include all infectious exposures that had been documented in troops and consider their possible long-term adverse health outcomes. It further requested that the time and geographic dimensions of the committee's work be widened to include military personnel deployed as part of Operation Enduring Freedom (OEF) in Afghanistan and Operation Iraqi Freedom (OIF) in the Persian Gulf region. OEF began in 2001, and OIF in 2003; they continued as this report went to press. The number of military personnel involved in the more recent conflicts now exceeds that in the 1991 Gulf War. Furthermore, they have remained for much longer periods on the average than in the Gulf War, and many have been deployed for more than one tour in this region. Thus, the potential for exposure to endemic pathogens is greater in these troops than in those deployed to the Gulf War. Because the possible exposures are relatively recent, there has been only a short time to observe long-term adverse health outcomes. The committee needed to rely on observations from the Gulf War, information on infectious diseases in OEF and OIF, and evidence in the scientific literature to allow conclusions to be drawn on possible long-term adverse health outcomes. With further time to observe the possible consequences of infectious exposures, the knowledge base will increase. Given the continuing presence of troops in the areas and the variable nature of infectious diseases, the exposures may change.

Valuable contributions were made to this study by a number of people who shared their expertise on infectious diseases. On behalf of the committee, I thank several of them—K. Craig Hyams, MD, MPH, chief consultant, Occupational and Environmental Health Strategic Healthcare Group, VA; Michael Kilpatrick, MD, deputy director, Deployment Health Support, Department of Defense (DOD); and Alan Magill, MD, science director, Walter Reed Army Institute of Research, for presenting information on infectious diseases that have been diagnosed in military personnel during the Gulf War, OIF, and OEF and Richard Reithinger, PhD, infectious diseases consultant, for presenting information on infectious diseases that are endemic in southwest and south-central Asia to the committee at its May 26, 2005 meeting. I also thank William Winkenwerder, Jr., MD, MBA, assistant secretary for defense for health affairs, and his staff at DOD's Deployment Health Support for expeditiously providing information to the committee on DOD health-related policies. Finally, the committee is grateful for the insight provided by representatives of veteran service organizations, veterans, and others who spoke with the committee or sent in written testimony.

I am grateful for the great expertise the committee members brought to bear on this subject. Furthermore, the report would not have been successfully completed without the diligent and expert contributions of the IOM staff, led by Abigail Mitchell and including Laura Sivitz, Deepali Patel, Michael Schneider, Peter James, Damika Webb, David Tollerud, and Renee Wlodarczyk.

Robert E. Black, MD, MPH, Chair

CONTENTS

SUMMARY

Thousands of US veterans of the Persian Gulf War have reported an array of unexplained illnesses since the war ended in 1991. Many veterans have believed that the illnesses were associated with their military service in southwest Asia during the war. In response, the US Congress legislated in 1998 that the Department of Veterans Affairs (VA) use a specific procedure to determine the illnesses that warrant presumption of a connection to Gulf War service (Public Law [PL] 105-277, Persian Gulf War Veterans Act). Moreover, VA must financially compensate Gulf War veterans in whom the determined illnesses are diagnosed (PL 105-368, Veterans Programs Enhancement Act). To reach those determinations, the law states, VA must obtain independent evaluations of the scientific evidence of associations between illnesses and exposures to various chemical, physical, and biologic substances connected to military service in southwest Asia during the war. The law instructs VA to obtain the scientific evaluations from the National Academy of Sciences (NAS). NAS assigned the task of evaluating the associations to the Institute of Medicine (IOM).

This report is the fifth volume produced by IOM for VA in response to the congressional mandate.[1] A committee of nationally recognized experts in infectious diseases was appointed and charged with evaluating the scientific and medical literature on long-term adverse human health outcomes associated with selected infectious diseases pertinent to Gulf War veterans. The conclusions herein characterize the long-term adverse health outcomes associated with infection by the following pathogens: *Brucella* species (spp.), the cause of brucellosis; *Campylobacter* spp., nontyphoidal *Salmonella* spp. and *Shigella* spp., which cause diarrheal disease; *Coxiella burnetii*, the cause of Q fever; *Leishmania* spp., the cause of leishmaniasis; *Mycobacterium tuberculosis*, which causes tuberculosis; *Plasmodium* spp., the cause of malaria; and West Nile virus, the cause of West Nile fever. The committee identified those pathogens through the process outlined below. The committee then developed conclusions by studying the relevant published evidence, deliberating to reach consensus, and responding to a formal process of peer review.[2]

METHODOLOGY

IOM appointed the Committee on Gulf War and Health: Infectious Diseases in January 2005. The committee considered infections that US troops might have contracted in southwest Asia during the Persian Gulf War. At VA's request, the committee also examined infections that might have afflicted US military personnel deployed to south-central and southwest Asia for Operation Enduring Freedom (OEF)[3] and Operation Iraqi Freedom (OIF).[4] Thus, the committee's deliberations covered infectious diseases known to occur in Saudi Arabia, Kuwait, Iraq, Afghanistan, and most countries along their borders (Yemen, Oman, United Arab Emirates,

[1] Earlier IOM reports in this series present conclusions about long-term adverse health outcomes associated with exposure to depleted uranium, pyridostigmine bromide, sarin, vaccines, insecticides, solvents, propellants, combustion products, and fuels.

[2] A detailed description of how IOM studies are conducted appears at www.iom.edu/?id=32248.

[3] OEF began on October 7, 2001, in Afghanistan.

[4] OIF began on March 19, 2003.

Qatar, Bahrain, Jordan, Israel, Lebanon, Syria, Iran, Turkmenistan, Uzbekistan, Tajikistan, Kyrgyzstan, and Pakistan).

Identifying the Pathogens to Study

The committee first identified about 100 naturally occurring pathogens that could potentially have infected US troops during their service in the Gulf War, OEF, or OIF. The identified pathogens comprise viruses, bacteria, helminths, and protozoa that have been reported in southwest and south-central Asia, have historically caused outbreaks of illness in military populations, or have generated particular concern among US veterans of the Persian Gulf War. As required by PL 105-277 and PL 105-368, the pathogens include *Escherichia coli*, *Shigella* spp., *Leishmania* spp., and the *Phlebovirus* pathogens that cause sand fly fever.

Definition of Long-Term Adverse Health Outcome

The committee then developed a set of criteria for determining which infectious diseases to evaluate for strength of association with specific long-term adverse health outcomes. Long-term adverse health outcomes include secondary diseases or conditions (sequelae) caused by primary diseases, reactivation or recrudescence of diseases, and delayed presentation of diseases. A long-term adverse health outcome, the committee agreed, should have one or more of the following characteristics:

- Significant interruption of normal physical and mental function outside the timeframe of acute infection.
- Persistent organ dysfunction or damage.
- Reproductive effects in military personnel, including birth defects in their offspring.

In addition, a long-term adverse health outcome could be reversible, related to secondary transmission,[5] or both.

Development of Inclusion Criteria

Given that definition, the committee identified about 90 infectious diseases that have long-term adverse health outcomes and that were any of the following:

- Endemic in southwest or south-central Asia during the period in question.
- Diagnosed in US troops during the three deployments under study.
- Of special concern to Gulf War, OIF, or OEF veterans.
- Historically reported among military populations.

Many of the diseases have never been reported in US military personnel in close temporal relationship to deployment to southwest or south-central Asia for the Gulf War, OEF, or OIF. Even so, the committee could not rule out the possibility that one or more people contracted an unreported disease during deployment. Consequently, the committee created a tabular summary of such diseases' acute and long-term characteristics.

---

[5] In this context, secondary transmission means the spread of a pathogen directly from a primary human host to one or more other humans.

The committee further defined its infections of focus according to the likelihood that the primary infection would be subacute or the infected person would be asymptomatic for days to years, and the adverse health outcome would begin months to years after infection. In such cases, diagnosis of the long-term adverse health outcome during military service in Asia would be unlikely, and such infections were candidates for in-depth review and conclusions. In contrast, military medical personnel would probably diagnose adverse health outcomes that are manifest during the acute illness or shortly after a person's deployment.

Finally, the committee examined the likelihood that the candidate infections would have occurred specifically during military deployment to southwest and south-central Asia during the three operations in question. The risk of contracting the disease in the theater of operations must have been equal to or greater than the risk of contracting it in the United States. Moreover, given the natural history of the disease or infection, it must have been diagnosed in US troops in appropriate temporal relationship to deployment.

By applying those criteria to the dozens of infectious diseases recognized initially, the committee identified the group that required in-depth evaluation and conclusions: brucellosis, *Campylobacter* infection, leishmaniasis, malaria, Q fever, salmonellosis, and shigellosis. Two other diseases did not meet all the criteria but still merited in-depth evaluation: tuberculosis and West Nile virus infection.

Tuberculosis (TB) could cause long-term adverse health outcomes in US troops and veterans deployed to southwest and south-central Asia, where TB is highly endemic. TB has a long history of activation and transmission in military settings. Moreover, about 2.5% of military personnel deployed to OEF and OIF and given predeployment and postdeployment skin tests for TB converted from negative to positive; that is, these troops acquired new TB infections during deployment.[6] Therefore, although the committee found no published reports of active TB cases among the troops in question, conclusions about the long-term adverse health outcomes of TB infection are quite pertinent.

Unlike TB, West Nile virus (WNV) has been reported in troops deployed to southwest and south-central Asia, where the virus is endemic. The long-term adverse health outcomes associated with WNV infection are usually manifest during the acute illness—a characteristic that disqualified other diseases from comprehensive evaluation in this report. Nevertheless, dramatic changes in the epidemiology of WNV since the mid-1990s led the committee to make an exception for WNV and to review it in depth.

In addition, a small set of biologic agents, infections, and diseases that failed to meet the committee's inclusion criteria nevertheless raised serious questions that merited discussion: Al Eskan disease, biowarfare agents, idiopathic acute eosinophilic pneumonia, mycoplasmal infection, and wound infection (including wound infection caused by *Acinetobacter baumanii*, the most notable pathogenic colonizer of wounds during OEF and OIF).

Development of Conclusions

Identifying the Literature to Review and Evaluate

Conducting extensive searches of the biomedical and epidemiologic peer-reviewed literature on the diseases identified for study yielded about 20,000 potentially relevant

---

[6] Kilpatrick ME. 2005. Presentation to IOM Committee on Gulf War and Health: Infectious Diseases. Washington, DC.

references. On closer examination, some 1,200 references appeared to provide the requisite types and quality of scientific evidence for this study.

Assessing the Strength of the Evidence

By evaluating the evidence in the published scientific literature, the committee determined the relationships between each of the nine diseases of interest and specific adverse health outcomes that might appear weeks to years after the primary infection. Those relationships are conceived in terms of the strength of association between the primary infection and a specific long-term adverse health outcome.

The committee framed its conclusions in categories, described below, that qualitatively rank the strength of the evidence of an association. Used by many previous IOM committees, including those in the *Gulf War and Health* series, this five-tier framework was adapted from the system used by the International Agency for Research on Cancer to evaluate evidence of the carcinogenicity of various agents.

SUMMARY OF CONCLUSIONS

Sufficient Evidence of a Causal Relationship

> The evidence is sufficient to conclude that there is a causal relationship between exposure to a specific agent and a specific health outcome in humans. The evidence is supported by experimental data and fulfills the guidelines for sufficient evidence of an association (defined below). The evidence must be biologically plausible and must satisfy several of the guidelines used to assess causality, such as strength of association, a dose–response relationship, consistency of association, and a temporal relationship.

The committee concludes that there is sufficient evidence of a causal relationship between

- *Coxiella burnettii* infection (Q fever) and osteomyelitis.
- Malarial infection and
    - Ophthalmologic manifestations, particularly retinal hemorrhage and scarring, recognized for the first time months or years after the infection.
    - Hematologic manifestations weeks or months later, particularly anemia after falciparum malaria and splenic rupture after vivax malaria.
    - Renal disease, especially the nephrotic syndrome that may occur weeks to months after acute infection.
    - Late presentation of disease (*Plasmodium malariae*) or relapse of disease (*Plasmodium ovale or Plasmodium vivax*) months to years after acute infection.
- *Mycobacterium tuberculosis* infection and occurrence of active TB months to decades after infection.

Sufficient Evidence of an Association

> The evidence from available studies is sufficient to conclude that there is an association. A consistent association has been observed between exposure to a specific agent and a specific health outcome in human studies in which chance and bias, including confounding, could be ruled out with reasonable confidence. For example, several high-quality studies report consistent associations and are sufficiently free of bias, including adequate control for confounding.

The committee concludes that there is sufficient evidence of an association between

- Brucellosis and
    - Arthritis and spondylitis; arthritis usually is manifest within 12 months of the acute illness, and spondylitis might be manifest later.
    - Hepatic abnormalities, including granulomatous hepatitis.
    - Chronic meningitis and meningoencephalitis.
    - Uveitis.
    - Orchioepididymitis and infections of the genitourinary system.
    - Cardiovascular, nervous, and respiratory system infections.
- *Campylobacter jejuni* infection and Guillain-Barré syndrome (GBS) if GBS is manifest within 2 months of the infection.
- *Campylobacter* infection and reactive arthritis (ReA) if ReA is manifest within 3 months of the infection; most cases of ReA are manifest within 1 month of the infection.
- *Coxiella burnetii* infection (Q fever) and
    - Endocarditis years after primary infection.
    - Vascular infection years after primary infection.
    - Chronic hepatitis years after primary infection.
- *Plasmodium malariae* infection and manifestation of immune-complex glomerulonephritis years to decades later.
- *Plasmodium falciparum* infection and recrudescence weeks to months after the primary infection, but only in the case of inadequate therapy.
- Nontyphoid *Salmonella* infection and ReA if ReA is manifest within 3 months of the infection.
- *Shigella* infection and
    - Hemolytic-uremic syndrome (HUS) if HUS is manifest within 1 month of the infection; most cases of HUS are manifest within 10 days of the infection.
    - ReA if ReA is manifest within 3 months of the infection; most cases of ReA are manifest within 1 month of the infection.
- Active TB and long-term adverse health outcomes due to irreversible tissue damage from severe forms of pulmonary and extrapulmonary TB.
- Visceral leishmaniasis (kala-azar) and
    - Delayed presentation of the acute clinical syndrome.
    - Reactivation of visceral leishmaniasis in the context of future immunosuppression.
    - Post-kala-azar dermal leishmaniasis (PKDL) if PKDL occurs generally within 2 years of the initial infection.

- West Nile virus infection and variable physical, functional, or cognitive disability, which may persist for months or years or be permanent.

Limited or Suggestive Evidence of an Association

> The evidence from available studies suggests an association between exposure to a specific agent and a specific health outcome in human studies, but the body of evidence is limited by the inability to rule out chance and bias, including confounding, with confidence. For example, at least one high-quality study reports an association that is sufficiently free of bias, including adequate control for confounding. Other corroborating studies provide support for the association, but they were not sufficiently free of bias, including confounding. Alternatively, several studies of less quality show consistent associations, and the results are probably not due to bias, including confounding.

The committee concludes that there is limited or suggestive evidence of an association between

- Brucellosis and
    - Myelitis-radiculoneuritis, demyelinating meningovascular syndromes, deafness, sensorineural hearing loss, and GBS.
    - Papilledema, optic neuritis, episcleritis, nummular keratitis, and multifocal choroiditis.
    - Fatigue, inattention, amnesia, and depression.
- *Campylobacter jejuni* infection and development of uveitis if uveitis is manifest within 1 month of infection.
- *Coxiella burnetii* infection and post-Q-fever chronic fatigue syndrome years after the primary infection.
- *Plasmodium falciparum* infection and neurologic disease, neuropsychiatric disease, or both months to years after the acute infection.
- *Plasmodium vivax* and *Plasmodium falciparum* infections and demyelinating polyneuropathy and GBS.

Inadequate or Insufficient Evidence to Determine Whether an Association Exists

> The evidence from available studies is of insufficient quantity, quality, or consistency to permit a conclusion regarding the existence of an association between exposure to a specific agent and a specific health outcome in humans.

For some potential long-term adverse health outcomes of the nine identified diseases, the evidence of an association is inadequate, insufficient, or both. The committee presents these potential long-term adverse health outcomes and their characteristics in tabular form in the body of the report.

Limited or Suggestive Evidence of No Association

> Evidence from well-conducted studies is consistent in not showing an association between exposure to a specific agent and a specific health outcome after exposure of any magnitude. A conclusion of no association is inevitably limited to the conditions, magnitudes of exposure, and length of observation in the available studies. The possibility of a very small increase in risk after exposure cannot be excluded.

For many potential long-term adverse health outcomes of the nine identified diseases, there is no evidence of an association. In this report, the committee focused on identifying positive associations between specific infectious diseases and specific long-term adverse health outcomes and did not present the numerous long-term adverse health outcomes for which there is no association.

DEPARTMENT OF DEFENSE POLICIES ON TUBERCULIN SKIN TESTING AND PREDEPLOYMENT AND POSTDEPLOYMENT SERUM COLLECTION

Each branch of the US military has polices regarding tuberculin skin testing and treatment of latent TB infection (LTBI). The most effective way to mitigate TB transmission and activation is to identify and treat for LTBI. In addition, the only way to determine whether military personnel and reservists have become infected with *M. tuberculosis* during their service is to test all personnel for TB shortly before and after deployment. Such testing would make it possible to trace cases of active TB to periods of military service if that is when infection occurred.

Department of Defense (DOD) policy specifies that predeployment serum specimens for medical examinations will routinely be collected within 1 year of deployment and that postdeployment serum specimens for medical examinations will be collected no later than 30 days after arrival at the demobilization site, home station, or in-patient medical treatment facility. The committee agrees with DOD's overall policy regarding collection and use of serum specimens. However, for banked serum specimens to be most useful for determining whether infectious exposures occurred during deployment, the predeployment specimens need to be collected before travel. Current policy allows for collection of predeployment serum specimens up to 1 year after deployment. If the collection of serum is not done until after deployment, it would be difficult to ascertain whether any signs of infection found in the "predeployment" specimen are due to exposure during the current deployment or before it.

1

INTRODUCTION

Five days after the Iraqi invasion of Kuwait on August 2, 1990, the United States deployed troops to Operation Desert Shield (ODSh). The United States attacked Iraqi armed forces by air on January 16, 1991, and this marked the beginning of Operation Desert Storm (ODSt). The ground war began on February 24, 1991, and ended 4 days later. The official cease-fire took effect on April 11, 1991, and the last troops to participate in the ground war arrived back in the United States on June 13, 1991. In this report, ODSh and ODSt are also referred to collectively as the Gulf War.

About 697,000 US troops were deployed to the Persian Gulf during ODSh and ODSt. Figure 1.1 depicts the size of the US military presence in the Persian Gulf from August 1990 through June 1991. The war was considered to be a successful military operation, and there were few injuries and deaths.

Shortly after returning to the United States, a number of veterans started reporting a variety of symptoms—fatigue, headache, muscle and joint pain, sleep disturbances, and cognitive difficulties (Persian Gulf Veterans Coordinating Board 1995). The veterans were concerned that they might have been exposed to chemical, biologic, or physical agents during their deployment to the Persian Gulf and that those exposures might be responsible for their unexplained illnesses.

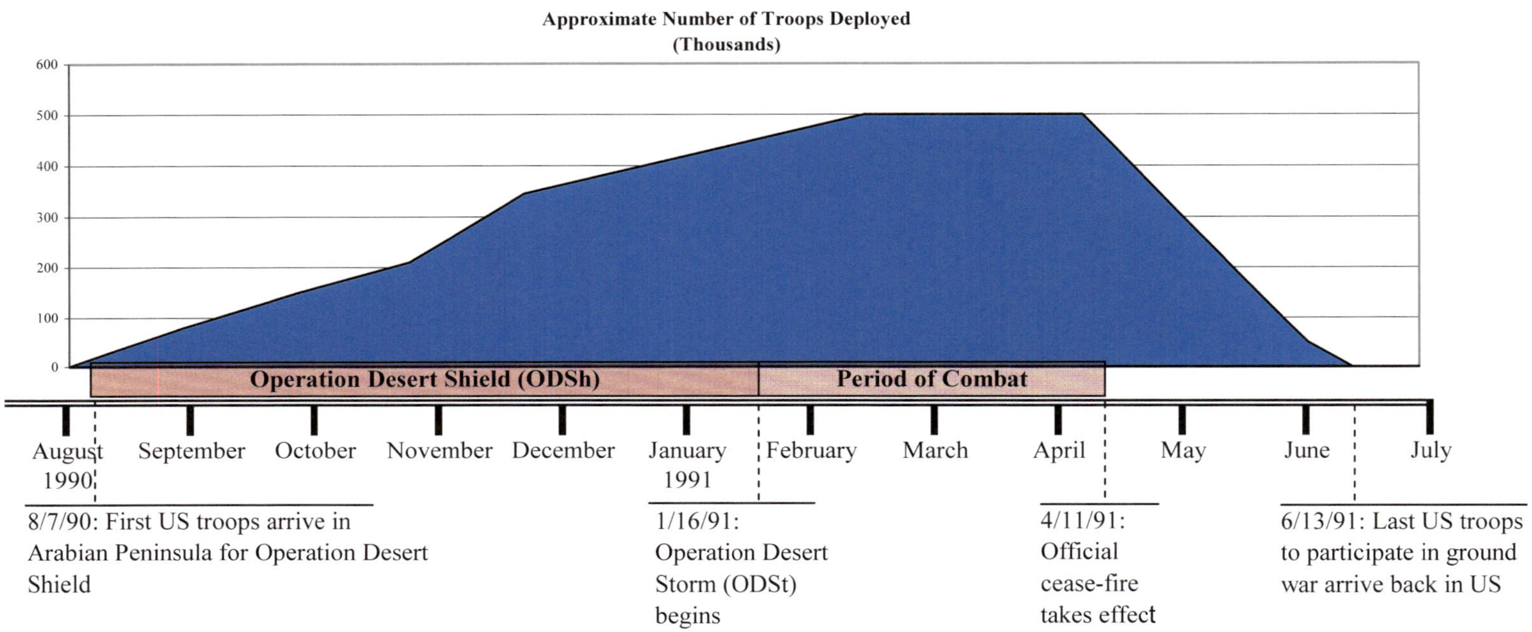

FIGURE 1.1 Operation Desert Shield and Operation Desert Storm: key dates and size of US military presence in theater.
SOURCE: DOD 2006; IOM 2000; PAC 1996.

In response to the concerns of the Gulf War veterans about their unexplained illnesses, the US Department of Veterans Affairs (VA) asked the Institute of Medicine (IOM) to conduct a study to evaluate the scientific literature on chemical, biologic, and physical agents to which military personnel in the gulf were potentially exposed and possible long-term adverse health outcomes. In addition, Congress passed two laws in 1998—the Persian Gulf War Veterans Act (PL 105-277) and the Veterans Programs Enhancement Act (PL 105-368)—that called for the review of the scientific literature on specified agents with regard to long-term adverse health outcomes. That legislation directs IOM to study a number of diverse chemical, biologic, and physical agents (listed in Box 1.1). IOM divided the task into several reviews. It has completed four reports: *Gulf War and Health, Volume 1: Depleted Uranium, Pyridostigmine Bromide, Sarin, Vaccines* (IOM 2000); *Gulf War and Health, Volume 2: Insecticides and Solvents* (IOM 2003); *Gulf War and Health Volume 3: Fuels, Combustion Products, and Propellants* (IOM 2005); and *Gulf War and Health, Volume 4: Health Effects of Serving in the Gulf War* (IOM 2006). The present report is the fifth volume in the series. An additional, related report has also been published: *Gulf War and Health: Updated Literature Review of Sarin* (IOM 2004).

Since VA asked IOM to conduct the above-mentioned study and PL 105-277 and PL 105-368 were enacted, the United States has again entered into military conflicts in southwest and south-central Asia—Operation Enduring Freedom (OEF) and Operation Iraqi Freedom (OIF). Therefore, VA has asked IOM to make this report relevant to the military personnel serving in OEF and OIF in addition to those who served in the 1991 Gulf War.

BOX 1-1 Agents Specified in PL 105-277 and PL 105-368

- The following organophosphorus pesticides:
    - Chlorpyrifos
    - Diazinon
    - Dichlorvos
    - Malathion
- The following carbamate pesticides:
    - Proxpur
    - Carbaryl
    - Methomyl
- The carbamate pyridostigmine bromide used as nerve-agent prophylaxis
- The following chlorinated hydrocarbons and other pesticides and repellents:
    - Lindane
    - Pyrethrins
    - Permethrins
    - Rodenticides (bait)
    - DEET (repellent)
- The following low-level nerve agents and precursor compounds at exposures below those which produce immediately apparent incapacitating symptoms:
    - Sarin
    - Tabun
- The following synthetic chemical compounds:
    - Mustard agents at exposures below those which cause immediate blistering
    - Volatile organic compounds
    - Hydrazine
    - Red fuming nitric acid
    - Solvents
- The following sources of radiation:
    - Depleted uranium
    - Microwave radiation
    - Radio frequency radiation
- The following environmental particulates and pollutants:
    - Hydrogen sulfide
    - Oil fire byproducts
    - Diesel heater fumes
    - Sand micro-particles
- Diseases endemic to the region (including the following):
    - Leishmaniasis
    - Sand fly fever
    - Pathogenic *Escherichia coli*
    - Shigellosis
- Time compressed administration of multiple live, ''attenuated'' and toxoid vaccines

IDENTIFYING THE INFECTIOUS DISEASES TO STUDY

In accordance with PL 105-277 and PL 105-368, IOM appointed the Committee on Gulf War and Health: Infectious Diseases and tasked it to review, evaluate, and summarize the peer-reviewed scientific and medical literature on long-term adverse health outcomes associated with selected infectious diseases pertinent to service in the Gulf War. The infectious diseases can include, but are not limited to, pathogenic *Escherichia coli* infection, shigellosis, leishmaniasis, and sand fly fever.

VA is also concerned about potential long-term adverse health outcomes of infectious diseases in veterans of OEF and OIF. As of October 2005, about 1.2 million US troops have been deployed to OEF or OIF (see Figure 1.2). VA asked IOM to evaluate infectious diseases pertinent to service in OEF and OIF.

It should be noted that the charge to IOM was not to determine whether a unique Gulf War syndrome or Gulf War illness exists or to make judgments about whether individual veterans were exposed to specific pathogens. Nor was the charge to focus on broader issues, such as the potential costs of compensation for veterans or policy regarding compensation; such decisions are the responsibility of the secretary of veterans affairs.

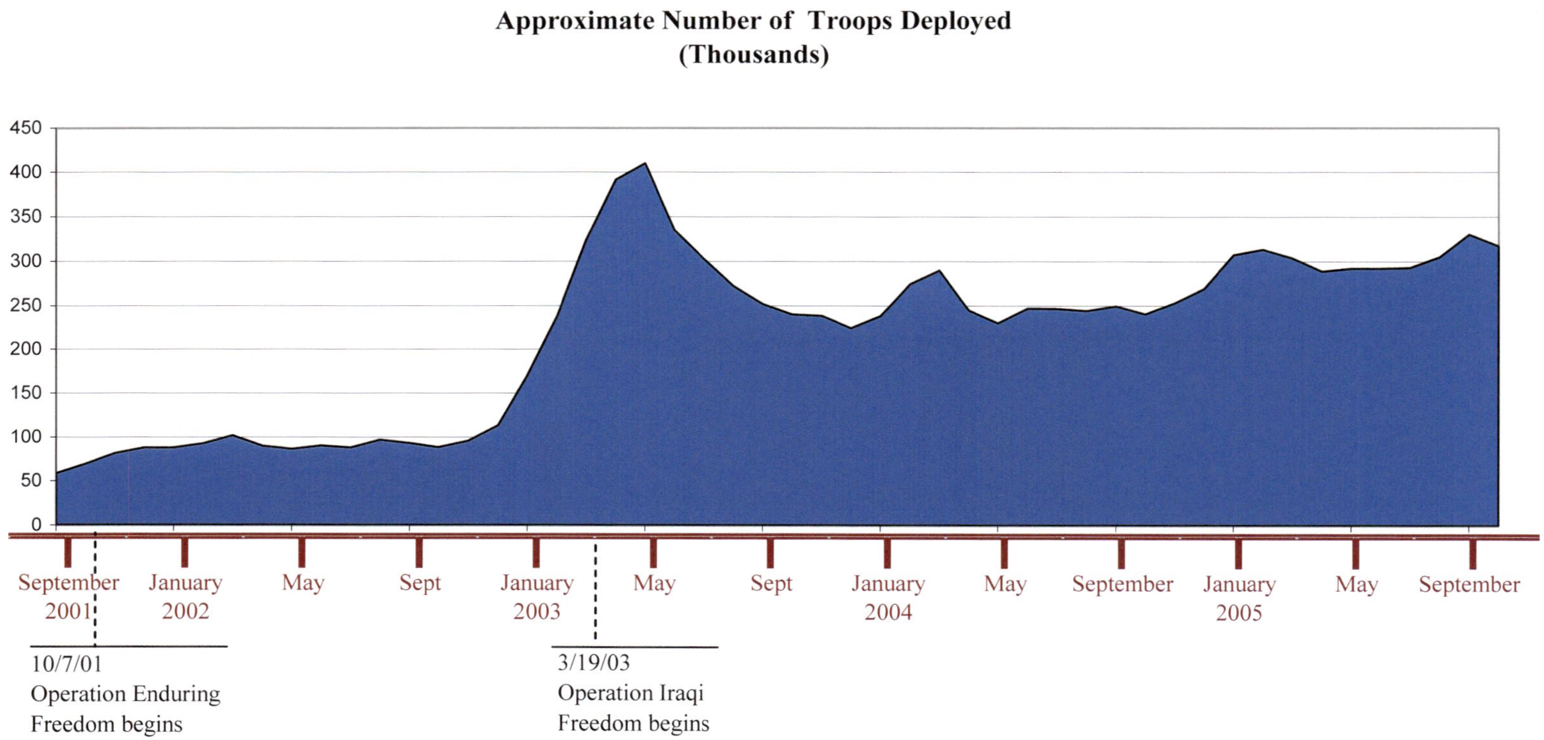

FIGURE 1.2 Operation Enduring Freedom and Operation Iraqi Freedom: key dates and size of US military presence in theater.
SOURCE: Personal Communication, Michelle Rudolph, Branch Chief, Defense Manpower Data Center, December 15, 2005.

THE COMMITTEE'S APPROACH TO ITS CHARGE

A brief overview of how the committee approached its charge is presented here. A more comprehensive explanation is provided in Chapter 2.

The committee identified numerous infectious diseases to which Gulf War, OIF, and OEF military personnel might have been exposed during their deployment. Dozens of infectious diseases are endemic to southwest and south-central Asia, which includes Iraq, Kuwait, and Afghanistan. The committee then determined which of the endemic infectious diseases are known to have long-term adverse health outcomes. To determine which infectious diseases to review in depth, the committee took several factors into account, including which ones were diagnosed in military personnel who served in the Gulf War, OEF, or OIF and in veterans after they returned home, as well as the prevalence of the infectious diseases in southwest and south-central Asia compared with their prevalence in the United States.

Overall, the incidence of infectious diseases among Gulf War military personnel was low (Hyams et al. 1995). Acute diarrheal and acute respiratory diseases were the major causes of morbidity from infectious diseases (Hyams et al. 1995; Hyams et al. 2001). The outbreaks of diarrhea were due primarily to enterotoxigenic *Escherichia coli* and *Shigella sonnei*. Some 12 cases of viscerotropic leishmaniasis and 20 cases of cutaneous leishmaniasis were diagnosed in Gulf War military personnel (Hyams et al. 1995; Hyams et al. 2001). Other reported infectious diseases included Q fever (three cases), West Nile fever (one case), and malaria (seven cases) (Hyams et al. 1995; Hyams et al. 2001).

Infectious diseases reported in troops who served in OEF and OIF as of December 2005 are visceral and cutaneous leishmaniasis, malaria, diarrheal disease, respiratory disease, tuberculosis infection (but not active tuberculosis), Q fever, brucellosis, and *Acinetobacter baumannii* infection (Kilpatrick 2005). Chapter 4 reviews the literature on infectious diseases that have been diagnosed in military personnel during or shortly after returning from the Gulf War, OIF, or OEF.

The committee identified for comprehensive evaluation nine infectious diseases known to have long-term adverse health outcomes that were diagnosed in military personnel who served in the Gulf War, OEF, or OIF. Some information is presented on a number of other infectious diseases as well because they are endemic to southwest and south-central Asia, although there have been no reported cases in military personnel through December 2005. It is possible that military personnel have become infected but that no diagnosis was made either because no acute symptoms were present or because the symptoms were mild and the soldier who had them did not seek medical care. We also present information on diseases and agents of special concern to veterans of the Gulf War, OEF, and OIF (Al Eskan disease, acute eosinophilic pneumonia, *Acinetobacter baumannii* infection, mycoplasmas, and biological warfare agents).

After determining which infectious diseases it would evaluate, the committee had to identify the relevant literature for review. The committee relied primarily on peer-reviewed published literature in developing its conclusions. It also consulted other material, such as surveillance reports, technical reports, and textbooks, and it obtained additional information from experts in infectious diseases of southwest and south-central Asia, from Deployment Health Support at the Department of Defense (DOD), from Walter Reed Army Institute of Research, from the VA Occupational and Environmental Health Strategic Healthcare Group, and from veteran service organizations and Gulf War veterans. The committee focused on medical and scientific data on long-term adverse health outcomes related to the infectious diseases it selected for study.

The final step in the committee's evaluation process was to weigh the evidence on the infectious diseases and their long-term adverse health outcomes and to develop conclusions about the strength of the evidence. The conclusions are assigned to categories of association, which range from sufficient evidence of a causal relationship to insufficient or inadequate evidence of an association.

This report includes discussion of acute diseases with potential long-term adverse health outcomes caused by known pathogens. The committee acknowledges that there might be clinically important pathogens that cannot be detected with available cultivation techniques (Relman 2002). Because the extent to which such pathogens might contribute to acute illnesses in military personnel is unknown, it is not possible to define a relationship between them and an acute illness or long-term adverse health outcome.

ORGANIZATION OF THE REPORT

Chapter 2 lays out the committee's process for selecting the infectious diseases to study and reviewing and evaluating the evidence on them. Chapter 3 presents, in tabular format, the endemic infectious diseases of southwest and south-central Asia that are known to have long-term adverse health outcomes. Chapter 4 summarizes the body of literature on infectious diseases that have been diagnosed in military personnel serving in the Gulf War, OIF, and OEF. The committee's comprehensive evaluations of selected infectious diseases are presented in Chapter 5, which also contains the committee's conclusions. The final chapter, Chapter 6, presents information about diseases and agents of special concern to veterans of the Gulf War, OIF, and OEF that have an infectious component or have been implicated as a cause of "Gulf War illness".

REFERENCES

DOD (Department of Defense). 2006. *US Department of Defense Official Website*. [Online]. Available: http://www.defenselink.mil/ [accessed March 2006].

Hyams KC, Hanson K, Wignall FS, Escamilla J, Oldfield EC, 3rd. 1995. The impact of infectious diseases on the health of US troops deployed to the Persian Gulf during operations Desert Shield and Desert Storm. *Clinical Infectious Diseases* 20(6):1497-1504.

Hyams KC, Riddle J, Trump DH, Graham JT. 2001. Endemic infectious diseases and biological warfare during the Gulf War: A decade of analysis and final concerns. *American Journal of Tropical Medicine and Hygiene* 65(5):664-670.

IOM (Institute of Medicine). 2000. *Gulf War and Health, Volume 1: Depleted Uranium, Sarin, Pyridostigmine Bromide, Vaccines.* Washington, DC: National Academy Press.

IOM. 2003. *Gulf War and Health, Volume 2: Insecticides and Solvents.* Washington, DC: The National Academies Press.

IOM. 2004. *Gulf War and Health: Updated Literature Review of Sarin.* Washington, DC: The National Academies Press.

IOM. 2005. *Gulf War and Health, Volume 3: Fuels, Combustion Products, and Propellants.* Washington, DC: The National Academies Press.

IOM. 2006. *Gulf War and Health, Volume 4: Health Effects of Serving in the Gulf War.* Washington, DC: The National Academies Press.

Kilpatrick ME. 2005. *Presentation to IOM Committee on Gulf War and Health: Infectious Diseases*. Washington, DC.

PAC (Presidential Advisory Committee). 1996. *Presidential Advisory Committee on Gulf War Veterans' Illnesses: Final Report.* Washington, DC: US Government Printing Office.

Persian Gulf Veterans Coordinating Board. 1995. Unexplained illnesses among Desert Storm veterans. A search for causes, treatment, and cooperation. Persian Gulf Veterans Coordinating Board. *Archives of Internal Medicine* 155(3):262-268.

Relman DA. 2002. New technologies, human-microbe interactions, and the search for previously unrecognized pathogens. *Journal of Infectious Diseases* 186(2 Suppl):S254-S258.

2

METHODOLOGY

This chapter articulates the committee's approach to its task. Of the dozens of pathogens known to exist in southwest and south-central Asia, the committee identified the ones that are known to cause long-term adverse health outcomes and infected at least one US veteran who served in southwest or south-central Asia in the period 1991-December 2005. The committee then oversaw a formal, comprehensive literature review that identified about 1,200 peer-reviewed studies about the late complications and latent and chronic infections that might be associated with primary infection by each of the pathogens. Those studies constituted the evidence from which the committee drew conclusions about the relationship between each primary infection and specific long-term adverse health outcomes in humans. Finally, the committee ranked the strength of the relationships through the five-category system presented at the end of this chapter.

IDENTIFYING THE INFECTIOUS DISEASES TO STUDY

Geographic Boundaries

As required by law, the committee considered infectious diseases that might have afflicted US troops who served in the 1991 Gulf War (PL 105-277 and PL 105-368). Additionally, in response to a request by the Department of Veterans' Affairs, the committee considered infectious diseases that might have afflicted US troops during Operation Enduring Freedom (OEF) or Operation Iraqi Freedom (OIF). Thus, the committee's preliminary deliberations covered infectious diseases known to occur specifically in Iraq, Kuwait, and Afghanistan and in the geographic region that includes the Arabian Peninsula, Syria, Lebanon, Israel, Iran, Qatar, Pakistan, Tajikistan, Kyrgyzstan, Uzbekistan, and Turkmenistan (Figure 2.1). The term *southwest and south-central Asia* refers to that region throughout this report.

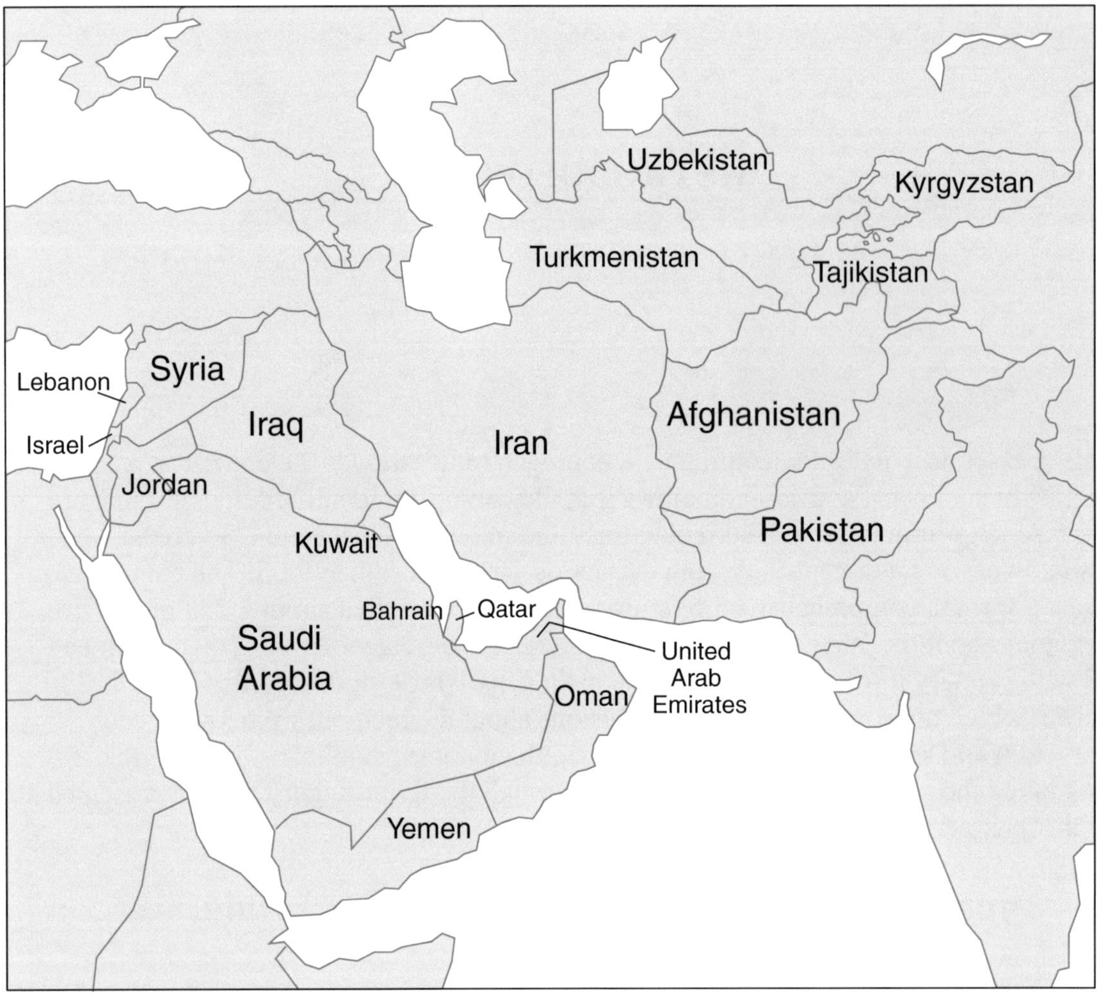

FIGURE 2.1 Southwest and South-Central Asia. The committee's preliminary deliberations covered infectious diseases known to occur specifically in Iraq, Kuwait, and Afghanistan and in the geographic region that includes the Arabian Peninsula, Syria, Iran, Qatar, Pakistan, Tajikistan, Kyrgyzstan, Uzbekistan, and Turkmenistan.
SOURCE: The National Academies Press.

Infectious Diseases Endemic to Southwest and South-Central Asia That Have Long-Term Adverse Health Outcomes

The committee approached its task by first identifying infectious diseases that could have affected US troops deployed to southwest and south-central Asia. The committee members drew upon their collective knowledge of infectious diseases, which stems from both professional experience (Appendix A) and information gathered specifically for this study. The committee acquired information from numerous sources about illnesses diagnosed in troops deployed to southwest and south-central Asia, infectious diseases known to occur in that region, and conditions of special interest to veterans. The information came from peer-reviewed journal articles, surveillance and technical reports, presentations by physicians and scientists, and veterans and representatives of veterans' groups.

Approximately 100 infectious diseases were identified for preliminary consideration (Table 2.1), including the four diseases specified in the legislation that directs the committee's work (Box 2.1).

TABLE 2.1 Diseases and Etiologic Agents Considered by the Committee for Evaluation

Disease	Etiologic Agent
Bacterial diseases	
Acinetobacter infection	*Acinetobacter baumanii* and other *Acinetobacter* species
Actinomycosis	*Actinomyces* spp.
Anthrax	*Bacillus anthracis*
Bartonellosis	*Bartonella* spp.
Cat-scratch disease	*B. henselae*
Trench fever	*B. quintana*
Botulism	*Clostridium botulinum*
Brucellosis	*Brucella* spp.
Campylobacteriosis	*Campylobacter* spp.
Capnocytophaga infection	*Capnocytophaga* spp.
Chlamydia	
Genital infections	*Chlamydia trachomatis*
Pneumonia	*Chlamydia pneumoniae*
Cholera (including vibrio infections)	*Vibrio* spp.
Diphtheria	*Corynebacterium diphtheriae*
E. coli gastroenteritis	*Escherichia coli*
	Enterotoxigenic *E. coli*
	Shiga toxin-producing *E. coli*
	Enteroaggregative *E. coli*
	Enteroinvasive *E. coli*
	Enterohemorrhagic *E. coli*
	Enteropathogenic *E. coli*
Ehrlichioses	*Ehrlichia* spp.
Enteric fever	
Paratyphoid fever	*Salmonella enterica* serovar Paratyphi A,B,C
Typhoid fever	*Salmonella enterica* serovar Typhi
Enterococcal infection (vancomycin-resistant)	*Enterococcus* spp.
Gas gangrene	*Clostridium perfringens*
Hemophilus meningitis	*Haemophilus influenzae*
*Helicobacte*r infection	*Helicobacter pylori*
Klebsiella infection	*Klebsiella* spp.
Legionnaire's disease	*Legionella* spp.
Leptospirosis	*Leptospira* spp.
Listeriosis	*Listeria monocytogenes*
Lyme disease	*Borrelia burgdorferi*
Melioidosis	*Burkholderia pseudomallei*
Meningococcal infection	*Neisseria meningitidis*
Moraxella infection	*Moraxella catarrhalis*

Disease	Etiologic Agent
Mycoplasma infection	*Mycoplasma* spp.
Nocardiosis	*Nocardia* spp. or aerobic actinomycetes
Nontuberculous mycobacterial infection	*Mycobacteria* spp. (except *M. tuberculosis* complex)
Pasteurella infection	*Pasteurella* spp.
Pertussis (whooping cough)	*Bordetella pertussis*
Plague	*Yersinia pestis*
Plesiomonas shigelloides infection	*Plesiomonas shigelloides*
Pneumococcal disease	*Streptococcus pneumoniae*
Pseudomonas infection	*Pseudomonas aeruginosa*
Q fever	*Coxiella burnetii*
Rat bite fever	*Spirillum minus*
Relapsing fever	*Borrelia spp.*
Rickettsioses	
Boutonneuse fever	*Rickettsia conorii*
Louse-borne typhus	*Rickettsia prowazekii*
Marine typhus	*Rickettsia typhi*
Ehrlichiosis	*Ehrlichia chafeensis*
Anaplasmosis	*Anaplasma phagocytophilum*
Salmonellosis (non-typhoid)	*Salmonella* spp. (except serovar Typhi)
Shigellosis	*Shigella* spp.
Staphylococcal infection	*Staphylococci* spp.
Methicillin-resistant *Staphylococcus aureus* (MRSA) infection	*S. aureus* (methicillin-resistant)
Stenotrophomonas infection	*Stenotrophomonas maltophilia*.
Streptococcal infection (group A)	*Streptococcus pyogenes*
Tetanus	*Clostridium tetani*
Tuberculosis	*Mycobacterium tuberculosis*
Tularemia	*Francisella tularensis*
Yaws (nonvenereal treponemal infection)	*Treponema pertenue*
Yersiniosis	*Yersinia enterocolitica*
Fungal diseases	
Aspergillosis	*Aspergillus* spp.
Cryptococcus	*Cryptococcus* spp.
Histoplasmosis	*Histoplasmosis capsulatum*
Mucormycosis	Fungi of the order Mucorales
Helminthic diseases	
Ascariasis	*Ascaris lumbricoides*
Echinococcosis	*Echinococcus* spp.
Enterobiasis	*Enterobius vermicularis*
Filariasis	*Wuchereria bancrofti*
Hookworm disease	*Necator americanus* and *Ancylostoma duodenale*
Onchocerciasis	*Onchocerca volvulus*
Schistosomiasis	*Schistosoma mansoni* and *S. haematobium*

Disease	Etiologic Agent
Strongyloidiasis	*Strongyloides stercoralis*
Tapeworm disease (taeniasis)	*Taenia* spp. and *Diphyllobothrium latum*
Cysticercosis	*T. solium (Cysticercus cellulosae)*
Trichinosis	*Trichinella spiralis*
Trichuriasis	*Trichuris trichiura*
Protozoan diseases	
Amebiasis	*Entamoeba histolytica*
Cryptosporidiosis	*Cryptosporidium parvum*
Cyclosporiasis	*Cyclospora cayetanensis*
Giardiasis	*Giardia lamblia*
Isosporiasis	*Isospora bella*
Leishmaniasis	*Leishmania* spp.
Malaria	*Plasmodium* spp.
Microsporidiosis	*Microsporidia* spp.
Toxoplasmosis	*Toxoplasma gondii*
Viral diseases	
Adenoviral infection	Adenovirus
Avian influenza	Influenza virus H5N1
Chickenpox (varicella)	Human herpesvirus 3 (varicella-zoster virus)
Crimean-Congo hemorrhagic fever	Crimean-Congo hemorrhagic fever virus, genus *Nairovirus*
Dengue	Dengue virus, genus *Flavivirus*
Dengue fever	
Dengue hemorrhagic fever, dengue shock syndrome	
Hantavirus hemorrhagic fever with renal syndrome and hantavirus pulmonary syndrome	genus *Hantavirus*
Influenza	Influenza virus
Rabies	Rabies virus
Retroviral diseases	Human T-cell lymphotropic virus I (HTLV-I), HTLV-II, human immunodeficiency virus (HIV)-1
Rift Valley fever	Rift Valley fever virus, genus *Phlebovirus*
Sand fly fever	Sand fly virus, genus *Phlebovirus*
Sindbis virus disease	Sindbis virus, genus *Alphavirus*
Viral enteritis	Various viruses
Rotavirus infection	group A Rotavirus
Norovirus infection	Norovirus
Viral hepatitis	Hepatitis viruses
West Nile fever	West Nile virus, genus *Flavivirus*
Miscellaneous diseases	
Acute eosinophilic pneumonia	Origin undetermined; not necessarily infectious
Idiopathic enteropathy	Origin undetermined; not necessarily infectious
Madura foot (mycetoma)	
Actinomycetoma	Various actinomycetes bacteria

Disease	Etiologic Agent
Eumycetoma	Various fungi
Nosocomial infection	*Acinetobacter baumannii* and other pathogens
Sexually transmitted diseases (STDs)	*Haemophilus ducreyi*, herpes simplex virus, HIV, human papillomavirus, HTLV, chancroid, *Chlamydia trachomatis*, *Neisseria gonorrhoeae*, *Treponema pallidum*, *Trichomonas vaginalis*, and others
Wound-associated bacterial infection	*Acinetobacter baumannii, Staphylococcus aureus,* and other pathogens

NOTE: The term *infection* refers to a primary infection that leads to disease.
SOURCE: CDC 2005; Heymann 2004; Mandell et al. 2005.

BOX 2.1 The Four Diseases Specified in PL 105-277 and PL 105-368

Leishmaniasis
Sand fly fever
Pathogenic *Escherichia coli* infection
Shigellosis

Though present in southwest or south-central Asia, some of the diseases on the committee's preliminary list do not have long-term adverse health outcomes. The committee's next step was to identify infectious diseases endemic in southwest and south-central Asia that have potential long-term adverse health outcomes, including secondary diseases or conditions (sequelae) caused by primary diseases, reactivation or recrudescence of diseases, and delayed presentation of diseases. Only diseases with known or possible long-term adverse health outcomes were selected from Table 2.1 for further evaluation.

The process began with the development of consensus on the meaning of *long-term adverse health outcomes*. Such health outcomes, the committee agreed, should have one or more of the following characteristics:

- Substantial interruption of normal physical and mental functioning occurring outside the timeframe of acute infection.
- Organ dysfunction or damage with a persistent effect.
- Reproductive effects in military personnel, including birth defects in offspring of military personnel.

A long-term adverse health outcome may be reversible. The committee also considered the potential for secondary transmission of the pathogen.

The application of these criteria to the infectious diseases listed in Table 2.1 generated the infectious diseases contained in Box 2.2: infectious diseases that are endemic to southwest and south-central Asia and have long-term adverse health outcomes.

Direct Attribution to Military Service in Southwest and South-Central Asia

The committee examined the likelihood that the candidate infections would have occurred specifically during military deployment to southwest and south-central Asia during the three operations in question. The risk of contracting a disease in the theater of operations must have been equal to or greater than the risk of contracting it in the United States. Moreover, given the natural history of the disease or infection, it must have been diagnosed in US troops in appropriate temporal relationship to deployment.

Chapter 4 comprises a review of infectious diseases that have been reported in US troops in close temporal relationship to the operations under study. On the basis of that review, the committee determined that many of the diseases in Box 2.2 have never been reported in US military personnel in close temporal relationship to deployment to southwest or south-central Asia during the Gulf War, OEF, or OIF. Nevertheless, it is impossible to prove that US troops did *not* contract any of the unreported diseases during deployment. Thus, the committee summarizes the acute and long-term characteristics of these unreported diseases in tabular form in Chapter 3 and excludes them from further analysis.

BOX 2.2 Infectious Diseases That Are Endemic in Southwest and South-Central Asia and Have Long-Term Adverse Health Outcomes

Type of Etiologic Agent			
Bacterium	**Virus**	**Protozoan**	**Helminth**
More prevalent in southwest or south-central Asia than in the United States	**More prevalent in southwest or south-central Asia than in the United States**	**More prevalent in southwest or south-central Asia than in the United States**	**More prevalent in southwest or south-central Asia than in the United States**
Anaplasmosis	Crimean-Congo hemorrhagic fever	Amebiasis	Ascariasis
Anthrax	Dengue fever	Cryptosporidiosis	Cysticercosis
Boutonneuse fever	Dengue hemorrhagic fever	Cyclosporiasis	Echinococcosis
Brucellosis	Dengue shock syndrome	Giardiasis	Enterobiasis
Campylobacter infection	Hepatitis A	Isosporiasis	Filariasis
Chancroid	Hepatitis B	Leishmaniasis	Hookworm disease
Cholera	Hepatitis C	Malaria	Onchocerciasis
E. coli gastroenteritis	Rift Valley fever	Microsporidiosis	Schistosomiasis
Ehrlichiosis	Sand fly fever	Toxoplasmosis	Strongyloidiasis
Enteric fever	Sindbis		
Helicobacter infection			
Leptospirosis	**Potentially more prevalent among troops in war theater than among US adult population**		
Lymphogranuloma venereum	Adenovirus infection		
Melioidosis	Avian influenza		
Plague	Hantaviral hemorrhagic fever with renal syndrome		
Q fever	Hantavirus pulmonary syndrome		
Rat bite fever	Influenza		
Relapsing fever	Viral enteritis		
Salmonellosis (nontyphoid)	West Nile fever		
Shigellosis			
Syphilis			
Tuberculosis			
Typhus group (louse-borne and murine)			
Yaws			
Yersinia enterocolitica infection			
Potentially more prevalent among troops in war theater than among US adult population			
Gonorrhea			
Trichomoniasis			

Bacterial diseases against which military personnel were immunized and for which vaccines are highly or fully protective
Diphtheria
Tetanus

Bacterial diseases against which military personnel were immunized and for which vaccines are partly protective
Meningococcal disease
Pertussis (whooping cough)

Bacterial diseases not more endemic in war theater than among US adult population
<u>Infections caused by</u>
Actinomyces
Bartonella
Capnocytophaga
Chlamydia pneumoniae
Clostridium botulinum
Clostridium perfringens
Francisella tularensis
Legionella
Listeria monocytogenes
Moraxella catarrhalis
Nocardia
Non-cholera *Vibrio*
Non-tuberculosis mycobacteria
Pasteurella
Plesiomonas shigelloides
Staphylococcus
Streptococcus
Streptococcus pneumoniae
Lyme disease

Antibiotic-resistant or common nosocomial infections
<u>Infections caused by</u>
Acinetobacter (Multiple drug-resistant)
Enterococcus (vancomycin-resistant)
Klebsiella (multiple drug-resistant)
Pseudomonas aeruginosa
Staphylococcus aureus (methicillin-resistant)
Stenotrophomonas maltophilia

Of special concern to US troops
Mycoplasma infection (atypical pneumonia)

Of special concern to US troops
Genital herpes
Human immunodeficiency virus-1
Human T-cell lymphotropic virus infection (I)
Human papillomavirus

Viral disease not more endemic in war theater than among U.S. adult population
Chickenpox (varicella)

NOTE: The term *infection* refers to a primary infection that leads to disease.

Timing of Appearance of Long-Term Adverse Health Outcomes

Next, the committee determined the likelihood that a disease's long-term adverse health outcomes would have been manifest and diagnosed during a person's term of military service.

If the onset of adverse health outcomes typically occurs during the acute illness, the committee reasoned, the long-term effects would probably be detected, diagnosed, and reported during the patient's term of military service. Likewise, diseases that have an acute phase—meaning that signs and symptoms become evident suddenly within hours or days of infection—are readily diagnosed during military service if the individual seeks medical care; in such cases, the physician would probably be cognizant of possible long-term adverse health outcomes. Finally, pre-existing conditions that were mild or latent before deployment but became reactivated or exacerbated during deployment also would probably be diagnosed during the patient's military service. Therefore, infectious diseases with one or both of the following characteristics were *not* comprehensively evaluated in this study; instead, their acute and long-term health outcomes are summarized in tabular form in Chapter 3:

- Onset of long-term adverse health outcomes typically occurs during the acute illness.
- The disease is a preexisting infection that becomes reactivated or exacerbated during deployment.

In contrast, the committee determined, there are other infectious diseases whose long-term adverse health outcomes were *unlikely* to be diagnosed during military service in southwest and south-central Asia. Such diseases have the following characteristics:

- The primary infection is subacute or the infected person is asymptomatic for days to years.
- Long-term adverse health outcomes begin months to years after infection.

Because a subacute infection may go unnoticed and undiagnosed, the committee reasoned, the primary disease might not be reported. Furthermore, if long-term adverse health outcomes begin months or even years after infection, the condition would be more likely to be diagnosed after the person completes military service, and the diagnosing physician may not attribute the patient's signs and symptoms to an infection acquired during deployment, particularly if the disease is uncommon in the United States, and thus more likely to be misdiagnosed. Infectious diseases that fit those criteria qualified for in-depth study.

The Infectious Diseases to Be Studied for Strength of Association with Long-Term Adverse Health Outcomes

The committee identified nine infectious diseases (Box 2.3) known to have long-term adverse health outcomes and to be potentially acquired by infected veterans during their military deployment to southwest and south-central Asia from 1991 to 2005. The committee conducted comprehensive reviews of the literature on the potential long-term adverse health outcomes of these diseases to determine the strength of association between the primary infection and the health outcome in humans.

BOX 2.3 Infectious Diseases with Long-Term Adverse Health Outcomes Studied for Strength of Association

Brucellosis
Campylobacteriosis
Leishmaniasis
Malaria
Q fever
Salmonellosis
Shigellosis
Tuberculosis
West Nile fever

Reasons for Excluding *E. coli* and Sand Fly Fever from In-Depth Study

Two of the infectious diseases named in PL 105-277 and PL 105-368—*E. coli* and sand fly fever—do not fulfill the above criteria for in-depth evaluation.

E. coli

Diarrheal infections were among of the most common ailments diagnosed in military personnel in regional theaters, and pathogenic *E. coli* is a well-recognized cause of diarrheal syndromes. The committee considered various infections related to pathogenic *E. coli*, focusing its attention on the role of pathogenic *E. coli* in diarrheal diseases. The unifying clinical syndrome associated with the various *E. coli* infections is a diarrheal illness that in healthy adults is usually transient without long-term adverse health outcomes. Therefore, the committee summarizes the health outcomes of *E. coli* infections in Chapter 3.

Sand Fly Fever

There are no published reports of sand fly fever in military personnel who served in the Gulf War; however, results from a search, requested by the Institute of Medicine (IOM), of a Department of Defense Gulf War hospitalization database identified five cases of this disease (the database and the search results are described in Chapter 4). As of December 2005, sand fly fever has not been found in military personnel serving in OIF and OEF. Sand fly fever is associated with a long-term adverse health outcome; however, the onset of the health outcome typically occurs during the acute illness. Therefore, the committee summarizes the health outcomes of sand fly fever in Chapter 3.

Comments on Diseases and Agents of Special Interest to Gulf War, OEF, and OIF Veterans

Several diseases and agents are of special interest to veterans of the Gulf War, OEF, and OIF. There is concern among Gulf War veterans that their symptoms might be connected to infection with *Mycoplasma fermentans* from contaminated vaccines (Nicolson et al. 2003) or exposure to biologic-warfare agents. In addition, during the Gulf War, troops stationed at Al Eskan Village, Saudi Arabia, developed respiratory illnesses at a high rate (Korenyi-Both et al. 1997; Korenyi-Both et al. 1992). The disease was termed Al Eskan disease and it has been hypothesized that a pathogen might be the cause. More recently, idiopathic acute eosinophilic pneumonia (IAEP) has been diagnosed in 18 military personnel serving in OIF or OEF (Shorr et al. 2004). IAEP is a syndrome characterized by febrile illness, diffuse pulmonary infiltrates, and pulmonary eosinophila (Allen et al. 1989; Badesch et al. 1989; Philit et al. 2002). There is also a discussion of wound-associated infections (for example, infections caused by *Acinetobacter baumannii*) that appear to be more prevalent in OIF and OEF personnel than in civilian populations (Davis et al. 2005). Chapter 6 discusses Al Eskan disease, IAEP, wound-associated infections, mycoplasmas, and biologic-warfare agents.

REVIEW AND EVALUATION OF THE LITERATURE

Selection of the Literature

The committee adopted a policy of basing its conclusions primarily on peer-reviewed, published literature. Non-peer-reviewed publications provided additional information for the committee and raised issues that were researched further in the peer-reviewed literature.

Although the process of peer review by fellow professionals ensures high standards of quality, it does not guarantee the validity of a study or the generalizability of its results. Accordingly, committee members read each study critically and considered its relevance and quality.

Amassing the Literature

The committee oversaw a multistep process for amassing a robust collection of scientific literature about the long-term adverse health outcomes of the diseases listed in Box 2.3. The process began with a search of PubMed, a database created and managed by the National Library of Medicine that includes more than 15 million citations of biomedical publications from the 1950s to the present. The PubMed search focused on journal articles published through December 2005 that contain information about late complications, long-term sequelae, and latent infections related to the relevant infectious diseases and etiologic agents identified by the committee. Additional studies were identified from the reference lists of topical technical reports, textbooks, and other documents. Further PubMed searches identified pertinent articles on Al Eskan disease, IAEP, wound-associated infections, mycoplasmas, and biologic-warfare agents. Those initial searches generated about 20,000 articles.

Reviewing the Literature

On closer examination of that large body of literature, a subset of about 1,200 articles appeared to provide the types and quality of scientific evidence that the committee needed to accomplish its task. After securing the full text of those articles, the committee reviewed and assessed them for evidence of associations between primary infections by the etiologic agents of interest and specific long-term adverse health outcomes in humans.

The committee included several types of studies, including epidemiologic studies, case reports, and case series. Ideally, epidemiologic studies should have methodologic details, a control or reference group, reasonable adjustment for confounders, and statistical power to detect effects. Review articles, technical reports, and textbooks were used for background information.

The committee relied heavily on studies that focused on human adult populations. Because the IOM task concerns adults who may have become infected during military service, studies of children were generally excluded unless the studies dealt with reproductive outcomes. One exception is that studies of children were included if they provided information about adult diseases; for example, a study on cerebral malaria in children might be reviewed if it provided information about the disease in adults.

CATEGORIES OF STRENGTH OF ASSOCIATION

The committee's goal was to use the evidence in the medical and scientific literature to determine the relationships between the infectious diseases of interest and specific adverse health outcomes that might appear months to years after primary infections. Those relationships, presented in Chapter 5, are conceived in terms of the "strength of association" between a primary infection and a specific long-term adverse health outcome. The committee ranks strength of association qualitatively using a five-tier system, presented below in full.

Origin and Evolution of the Categories

A brief historical overview of the committee's categories of association will elucidate their scientific roots. The International Agency for Research on Cancer (IARC), part of WHO, established criteria in 1971 to evaluate the human carcinogenic risk posed by chemicals (IARC 1998). First published in 1972, IARC's evaluations are scientific, qualitative judgments by ad hoc working groups about the evidence of carcinogenicity or noncarcinogenicity provided by the available data. The working groups express their qualitative judgments in terms of five categories of the relative strength of the evidence that a substance or exposure is carcinogenic (IARC 1999a). Agencies in 57 countries use IARC's published evaluations—a reflection of the widespread acceptance of the categorization scheme as it has been updated and applied to about 900 agents, mixtures, and exposures (IARC 1999b; IARC 2005).

In the early 1990s, an IOM committee adopted IARC's categories in evaluating the adverse health outcomes of pertussis and rubella vaccines (IOM 1991). Later IOM committees used the categories, with some modifications, in evaluating the safety of childhood vaccines (IOM 1994a), the health outcomes of herbicides used in Vietnam (IOM 1994b; IOM 1996; IOM 1999; IOM 2001; IOM 2003b), and the relationship between indoor pollutants and asthma (IOM 2000a). The present committee's predecessors also adapted and used the categories in evaluating the health effects of outcomes given to US troops and of chemical exposures that may have occurred during the Gulf War (IOM 2000b; IOM 2003a; IOM 2004; IOM 2005).

The five categories of strength of association used in this report are presented and defined below.

Sufficient Evidence of a Causal Relationship

Evidence from available studies is sufficient to conclude that there is a causal relationship between exposure to a specific agent and a specific health outcome in humans. The evidence includes supporting experimental data and fulfills the guidelines for sufficient evidence of an association (see next category). The association is biologically plausible, and the evidence satisfies several of the guidelines used to assess causality, such as strength of association, dose-response relationship, consistency of association, and a temporal relationship.

Sufficient Evidence of an Association

Evidence from available studies is sufficient to conclude that there is an association. A consistent association has been observed between exposure to a specific agent and a specific health outcome in several high-quality human studies in which chance and bias, including confounding, could be ruled out with reasonable confidence.

Limited or Suggestive Evidence of an Association

Evidence from available studies suggests an association between exposure to a specific agent and a specific health outcome, but the body of evidence is limited by the inability to rule out chance and bias, including confounding, with confidence. For example, at least one high-quality study that is sufficiently free of bias, including adequate control for confounding, reports an association, while other studies provide support for the association but are not sufficiently free of bias, including confounding. Alternatively, several studies of lesser quality are consistent in showing an association, and the results are probably not due to bias, including confounding.

Inadequate or Insufficient Evidence to Determine Whether an Association Exists

Evidence from available studies is of insufficient quantity, quality, or consistency to permit a conclusion regarding the existence of an association between exposure to a specific agent and a specific health outcome in humans.

Limited or Suggestive Evidence of No Association

Evidence from well-conducted studies is consistent in not showing an association between exposure of any magnitude to a specific agent and a specific health outcome in humans. A conclusion of no association is inevitably limited to the conditions, magnitudes of exposure, and length of observation in the available studies. The possibility of a very small increase in risk after the exposure studied cannot be excluded.

REFERENCES

Allen JN, Pacht ER, Gadek JE, Davis WB. 1989. Acute eosinophilic pneumonia as a reversible cause of noninfectious respiratory failure. *New England Journal of Medicine* 321(9):569-574.

Badesch DB, King TE Jr., Schwarz MI. 1989. Acute eosinophilic pneumonia: A hypersensitivity phenomenon? *American Review of Respiratory Disease* 139(1):249-252.

CDC (Centers for Disease Control and Prevention). 2005. *Health Information for International Travel 2005-2006.* Centers for Disease Control and Prevention. Atlanta, GA: US Department of Health and Human Services, Public Health Service.

Davis KA, Moran KA, McAllister CK, Gray PJ. 2005. Multidrug-resistant Acinetobacter extremity infections in soldiers. *Emerging Infectious Diseases* 11(8):1218-1224.

Heymann DL. 2004. *Control of Communicable Diseases Manual.* Washington, DC: American Public Health Association.

IARC (International Agency for Research on Cancer). 1998. *Preamble to the IARC Monographs*. [Online]. Available: http://www-cie.iarc.fr/monoeval/background.html [accessed July 19, 2005].

IARC. 1999a. *Evaluation. Preamble to the IARC Monographs.* [Online]. Available: http://www-cie.iarc.fr/monoeval/eval.html [accessed August 3, 2005].

IARC. 1999b. *Objective and Scope. Preamble to the IARC Monographs*. [Online]. Available: http://www-cie.iarc.fr/monoeval/objectives.html [accessed August 3, 2005].

IARC. 2005. *Monographs on the Evaluation of Carcinogenic Risks to Humans*. [Online]. Available: http://www-cie.iarc.fr/ [accessed August 3, 2005].

IOM (Institute of Medicine). 1991. *Adverse Effects of Pertussis and Rubella Vaccines*. Washington, DC: National Academy Press.

IOM. 1994a. *Adverse Events Associated With Childhood Vaccines: Evidence Bearing on Causality*. Washington, DC: National Academy Press.

IOM. 1994b. *Veterans and Agent Orange: Health Effects of Herbicides Used in Vietnam.* Washington, DC: National Academy Press.

IOM. 1996. *Veterans and Agent Orange: Update 1996*. Washington, DC: National Academy Press.

IOM. 1999. *Veterans and Agent Orange: Update 1998*. Washington, DC: National Academy Press.

IOM. 2000a. *Clearing the Air: Asthma and Indoor Air Exposures.* Washington, DC: National Academy Press.

IOM. 2000b. *Gulf War and Health, Volume 1: Depleted Uranium, Sarin, Pyridostigmine Bromide, Vaccines.* Washington, DC: National Academy Press.

IOM. 2001. *Veterans and Agent Orange: Update 2000*. Washington, DC: National Academy Press.

IOM. 2003a. *Gulf War and Health, Volume 2: Insecticides and Solvents.* Washington, DC: The National Academies Press.

IOM. 2003b. *Veterans and Agent Orange: Update 2002*. Washington, DC: The National Academies Press.

IOM. 2004. *Gulf War and Health: Updated Literature Review of Sarin.* Washington, DC: The National Academies Press.

IOM. 2005. *Gulf War and Health, Volume 3: Fuels, Combustion Products, and Propellants.* Washington, DC: The National Academies Press.

Korenyi-Both AL, Korenyi-Both AL, Molnar AC, Fidelus-Gort R. 1992. Al Eskan disease: Desert Storm pneumonitis. *Military Medicine* 157(9):452-462.

Korenyi-Both AL, Korenyi-Both AL, Juncer DJ. 1997. Al Eskan disease: Persian Gulf syndrome. *Military Medicine* 162(1):1-13.

Mandell GL, Bennett JE, Dolin R. 2005. *Principles and Practice of Infectious Diseases*. 6th ed. Philadelphia, PA: Elsevier Churchill Livingstone.

Nicolson GL, Nasralla MY, Nicolson NL, Haier J. 2003. High prevalence of mycoplasma infections in symptomatic (Chronic Fatigue Syndrome) family members of mycoplasma-positive Gulf War illness patients. *Journal of the Chronic Fatigue Syndrome* 11(2):21-36.

Philit F, Etienne-Mastroianni B, Parrot A, Guerin C, Robert D, Cordier JF. 2002. Idiopathic acute eosinophilic pneumonia: A study of 22 patients. *American Journal of Respiratory and Critical Care Medicine* 166(9):1235-1239.

Shorr AF, Scoville SL, Cersovsky SB, Shanks GD, Ockenhouse CF, Smoak BL, Carr WW, Petruccelli BP. 2004. Acute eosinophilic pneumonia among US Military personnel deployed in or near Iraq. *Journal of the American Medical Association* 292(24):2997-3005.

3

INFECTIOUS DISEASES ENDEMIC TO SOUTHWEST AND SOUTH-CENTRAL ASIA THAT HAVE LONG-TERM ADVERSE HEALTH OUTCOMES

In Chapter 2, the committee developed an extensive list of infectious diseases that are endemic to southwest and south-central Asia (Table 2.1) and then narrowed the list to diseases or syndromes with known long-term adverse health outcomes (Box 2.2). Although most diseases in that subset have not been reported in military personnel deployed to southwest and south-central Asia, they have historically been diagnosed in local populations and thus pose a theoretical risk to US troops deployed to the region. Also, given the nature and duration of Operation Iraqi Freedom and Operation Enduring Freedom, some of the diseases in Box 2.2 could be diagnosed after a person's deployment or period of military service.

The committee decided that the most effective way to give additional information on the diseases listed in Box 2.2 would be to present them in tables containing

- A description of the acute syndrome in adults,
- A description of the potential long-term adverse health outcomes in adults with clinical disease,
- The frequency with which the long-term adverse health outcomes occur in adults with clinical disease,
- The delay, if any, between acute infection and onset of long-term adverse health outcomes.

Tables 3.1-3.4 categorize the infections of interest by type of pathogen (viral, bacterial, helminthic, or protozoan), and Table 3.5 describes sexually transmitted diseases. The infectious diseases with long-term adverse health outcomes that have been diagnosed in military personnel and that the committee reviewed in depth (see Chapter 5) are also included here.

TABLE 3.1 Bacterial Diseases That Are Endemic to Southwest and South-Central Asia and Have Potential Long-Term Adverse Health Outcomes

		Potential Long-Term Outcomes in Adults with Clinical Disease		
Disease or Syndrome	**Acute Syndrome(s) in Adults**	**Disease(s), Syndrome(s), or Clinical Features**	**Frequency of Occurrence of Outcomes[a]**	**Delay Between Acute Infection and Onset of Outcomes[b]**
	More Prevalent in Southwest and South-Central Asia Than in the United States			
Anthrax (*Bacillus anthracis*)	*Abdominal anthrax*: initially fever, acute gastroenteritis, vomiting, bloody diarrhea; hemorrhagic lesions of intestinal lumen followed by massive infected ascites, septicemia, death	Sepsis or infection-related organ damage	Frequent	No
	Inhalational anthrax: fever, chills, malaise, cough, nausea or vomiting, dyspnea, sweats, chest discomfort or pleuritic pain, muscle aches, headache followed by respiratory distress due to hemorrhagic mediastinitis and mediastinal lymphadenitis with pleural effusions; often terminates in respiratory damage, shock, death	Sepsis or infection-related organ damage	Frequent	No
	Oropharyngeal anthrax: fever, lesion in oral cavity, pharyngeal pain, cervical edema, local lymphadenitis	Sepsis or infection-related organ damage	Frequent	No
	Cutaneous anthrax: eschar with surrounding edema, regional lymphadenopathy, fever, malaise, headache; bacteremia in 5% of untreated persons	Sepsis or infection-related organ damage	Rare	No
Brucellosis[c] (*Brucella* spp) (see Chapter 5 for detailed discussion)	Fever, headache, myalgia, hepatosplenomegaly, arthritis, meningoencephalitis	Arthritis	Common (if untreated)	Yes (weeks to years)
		Fatigue	Common	Yes (weeks to years)
		Hepatic abnormalities	Rare	Yes (weeks to years)
		Mental inattention	Rare	Yes (weeks to years)
		Neurologic disease	Rare	Yes (weeks to years)

Disease or Syndrome	Acute Syndrome(s) in Adults	Potential Long-Term Outcomes in Adults with Clinical Disease		
		Disease(s), Syndrome(s), or Clinical Features	**Frequency of Occurrence of Outcomes[a]**	**Delay Between Acute Infection and Onset of Outcomes[b]**
		Osteomyelitis; cardiovascular, splenic, renal, hepatic, respiratory, nervous system, other abscesses	Rare	Yes (weeks to years)
		Sepsis or infection-related organ damage	Very rare	No
		Chronic meningitis and meningoencephalitis	Very rare	Yes (weeks to years)
		Eye involvement (including uveitis)	Very rare	Yes (weeks to years)
Enteric fever (typhoid fever, *Salmonella enterica* serovar Typhi; paratyphoid fever, *S. enterica* serovars Paratyphi A, B, C)	Fever, bacteremia, headache, lymphadenopathy, enlarged liver or spleen, encephalopathy, intestinal rupture and hemorrhage	Endovascular infection	Rare	No
		Postinfection enteropathy[d]	Rare	No
		Sepsis or infection-related organ damage	Rare	No
		Chronic intestinal carriage	Rare	Yes (months to years)
		Infection of gall bladder or gall stones	Rare	Yes (months to years)
		Focal infections or abscesses	Very rare	Yes (weeks to months)
Helicobacter pylori infection	Usually asymptomatic; occasionally gastritis	Atrophic gastritis	Common	Yes (years to decades)
		Duodenal ulcer disease	Rare	Yes (months to years)
		Gastric ulcer disease	Rare	Yes (months to years)
		Gastric cancer	Very rare	Yes (years to decades)
Plague (*Yersinia pestis*)	*Bubonic plague*: sudden onset of high fever, enlarged and tender lymph nodes; patchy bleeding under skin, may progress to pneumonia or septicemic forms	Sepsis or infection-related organ damage	Frequent	No
	Pneumonic plague: headache, fever, malaise, muscle pain, pneumonia with cough and bloody sputum; often terminates in respiratory collapse, hemodynamic collapse, death	Sepsis or infection-related organ damage	Frequent	No

Disease or Syndrome	Acute Syndrome(s) in Adults	Potential Long-Term Outcomes in Adults with Clinical Disease: Disease(s), Syndrome(s), or Clinical Features	Frequency of Occurrence of Outcomes[a]	Delay Between Acute Infection and Onset of Outcomes[b]
	Septicemic plague: skin infection leads to bacteremia and severe endotoxemia, often followed by shock, disseminated intravascular coagulation, acute respiratory distress syndrome; fatal if untreated	Sepsis or infection-related organ damage	Frequent	No
Q fever[c] (*Coxiella burnetti*) (see Chapter 5 for detailed discussion)	Fever, headache, myalgia, pneumonitis, hepatosplenomegaly, meningoencephalitis	Neurologic residua of meningoencephalitis	Very rare	No
		Endovascular infections, osteomyelitis	Very rare	Yes (weeks to months)
		Chronic hepatitis	Very rare	Yes (weeks to months)
		Post-Q fever fatigue syndrome	Unknown	Unknown
Tuberculosis[c] (*Mycobacterium tuberculosis*) (see Chapter 5 for detailed discussion)	Initial infection asymptomatic (positive tuberculosis skin test or gamma interferon release assay); progression to active tuberculosis in 1-5%	Tuberculosis of lungs, pleura, lymph nodes; meningitis; musculoskeletal, genitourinary, other system effects	Common	Yes (months to decades)
		Long-term adverse health outcomes of active tuberculosis	Common	Yes (months to decades)
Enteric infections				
Campylobacter infection[c] (*Campylobacter jejuni*) (see Chapter 5 for detailed discussion)	Diarrhea, fever, abdominal pain	Postinfection enteropathy[d]	Very rare	No
		Guillain-Barré syndrome	Very rare	Yes (weeks)
		Reactive arthritis	Very rare	Yes (weeks)
		Uveitis	Very rare	Yes (weeks)
		Ankylosis spondylitis	Very rare	Yes (months)
Cholera (*Vibrio cholerae*)	Watery diarrhea, may be severe	Shock-related organ damage	Rare	No
Escherichia coli gastroenteritis				
Enterohemorrhagic *E. coli*	Bloody diarrhea, low or absent fever, hemolytic uremic syndrome, 5-10 days after onset of gastroenteritis	Renal damage	Common	No

Disease or Syndrome	Acute Syndrome(s) in Adults	Potential Long-Term Outcomes in Adults with Clinical Disease		
		Disease(s), Syndrome(s), or Clinical Features	Frequency of Occurrence of Outcomes[a]	Delay Between Acute Infection and Onset of Outcomes[b]
Other pathogenic strains of *E. coli*	Watery diarrhea, may be severe	Postinfection enteropathy[d]	Very rare	No
		Shock-related organ damage	Very rare	No
Melioidosis (*Burkholderia pseudomallei*)	Fever, chills, pneumonia, cellulitis, osteomyelitis, abscesses, bacteremia	Sepsis or infection-related organ damage	Rare	No
		Abscesses, osteomyelitis	Rare	Yes (weeks to years)
		Relapses of pulmonary disease	Rare	Yes (weeks to years)
Plesiomonas shigelloides infection	Intestinal manifestations—watery diarrhea or colitis-like dysentery; fever	Chronic diarrhea	Rare	No
		Sepsis or infection-related organ damage	Very rare	No
Salmonellosis (nontyphoid)[c] (*Salmonella* spp.) (see Chapter 5 for detailed discussion)	Diarrhea, abdominal pain, nausea, fever	Endovascular infection	Very rare	No
		Postinfection enteropathy[d]	Very rare	No
		Prosthesis infection	Very rare	No
		Sepsis or infection-related organ damage	Very rare	No
		Reactive arthritis	Very rare	Yes (weeks)
		Reiter's syndrome (inflammatory arthritis, conjunctivitis, urethritis)	Very rare	Yes (weeks)
		Abscesses, local infection	Very rare	No
		Chronic intestinal colonization	Very rare	No
		Gall bladder infection	Very rare	No
Shigellosis[c] (*Shigella* spp.) (see Chapter 5 for detailed discussion)	Diarrhea (may be bloody), fever, abdominal pain	Postinfection enteropathy[d]	Very rare	No
		Sepsis or infection-related organ damage	Very rare	No
	S. dysenteriae: hemolytic uremic syndrome (HUS)	Renal failure (HUS-related)	Very rare	Yes (days)
		Reactive arthritis	Very rare	Yes (weeks)
		Uveitis	Very rare	Yes (weeks)
		Ankylosis spondylitis	Very rare	Yes (months)
Yersinia enterocolitica infection	Diarrhea, abdominal pain, fever, mesenteric lymphadenopathy, intestinal obstruction,	Reactive arthritis	Common	Yes (weeks)

Disease or Syndrome	Acute Syndrome(s) in Adults	Potential Long-Term Outcomes in Adults with Clinical Disease: Disease(s), Syndrome(s), or Clinical Features	Frequency of Occurrence of Outcomes[a]	Delay Between Acute Infection and Onset of Outcomes[b]
	hemorrhage perforation, sepsis			
		Abscesses, local infections	Very rare	No
		Sepsis or infection-related organ damage	Very rare	No
		Reiter's syndrome	Very rare	Yes (weeks)
		Ankylosing spondylitis	Very rare	Yes (weeks to months)
Rickettsioses				
Boutonneuse fever (*Rickettsia conorii* and related species)	Dermal eschar followed by fever; headache; myalgias; rash on trunk, extremities, and face; disseminated vascular infection and vascular leakage; focal hepatocellular necrosis; granuloma-like lesions	Shock or infection-related organ damage	Rare	No
Ehrlichiosis (*Ehrlichia chaffeensis*) and anaplasmosis (*Anaplasma phagocytophilum*)	Abrupt onset of fever, severe headache, myalgia, vomiting, nausea, rash, lymphadenopathy, confusion, decreased blood counts, liver abnormalities	Shock or infection-related organ damage	Very rare	No
Louse-borne typhus (*R. prowazekii*)	Abrupt onset of headache, fever, chills, myalgia; rash begins at axillary folds of trunk and spreads to extremities; sometimes also non-productive cough, deafness, tinnitus; high fever causes altered mental state	Shock or infection-related organ damage	Rare	No
		Recurrence of acute symptoms, sometimes without rash (Brill-Zinnser disease)	Very rare	Yes (years to decades)
Murine typhus (*R. typhi*)	Abrupt onset of fever, severe headache, chills, myalgia, nausea, rash, enlarged liver and spleen, cough, confusion, mental-status changes	Shock or infection-related organ damage	Rare	No
Spirochetal illnesses				
Leptospirosis (*Leptospira interrogans* and	Wide range of symptoms from subclinical to severe; abrupt onset of flu-like illness,	Sepsis or infection-related organ damage	Rare	No

		Potential Long-Term Outcomes in Adults with Clinical Disease		
Disease or Syndrome	**Acute Syndrome(s) in Adults**	**Disease(s), Syndrome(s), or Clinical Features**	**Frequency of Occurrence of Outcomes**[a]	**Delay Between Acute Infection and Onset of Outcomes**[b]
others)	lymphadenopathy, jaundice, hepatosplenomegaly, conjunctival suffusion, aseptic meningitis, uveitis, pneumonitis, bleeding, diathesis, sepsis			
Rat-bite fever (*Spirillum minus*)	Painful, swollen, ulcerated bite site; swollen lymph nodes, fever, headache, rash, relapses if untreated	Relapses (if acute syndrome untreated)	Rare	No
		Sepsis or infection-related organ damage	Rare	No
		Endocarditis	Very rare	No
Relapsing fever (*Borrelia recurrentis* louse-borne; other species, tick-borne)	Range of severity; fever, headache, myalgia, jaundice, enlarged liver and spleen, rash, central nervous system infection, iritis, iridocyclitis, hemorrhage, mycocarditis, relapses	Sepsis or infection-related organ damage	Rare	No
Yaws (nonvenereal treponemal infection, *Treponema pertenue*)	Rash, osteitis	Rash (if untreated)	Very rare	No
Of special concern to US troops or veterans				
Mycoplasmal infection (primary atypical pneumonia)	Fever, malaise, cough, headache, rash, cryoglobulinemia, myocarditis, arthritis, meningitis, myelitis, encephalitis, hemolytic anemia, glomerulonephritis, Stevens-Johnson syndrome, arthritis	Sepsis or infection-related organ damage	Very rare	No
Bacterial diseases against which all military personnel were immunized and vaccines are highly or fully protective				
Diphtheria (*Corynebacterium diphtheriae*)	Pharyngeal or wound infection with necrotic membrane formation, respiratory damage, myocarditis	Sepsis or infection-related organ damage	Frequent	No
Haemophilus influenzae type B infection	Meningitis, epiglottitis, arthritis, osteomyelitis	Sepsis or infection-related organ damage	Rare	No

Disease or Syndrome	Acute Syndrome(s) in Adults	Potential Long-Term Outcomes in Adults with Clinical Disease		
		Disease(s), Syndrome(s), or Clinical Features	Frequency of Occurrence of Outcomes[a]	Delay Between Acute Infection and Onset of Outcomes[b]
Tetanus (*Clostridium tetani*)	Wound infection leading to muscle spasm, respiratory damage, autonomic instability	Sepsis or infection-related organ damage, lockjaw	Frequent	No
Bacterial diseases against which all military personnel were immunized and vaccines are partly protective				
Meningococcal disease (*Neisseria meningitidis*)	Meningitis, sepsis	Sepsis or infection-related organ damage	Frequent	No
Pertussis (whooping cough, *Bordetella pertussis*)	Respiratory tract infection, secondary infections, encephalopathy	Trauma from severe cough	Rare	No
Bacterial diseases not more prevalent in Southwest and South-Central Asia than in the United States				
Actinomycosis (*Actinomyces*)	Abscesses, soft-tissue infection	Orofacial, pulmonary, genitourinary disease; osteomyelitis	Common	Yes (months)
Bartonellosis (*Bartonella*)	Cat-scratch disease, systemic infection, encephalopathy, retinopathy	Sepsis or infection-related organ damage	Rare	No
Capnocytophaga infection	Bite-site infection (dogs), bacteremia, sepsis	Sepsis or infection-related organ damage	Rare	No
Chlamydia pneumoniae infection	Respiratory tract infections	Sepsis or infection-related organ damage, focal infection	Rare	No
Botulism (*Clostridium botulinum*)	Neurotoxicity, cranial nerve palsies, respiratory damage	Sepsis or infection-related organ damage	Rare	No
Gas gangrene (*Clostridium perfringens*)	Gas gangrene, wound infection	Sepsis or infection-related organ damage	Rare	No
Tularemia (*Francisella tularensis*)	Pneumonia, typhoidal illness, sepsis	Sepsis or infection-related organ damage	Rare	No

Disease or Syndrome	Acute Syndrome(s) in Adults	Potential Long-Term Outcomes in Adults with Clinical Disease: Disease(s), Syndrome(s), or Clinical Features	Frequency of Occurrence of Outcomes[a]	Delay Between Acute Infection and Onset of Outcomes[b]
Haemophilus influenzae infection	Exacerbation of chronic obstructive pulmonary disease	Pneumonia	Common	No
	Acute maxillary sinusitis	Chronic sinusitis	Common	No
		Empyema, brain abscess, cavernous sinus thrombosis	Very rare	No
	Community-acquired pneumonia	Infection-related organ damage	Very rare	No
	Middle-ear infection	Meningitis, brain abscess, sinus thrombosis, mastoiditis, acute petrositis, facial paralysis	Very rare	No
	Purulent conjunctivitis	Keratitis	Very rare	No
Legionnaire's disease (*Legionella*)	Respiratory tract infections	Sepsis or infection-related organ damage	Rare	No
Listeriosis (*Listeria monocytogenes*)	Diarrhea, meningoencephalitis, endocarditis	Sepsis or infection-related organ damage	Very rare	No
Lyme disease (*Borrelia burghdorferi*)	Fever, flu-like illness, arthritis, rash, myocarditis, meningoencephalitis	Chronic arthritis	Common (if untreated)	Yes (weeks to months)
Moraxella catarrhalis infection	Respiratory tract infection	Sepsis or infection-related organ damage	Common	No
Nocardiosis (*Nocardia*)	Soft-tissue infection, pneumonia, brain infection	Chronic and progressive tissue damage (Madura foot)	Rare	Yes (months)
Noncholera *Vibrio* infection	Wound infections, diarrhea, bacteremia, sepsis	Sepsis or infection-related organ damage	Rare	No
Nontuberculosis mycobacteria infection	Chronic soft-tissue infections	Chronic focal infections	Common	No
Pasteurella infection	Bite-site soft-tissue infection (from cats, dogs), bacteremia, sepsis	Sepsis or infection-related organ damage	Rare	No

Disease or Syndrome	Acute Syndrome(s) in Adults	Potential Long-Term Outcomes in Adults with Clinical Disease: Disease(s), Syndrome(s), or Clinical Features	Frequency of Occurrence of Outcomes[a]	Delay Between Acute Infection and Onset of Outcomes[b]
Staphylococcus infection	Focal infections, pneumonia, bacteremia	Sepsis or infection-related organ damage	Rare	No
Streptococcus infection	Pharyngitis, bacteremia, pneumonia, focal infections	Sepsis or infection-related organ damage	Rare	No
		Glomerulonephritis	Very rare	No
		Rheumatic fever	Very rare	No
Streptococcus pneumoniae infection	Respiratory tract infection, meningitis, bacteremia, sepsis	Sepsis or infection-related organ damage	Rare	No
Antibiotic-resistant or common nosocomial bacterial infections				
Acinetobacter infection[c] (multiple-drug-resistant)	Skin and soft-tissue infections, abscesses, pneumonia, bacteremia, urinary tract infections	Sepsis or infection-related organ damage	Rare	No
Enterococcus infection (vancomycin resistant)	Skin and soft-tissue infections, abscesses, bacteremia, urinary tract infections	Sepsis or infection-related organ damage, endocarditis	Rare	No
Klebsiella infection (multiple-drug-resistant)	Skin and soft-tissue infections, abscesses, pneumonia, bacteremia, urinary tract infections	Sepsis or infection-related organ damage	Rare	No
Pseudomonas aeruginosa infection	Skin and soft-tissue infections, abscesses, pneumonia, bacteremia, urinary tract infections	Sepsis or infection-related organ damage	Rare	No
Staphylococcus aureus infection (methicillin-resistant)	Skin and soft-tissue infections, abscesses, pneumonia, bacteremia	Sepsis or infection-related organ damage, endocarditis	Rare	No
		Osteomyelitis	Rare	Yes (months)
Stenotrophomonas maltophilia infection	Respiratory tract infection, bacteremia	Sepsis or infection-related organ damage	Very rare	No

NOTE: The term *infection* refers to a primary infection that leads to disease.
[a] Probability calculated as percentage of acute cases. Frequent, >50% of cases; common, >5-50% of cases; rare, 1-5% of cases; very rare, <1% of cases.
[b] Delay defined as adverse health outcome not evident at time of acute illness.
[c] Reported in military personnel in Gulf War, Operation Enduring Freedom, or Operation Iraqi Freedom as of December 2005.
[d] Postinfection enteropathy: syndrome of chronic or intermittent diarrhea and/or constipation that follows elimination of previous infectious enteropathy; poorly defined etiology and pathogenic mechanism; often self-limited over months to years.
SOURCE: GIDEON 2006; Heymann 2004; Mandell et al. 2005; Nester et al. 2004; Wilson 1991.

TABLE 3.2 Viral Diseases That Are Endemic to Southwest and South-Central Asia and Have Potential Long-Term Adverse Health Outcomes

		Potential Long-Term Outcomes in Adults with Clinical Disease		
Disease or Syndrome	**Acute Syndrome(s) in Adults**	**Disease(s), Syndrome(s), or Clinical Features**	**Frequency of Occurrence of Outcomes**[a]	**Delay Between Acute Infection and Onset of Outcomes**[b]
	More Prevalent in Southwest and South-Central Asia Than in the United States			
Crimean-Congo hemorrhagic fever (*Nairovirus* spp.)	Severe hemorrhagic fever with shock, disseminated intravascular coagulation, frequent extensive bleeding, severely decreased number of platelets	Organ failure	Common	No
Dengue fever (*Flavivirus* spp.)	Sudden onset of fever, intense headache, myalgia, arthralgia, retro-orbital pain, anorexia, nausea, vomiting, rash; lymphadenopathy and leukopenia with relative lymphocytosis	Prolonged fatigue and mental depression	Common	No
	In some cases: minor bleeding, early onset of generalized erythema			
	In some adults with underlying conditions: major bleeding phenomena			
	Rarely: increased transaminases			
Dengue hemorrhagic fever (DHF) and Dengue shock syndrome (*Flavivirus* spp.)	Fever, hemorrhagic manifestation, thrombocytopenia, evidence of plasma leakage; preceded by intense, continuous abdominal pain with persistent vomiting	Severe liver damage, sepsis, hemorrhage, disseminated intravascular coagulation	Common	No
	In severe cases: marked weakness, restlessness, facial pallor, often diaphoresis, severe abdominal pain, circumoral cyanosis, signs of shock			
Hepatitis B (hepatitis B virus [HBV])	*Severe cases*: acute hepatic necrosis	Clinically evident cases:		
	Most cases: no clinical signs	Chronic infection	Rare	Yes (months to years)

Disease or Syndrome	Acute Syndrome(s) in Adults	Potential Long-Term Outcomes in Adults with Clinical Disease: Disease(s), Syndrome(s), or Clinical Features	Frequency of Occurrence of Outcomes[a]	Delay Between Acute Infection and Onset of Outcomes[b]
	Clinically evident cases: insidious onset with anorexia, vague abdominal discomfort, jaundice, nausea, vomiting; sometimes arthralgias and rash	Cirrhosis	Rare	Yes (years)
		Hepatocellular carcinoma	Very rare	Yes (years to decades)
Hepatitis C (hepatitis C virus [HCV])	Asymptomatic or acute hepatitis; rarely, associated with arthritis when virus induces cryoglobulinemia	Cirrhosis	Common	Yes (years to decades)
		Hepatocellular carcinoma	Rare	Yes (years to decades)
Rift Valley fever (*Phlebovirus* spp.)	Acute, undifferentiated, febrile illness; retinitis; vasculitis; hepatitis (may be fulminant); encephalitis	Fulminant disease with infection-related organ dysfunction	Rare	No
		Macular and perimacular retinitis and blindness	Very rare	No
		Severe encephalopathy	Very rare	No
Sand fly fever (*Phlebovirus* spp.)	Headache, fever, injected sclerae, malaise, nausea, pain in limbs and back, leukopenia	Prolonged mental depression	Rare	No
Sindbis virus infection (*Alphavirus* spp.)	Fever, often with shaking chills; severe polyarticular arthralgia; rash with headache, photophobia, retro-orbital pain, sore throat, pharyngitis, nausea, vomiting	Arthralgia and myalgia	Frequent	No
Potentially More Prevalent Among Troops in Southwest and South-Central Asia Than Among US Population				
Adenovirus infection (*Adenovirus* spp.)	*Usually*: asymptomatic	Chronic hemorrhagic cystitis	Very rare	Yes (weeks to months)
	Sometimes: acute respiratory disease (most often tracheobronchitis) and atypical pneumonia, hemorrhagic cystitis	Keratitis	Rare	No
	Sometimes: epidemic keratoconjunctivitis			
Avian influenza (H5N1)	Fever, cough pneumonia, myalgia, headache, respiratory failure, encephalitis	Infection-related organ damage	Unknown	Unknown

Disease or Syndrome	Acute Syndrome(s) in Adults	Potential Long-Term Outcomes in Adults with Clinical Disease: Disease(s), Syndrome(s), or Clinical Features	Frequency of Occurrence of Outcomes[a]	Delay Between Acute Infection and Onset of Outcomes[b]
Hantaviral hemorrhagic fever with renal syndrome (*Bunyaviridae* spp.)	*Severe form* (due to Hantaan virus): toxic fever, severe shock, bleeding; sometimes renal failure, death	Renal failure: sepsis or hypertension-related organ dysfunction	Common	No
		Chronic hypertensive renal failure	Rare	No
	Renal insufficiency: can include anuria, oliguria, mucosal bleeding diathesis, electrolyte and acid-base abnormalities, hypertension, pneumotitis complicated by pulmonary edema	Renal failure, thrombocytopenia	Common	No
	Mild to moderately severe (due to Seoul virus): fever, bleeding, abdominal pain, hyposphenuria			
	Mild (due to Puumala virus): asymptomatic (90%); abdominal pain, hyposphenuria (10%) Headache, backache, myalgia, diarrhea, vomiting, conjunctivitis, hemorrhage, azotemia, proteinuria, decreased number of platelets			
Hantavirus pulmonary syndrome (*Hanta* spp.)	Fever of sudden onset and generalized myalgia, sometimes with abdominal pain, gastrointestinal disturbances	Renal failure	Very rare	No
	Within 1-10 days: onset of respiratory symptoms; these can progress from modest cough and dyspnea to florid pulmonary edema with respiratory failure in hours Shock In patients who survive shock, vascular leak reverses in a few days; recovery is apparently complete			
Influenza (influenza A, B, C spp.)	In healthy adults, infection may be asymptomatic, mild illness, or classic influenza	Exacerbation of chronic pulmonary disease (for example, asthma, cystic fibrosis, chronic	Common	No

Disease or Syndrome	Acute Syndrome(s) in Adults	Potential Long-Term Outcomes in Adults with Clinical Disease: Disease(s), Syndrome(s), or Clinical Features	Frequency of Occurrence of Outcomes[a]	Delay Between Acute Infection and Onset of Outcomes[b]
	Classic uncomplicated influenza: Systemic symptoms: abrupt onset of fever, chills, headache, myalgia, malaise, anorexia *Common*: arthralgias *More severe cases*: prostration Respiratory symptoms (overshadowed by systemic symptoms): dry cough, severe pharyngeal pain, nasal obstruction and discharge	bronchitis)		
		Lower respiratory tract infection	Common	No
		Cardiac complications	Common (in patients with cardiac disease)	Yes (days to months)
		Encephalitis	Rare	No
		Myositis and myoglobinuria with tender leg muscles and increased serum creatine kinase	Rare	No
		Secondary bacterial pneumonia	Rare	No
		Guillain-Barré syndrome	Rare	Yes (days to weeks)
		Transverse myelitis	Rare	Yes (days)
		Toxic shock syndrome	Very rare	No
Varicella (Varicella-zoster virus)	Generalized exanthemous rash, low-grade fever, malaise *In complicated cases*: acute cerebellar ataxia, encephalitis, pneumonitis, meningitis, transverse myelitis, Reye's syndrome, myocarditis, nephritis, bleeding diatheses, hepatitis	In all cases:		
		Herpes zoster (shingles)	Common	Yes (years to decades)
		Posttherapeutic neuralgia	Common	No delay after herpes zoster
		Ophthalmicus	Rare	No delay after herpes zoster
		Ramsey-Hunt syndrome	Very Rare	No delay after herpes zoster
		Meningoencephalitis or encephalitis	Very Rare	No delay after herpes zoster
		Guillain-Barré syndrome	Very Rare	No delay after herpes

Disease or Syndrome	Acute Syndrome(s) in Adults	Potential Long-Term Outcomes in Adults with Clinical Disease: Disease(s), Syndrome(s), or Clinical Features	Frequency of Occurrence of Outcomes[a]	Delay Between Acute Infection and Onset of Outcomes[b]
				zoster
		Varicella pneumonitis	Very Rare	No delay after herpes zoster
		Hepatitis	Very Rare	No delay after herpes zoster
		In complicated cases: Infection-related organ damage	Rare	No
Viral enteritis (*Enterovirus* spp.)	Fever and pharyngitis, rash, aseptic meningitis, epidemic conjunctivitis, herpangina, hand-foot-and-mouth disease, myocarditis, pericarditis, pleurodynia, acute flaccid paralysis, conjunctivitis	Heart failure due to myocarditis	Very rare	No
		Chronic meningoencephalitis	Very rare	No
West Nile fever[c] (*Flavivirus* spp.) (see Chapter 5 for detailed discussion)	*Usually*: asymptomatic *Sometimes*: fever, headache, body aches, nausea, vomiting, swollen lymph glands, rash *Uncommon*: high fever, headache, neck stiffness, stupor, disorientation, coma, tremors, convulsions, muscle weakness, vision loss, numbness and paralysis	If symptomatic: West Nile neurologic disease	Very rare	No
		Acute flaccid paralysis	Very rare	No
		Cognitive, physical, or functional impairment	Very rare	No

NOTE: The term *infection* refers to a primary infection that leads to disease.
[a] Probability calculated as percentage of acute cases. Frequent, >50% of cases; common, >5- 50% of cases; rare, 1-5% of cases; very rare, <1% of cases.
[b] Delay defined as adverse health outcome not evident at time of acute illness.
[c] Reported in military personnel in Gulf War, Operation Enduring Freedom, or Operation Iraqi Freedom as of December 2005.
SOURCE: GIDEON 2006; Heymann 2004; Mandell et al. 2005; Nester et al. 2004; Wilson 1991.

TABLE 3.3 Protozoan Diseases That Are Endemic to Southwest and South-Central Asia and Have Potential Long-Term Adverse Health Outcomes

		Potential Long-Term Outcomes in Adults with Clinical Disease		
Disease or Syndrome	**Acute Syndrome(s) in Adults**	**Disease(s), Syndrome(s), or Clinical Feature**	**Frequency of Occurrence of Outcomes**[a]	**Delay Between Acute Infection and Onset of Outcomes**[b]
Amebiasis (*Entamoeba histolytica*)	Diarrhea, fever, abdominal pain, intestinal perforation and hemorrhage, fulminant colitis, hepatomegaly, liver abscesses, fistulae, rarely amebic empyema or amebic pericarditis	Postinfection enteropathy[c]	Rare	No
		Liver abscesses	Rare	Yes (weeks to years)
		Empyema, pericarditis	Very rare	Yes (weeks to years)
		Intra-abdominal and cutaneous fistulae	Very rare	Yes (weeks to years)
Cryptosporidiosis (*Cryptosporidium* spp.)	Diarrhea (may last 1-4 weeks), nausea, fever, myalgia	Chronic diarrhea (in people immunocompromised at time of infection, diarrhea may be persistent despite treatment)	Rare	No
		Postinfection enteropathy[c]	Rare	No
		Cryptosporidial cholangitis and acalculous cholecystitis (only in people immunocompromised at time of initial infection)	Very rare	Yes (weeks to months)
Cyclosporiasis (*Cyclospora cayetanensis*)	Diarrhea, nausea	Postinfection enteropathy[c]	Rare	No
Giardiasis (*Giardia lamblia*)	Diarrhea, abdominal cramps, bloating, flatulence, malaise, nausea, anorexia	Chronic diarrhea, malabsorption, weight loss	Common (if untreated)	No
		Postinfection enteropathy[c]	Rare	No
Isosporiasis (*Isospora belli*)	Diarrhea, nausea, eosinophilia	Persistent diarrhea (if untreated)	Rare	No
		Postinfection enteropathy[c]	Rare	No
Leishmaniasis[d] (*Leishmania* spp.) (see Chapter 5 for detailed discussion)	*Cutaneous leishmaniasis* (CL): any of variety of skin lesions ranging from small, dry, crusted areas to large, deep, disfiguring ulcers	CL:		
		Lesions may persist 3-24 months	Common	No
		Scarring	Common	No
		Contractures over joints	Very rare	Yes (weeks to months)

Disease or Syndrome	Acute Syndrome(s) in Adults	Potential Long-Term Outcomes in Adults with Clinical Disease		
		Disease(s), Syndrome(s), or Clinical Feature	**Frequency of Occurrence of Outcomes[a]**	**Delay Between Acute Infection and Onset of Outcomes[b]**
	Visceral leishmaniasis (VL [kala-azar]): fever, chills, weight loss, hepatosplenomegaly, anemia, leukopenia, hypergammaglobulinemia	VL:		
		Reactivation (if immunosuppressed)	Common	Yes (months to years)
		Delayed presentation of acute syndrome	Rare	Yes (months to years)
	Viscerotropic leishmaniasis: fever, chills, weight loss, headache, splenomegaly, lymphadenopathy	Post-kala-azar dermal leishmaniasis (disseminated nodular infiltration of skin with parasites after treatment of visceral leishmaniasis)	Very rare	Yes (weeks to years)
Malaria[d] (*Plasmodium* spp.) (see Chapter 5 for detailed discussion)	*P. falciparum*: fever, chills, anemia, headache, myalgia, cerebral malaria (including seizures, coma, neurologic complications), hypoglycemia, acidosis, severe anemia, splenic disease, renal failure, respiratory failure	*P. falciparum*:		
		Anemia	Common	Yes (months)
		Shock or hypoperfusion-related organ damage	Rare	No
		Recrudescence	Rare	Yes (months)
		Ophthalmologic manifestations	Very rare	Yes (months to years)
	P. ovale and *P. vivax*: fever, chills, headache, myalgia, anemia, splenic disease, rarely respiratory failure	Persistent neurologic deficits (consequence of cerebral malaria)	Very rare	Yes (months to years)
	P. malariae: Fever, chills, headache, myalgia, anemia, splenomegaly; if untreated, infection may be chronic	*P. ovale* and *P. vivax*:		
		Relapse of acute syndrome	Common (if untreated)	Yes (weeks to years)
		Splenic rupture	Very rare	Yes (weeks to months)
		P. malariae:		
		Late presentation	Rare	Yes (years)
		Glomerulonephritis/nephrotic syndrome	Very rare	Yes (months to decades)
		Myelodysplastic syndrome	Very rare	Yes (months to decades)
Microsporidiosis (*Microsporidia* spp.)	Diarrhea (usually self-limited), kerato-conjunctivitis	Postinfection enteropathy[c]	Rare	No
	If immunocompromised: persistent diarrhea, sinusitis, acalculous cholecystitis, pneumonitis, nephritis, systemic infection	Self-limited diarrhea, unless immunocompromised at time of infection	Very rare	No

Disease or Syndrome	Acute Syndrome(s) in Adults	Potential Long-Term Outcomes in Adults with Clinical Disease		
		Disease(s), Syndrome(s), or Clinical Feature	Frequency of Occurrence of Outcomes[a]	Delay Between Acute Infection and Onset of Outcomes[b]
Toxoplasmosis (*Toxoplasma gondii*)	Range of symptoms: may be asymptomatic, fever, cervical lymphadenopathy, myositis, mononucleosis-like syndrome (pharyngitis, fever, hepatosplenomegaly, lymphadenopathy), encephalitis, myocarditis, chorioretinitis, rarely pneumonitis; congenital infection can occur if acute infection occurs during pregnancy	Reactivation of disease (if immunocompromised)	Common (if immuno-compromised)	Yes (years)
		Toxoplasmic brain abscesses (only in severely immunocompromised)	Rare	Yes (years)
		Chorioretinitis	Very rare (if infected as adult); Common (if infected in utero)	Yes (years)

[a] Probability calculated as percentage of acute cases. Frequent, >50% of cases; common, >5- 50% of cases; rare, 1-5% of cases; very rare, <1% of cases.
[b] Delay defined as adverse health outcome not evident at time of acute illness.
[c] Postinfection enteropathy: syndrome of chronic or intermittent diarrhea and/or constipation that follows elimination of previous infectious enteropathy; poorly defined etiology and pathogenic mechanism; often self-limited over months to years.
[d] Reported in military personnel in the Gulf War, Operation Enduring Freedom, or Operation Iraqi Freedom as of December, 2005.
SOURCE: GIDEON 2006; Heymann 2004; Mandell et al. 2005; Nester et al. 2004; Wilson 1991.

TABLE 3.4 Helminthic Diseases That Are Endemic to Southwest and South-Central Asia and Have Potential Long-Term Adverse Health Outcomes

		Potential Long-Term Outcomes in Adults with Clinical Disease		
Disease or Syndrome	**Acute Syndrome(s) in Adults**	**Disease(s), Syndrome(s), or Clinical Feature**	**Frequency of Occurrence of Outcomes**[a]	**Delay Between Acute Infection and Onset of Outcomes**[b]
Nematodes				
Ascariasis (*Ascaris* spp.)	Largely asymptomatic Transient respiratory symptoms associated with pulmonary infiltration and peripheral blood eosinophilia, intestinal obstruction or blockage	Biliary duct obstruction, ascending cholangitis, acute pancreatitis, obstructive jaundice, peritonitis	Very rare	Yes (months to years)
Enterobiasis (pinworm infection, *Enterobius vermicularis*)	Largely asymptomatic *Symptomatic*: perianal or perineal pruritus *Occasionally*: abdominal pain	Appendicitis	Very rare	Yes (months to years)
		Pelvic infection	Very rare	Yes (months to years)
Filariasis (*Wuchereria bancrofti*)	Lymphangitis, lymphadenitis, eosinophilia	Episodes of fever and lymphangitis, may recur over several years	Rare	Yes (years)
		Lymphedema	Rare	Yes (years)
		Persistent adenopathy	Rare	Yes (years)
		Epididymitis	Very rare	Yes (years)
		Chyluria	Very rare	Yes (years)
		Orchitis	Very rare	Yes (years)
Hookworm disease (*Ancylostoma duodenale* and *Necata americanus*)	Largely asymptomatic Pruritus at dermal site of larval penetration	Iron-deficiency anemia	Common	Yes (months to years)
Onchocerciasis (river blindness, *Onchocerca volvulus*)	Dermatitis, keratitis	Skin hyperpigmentation, depigmentation, chronic dermatitis, dermal atrophy	Common	Yes (years to decades)
		Sclerosing keratitis	Common (if untreated)	Yes (years to decades)

Disease or Syndrome	Acute Syndrome(s) in Adults	Potential Long-Term Outcomes in Adults with Clinical Disease		
		Disease(s), Syndrome(s), or Clinical Feature	Frequency of Occurrence of Outcomes[a]	Delay Between Acute Infection and Onset of Outcomes[b]
		Visual loss	Common (if untreated)	Yes (years to decades)
		Iridocyclitis	Rare	Yes (years to decades)
Strongyloidiasis (*Strongyloides stercoralis*)	Diarrhea, intestinal irregularities, gluteal or perineal pruritus and rash, eosinophilia	Hyperinfection syndrome, generalized strongyloidiasis	Common (in immunosuppressed patients on steroids)	Yes (months to decades)
Cestodes				
Cysticercosis (*Taenia solium* larvae [cysticerci])	Cerebral, ocular, or subcutaneous cysts usually without eosinophilia; involvement of central nervous system may present as seizures, increased intracranial pressure, altered mental status, eosinophilic meningitis, focal neurologic deficits, spinal-cord mass, or encephalitis	Chronic seizure disorder	Common	Yes (years)
		Recurrence of acute symptoms	Very rare	Yes (months to years)
Echinococcosis (*Echinococcus multilocularis*)	*Usually*: asymptomatic *Rarely*: abdominal pain with or without apalpable mass in right upper quadrant, fever, pruritus, urticaria, eosinophilia, anaphylactic shock, cough, hemoptysis, chest pain	Hepatic and metastatic cysts	Common	Yes (years to decades)
Trematodes				
Schistosomiasis (*Schistosoma haematobium*)	Often asymptomatic Bladder inflammation, urinary obstruction, scarring, eosinophilia	Recurrent urinary tract infection	Common (if untreated)	Yes (years)
		Cerebral mass, generalized encephalopathy, or focal epilepsy	Very rare	Yes (weeks to years)
		Transverse myelitis	Very rare	Yes (weeks to years)
		Bladder cancer (squamous-	Very rare	Yes (decades)

Disease or Syndrome	Acute Syndrome(s) in Adults	Potential Long-Term Outcomes in Adults with Clinical Disease: Disease(s), Syndrome(s), or Clinical Feature	Frequency of Occurrence of Outcomes[a]	Delay Between Acute Infection and Onset of Outcomes[b]
		cell)		
		Urinary obstruction (hydronephrosis)	Very rare	Yes (decades)
Schistosomiasis (*S. mansoni*)	Often asymptomatic Gastrointestinal symptoms, colonic polyps, hepatosplenomegaly, jaundice, cirrhosis, eosinophilia	Fatigue, abdominal pain, intermittent diarrhea or dysentery, moderate anemia	Common	Yes (weeks to years)
		Gastrointestinal symptoms	Common	Yes (weeks to years)
		Hepatosplenomegaly and variceal hemorrhage	Rare	Yes (years)
		Cirrhosis	Rare	Yes (years to decades)
		Portal hypertension	Rare	Yes (years to decades)
		Transverse myelitis	Very rare	Yes (weeks to years)
		Right ventricular congestion or cor pulmonale	Very rare	Yes (years)
		Cerebral masses	Very rare	Yes (years to decades)

[a] Probability calculated as percentage of acute cases. Frequent, >50% of cases; common, >5- 50% of cases; rare, 1-5% of cases; very rare, <1% of cases.
[b] Delay defined as adverse health outcome not evident at time of acute illness.
SOURCE: GIDEON 2006; Heymann 2004; Mandell et al. 2005; Nester et al. 2004; Wilson 1991.

TABLE 3.5 Sexually Transmitted Diseases That Are Endemic to Southwest and South-Central Asia and Have Potential Long-Term Adverse Health Outcomes

		Potential Long-Term Outcomes in Adults with Clinical Disease		
Disease or Syndrome	**Acute Syndrome(s) in Adults**	**Disease(s), Syndrome(s), or Clinical Feature**	**Frequency of Occurrence of Outcomes**[a]	**Delay Between Acute Infection and Onset of Outcomes**[b]
More prevalent in Southwest and South-Central Asia Than in the United States				
Chancroid (*Haemophilus ducreyi*)	Genital ulcers, inguinal lymphadenopathy	Scarring	Very rare	Yes (weeks)
Hepatitis A (hepatitis A virus [HAV])	Acute hepatitis (jaundice, nausea, anorexia, fever) if symptomatic	Liver failure	Very rare	No
Hepatitis B (hepatitis B virus [HBV])	*Severe cases*: acute hepatic necrosis	Chronic infection Cirrhosis Hepatocellular carcinoma	Rare Rare Very rare	Yes (months to years) Yes (years) Yes (years to decades)
	Most cases: no clinical signs			
	Clinically evident cases: insidious onset with anorexia, vague abdominal discomfort, nausea, vomiting Sometimes arthralgias and rash Jaundice: 30-50% of cases			
Lymphogranuloma venereum (*Chlamydia trachomatis* serovars L_1-L_3)	Genital ulcers, inguinal lymphadenopathy, proctitis	Genital scarring and fistulae; perirectal abscess	Unknown, but presumably rare	Yes (month to years)
Syphilis (*Treponema pallidum*)	Genital ulcers (primary stage) Rash, fever, meningitis, stroke, nephrotic syndrome, hepatitis (secondary stage) Spontaneous abortion (any stage)	Gummas, tabes dorsalis, dementia, meningovascular disease, generalized paresis, aortitis (tertiary stage)	Common (if untreated)	Yes (months to years)
Potentially More Prevalent Among Troops in Southwest and South-Central Asia Than Among US Adult Population				
Chlamydia (*Chlamydia trachomatis* serovars D-K)	*Usually*: asymptomatic	Chronic pelvic pain, tubal infertility, ectopic pregnancy	Common in untreated women	Yes (months to years)
	Sometimes: cervicitis, pelvic inflammatory	In infants born to infected		

Disease or Syndrome	Acute Syndrome(s) in Adults	Potential Long-Term Outcomes in Adults with Clinical Disease: Disease(s), Syndrome(s), or Clinical Feature	Frequency of Occurrence of Outcomes[a]	Delay Between Acute Infection and Onset of Outcomes[b]
	disease, urethritis, conjunctivitis In infants born to infected mothers: pneumonia, conjunctivitis	mothers: Reactive airways disease	Unknown	Yes (years)
Gonorrhea (*Neisseria gonorrhoeae*)	*Usually*: asymptomatic *Sometimes*: cervicitis, pelvic inflammatory disease, urethritis, conjunctivitis *Uncommon*: disseminated gonococcal infection (arthritis, tenosynovitis, rash, meningitis, endocarditis)	Chronic pelvic pain, tubal infertility, ectopic pregnancy	Common in untreated women	Yes (months to years)
Of Concern to US troops, but No Evidence of Increased Frequency or Association with Service in Southwest or South-Central Asia				
Genital herpes (herpes simplex virus [HSV])	*Usually*: asymptomatic *Sometimes*: genital ulcers *Uncommon*: meningitis, radiculitis	Recurrent genital herpes (HSV-2) Recurrent meningitis (Mollaret's)	Common Very rare	Yes (weeks to years) Yes (weeks to years)
Human immunodeficiency virus Type 1 (HIV-1)	Asymptomatic Primary infection syndrome (acute retroviral syndrome) Acquired immune deficiency syndrome (AIDS)	AIDS-related opportunistic infection HIV-related malignancies	Frequent if untreated Common	Yes (years to decades) Yes (years to decades)
Human papillomavirus infection	Asymptomatic Genital warts	Cervical neoplasia Genital squamous cell cancers (penis, anus) Tracheal infection in newborns of infected mothers	Rare Rare Very rare	Yes (months to years) Yes (years) Yes (months to years)
Human T-cell lymphotropic virus infection (I) (HTLV-I)	Asymptomatic Chronic persistent oligoarthritis	Adult T-cell leukemia or lymphoma HTLV-I-associated myelopathy	Rare Rare	Yes (years) Yes (years)

Disease or Syndrome	Acute Syndrome(s) in Adults	Potential Long-Term Outcomes in Adults with Clinical Disease		
		Disease(s), Syndrome(s), or Clinical Feature	Frequency of Occurrence of Outcomes[a]	Delay Between Acute Infection and Onset of Outcomes[b]
Trichomoniasis (*Trichomonas vaginalis*)	Asymptomatic Vaginitis Urethritis	Preterm delivery	Rare	No

NOTE: The term *infection* refers to a primary infection that leads to disease.
[a] Probability calculated as percentage of acute cases. Frequent, >50% of cases; common, >5- 50% of cases; rare, 1-5% of cases; very rare, <1% of cases.
[b] Delay defined as health outcomes not evident at time of acute illness.
SOURCE: Baum 2005; Holmes et al. 1999.

REFERENCES

Baum S. 2005. Introduction to Mycoplasma diseases. Mycoplasma Diseases. In: Mandell G, Bennett J, Dolin R, Editors. *Principles and Practice of Infectious Diseases*. 6th ed. Philadelphia, PA: Churchill Livingstone. Pp. 2269-2271.

GIDEON. 2006. *Global Infectious Disease and Epidemiology Network*. [Online]. Available: http://www.gideononline.com [accessed April 12, 2006].

Heymann DL. 2004. *Control of Communicable Diseases Manual*. Washington, DC: American Public Health Association.

Holmes KK, Sparling PF, Mardh P, Lemon SM, Stamm WE, Piot P, Wasserheit JN. 1999. *Sexually Transmitted Diseases*. 3rd ed. New York: McGraw-Hill.

Mandell GL, Bennett JE, Dolin R. 2005. *Principles and Practice of Infectious Diseases*. 6th ed. Philadelphia, PA: Elsevier Churchill Livingstone.

Nester EW, Anderson DG, Roberts JCE, Pearsall NN, Nester MT. 2004. *Microbiology: A Human Perspective*. 4th ed. New York: McGraw-Hill.

Wilson ME. 1991. *A World Guide to Infections: Diseases, Distribution, Diagnosis*. New York: Oxford University Press.

4

INFECTIOUS DISEASES DIAGNOSED IN US TROOPS WHO SERVED IN THE PERSIAN GULF WAR, OPERATION ENDURING FREEDOM, OR OPERATION IRAQI FREEDOM

Infectious diseases have accompanied war throughout recorded history; the clinical aspects of Operation Desert Shield (ODSh), Operation Desert Storm (ODSt), Operation Iraqi Freedom (OIF), and Operation Enduring Freedom (OEF) have been no different. Although medical and epidemiologic personnel in the US military can anticipate troops' exposure to many pathogens and mitigate their effects, naturally-occurring pathogens infected some troops during these operations. This chapter summarizes information about the infectious diseases and pathogens identified in US troops who served or are serving in ODSh, ODSt, OIF, or OEF. That information comes from several sources, including published scientific literature, medical surveillance monthly reports published by the Army Medical Surveillance Activity, the Centers for Disease Control and Prevention (CDC), and infectious disease experts at the Department of Defense (DOD) and the Department of Veterans Affairs. In Chapter 5, the committee evaluates the published scientific literature about the possible long-term adverse health outcomes of nine of the diseases discussed in this chapter.

Thriving on the troops' crowded and sometimes unsanitary living conditions, microbial pathogens have caused primarily diarrheal illnesses and acute upper respiratory infections during ODSt, ODSh, OEF, and OIF (Hyams et al. 2001a; Paparello et al. 1993; Richards et al. 1993a; Thornton et al. 2005; Wasserman et al. 1997). Smaller numbers of military personnel have had various insect-borne diseases, nosocomial infections, brucellosis, chickenpox, meningococcal disease, and Q fever.

Even this chapter's comprehensive review of public documents may not capture the full burden of infectious disease on US troops who have served in southwest and south-central Asia. Military medical investigators' primary mission is to apply their findings to maintain troops' health and they might not always publish summary reports in medical journals. In addition, field commanders may be reluctant to report illnesses perceived as trivial (such as vomiting and diarrhea) even when an outbreak of disease interferes with military operations (Matson 2005). Finally, a new policy purveyed by the DOD restricts the publication of some kinds of medical information that enemy combatants could use to gain an advantage over US troops (Department of the Army 2005b).

DIARRHEAL DISEASE

Enteric Infections in the Gulf War

The leading cause of morbidity among American forces deployed to the Persian Gulf region was diarrheal disease (Hyams et al. 1995a). From August 1990 to May 1991, about 50% of surveyed ground troops and personnel onboard the USNS Mercy experienced at least one episode of acute diarrhea (Haberberger et al. 1994; Hyams et al. 1991). Large outbreaks of watery diarrhea began in August 1990; outbreaks of more severe, bloody diarrhea began in the following month. In addition, gastroenteritis with vomiting as a primary symptom occurred both sporadically and epidemically throughout the war.

Ground Troops

Laboratory Analysis

Hyams and colleagues collected clinical and epidemiologic data from male US troops stationed in northeastern Saudi Arabia to determine the causes and prevalence of diarrheal disease among the troops, risk factors for diarrheal disease in the field, and the effectiveness of pharmacologic treatments (Hyams et al. 1991). From 432 soldiers who sought medical care and presented with gastroenteritis, stool samples were collected and examined for numerous enteropathogens, as described below and summarized in Table 4.1. The soldiers collectively represented all branches of the military, several regions of northeastern Saudi Arabia, and a variety of living conditions. Gastroenteritis was defined as diarrhea (three or more loose or watery stools within 24 hours), abdominal cramps, vomiting, or bloody stools.

The stool specimens were cultured for various pathogens: *E. coli*, *Salmonella, Shigella, Aeromonas, Plesiomonas, Yersinia, Vibrio spp*., and *Campylobacter*. Bacterial enteropathogens were identified with the methods described in *Manual of Clinical Biology*, 4th edition (Kelly et al. 1985). The specimens were also examined for parasites with direct microscopy and for group A rotavirus with a commercial monoclonal-antibody-based immunoassay. Stool specimens and serum from subsets of patients underwent other tests for adenovirus, astrovirus, calicivirus, coronavirus-like agents, group A rotavirus, and norovirus (also known as Norwalk virus). One or more bacterial enteropathogens were identified in 49.5% of the stool cultures, representing 214 patients. Enterotoxigenic *E. coli* (ETEC), *Shigella sonnei,* or both were found in cultures from 205 of those patients. The scientists also found nontyphoid *Salmonella* spp., enteroinvasive *E. coli*, and *Campylobacter*. Tests for viruses yielded positive results for norovirus and rotavirus. There was no evidence of parasitic infection.

TABLE 4.1 Summary of Test Results for Enteropathogens in Stool or Serum from 432 US Military Personnel with Gastroenteritis During Operation Desert Shield

Enteropathogen or Enterotoxin	Identified	
	Yes (No. patients)	**No (No. patients)**
Bacteria		
Aeromonas	--	x
Campylobacter spp.	x (2)	x (430)
Enteroinvasive *E. coli*	x (3)	x (429)
Enterotoxigenic *E. coli*	x (128)	x (304)
Plesiomonas	--	x

Enteropathogen or Enterotoxin	Identified	
	Yes (No. patients)	No (No. patients)
Salmonella spp. (not *S. typhi*)	x (7)	x (425)
Salmonella typhi	--	x
Shigella spp.	x (113)	x (319)
Vibrio cholerae	--	x
Yersinia spp.	--	x
Enterotoxins		
Circulating *Clostridium perfringens* enterotoxins	--	x
Circulating staphylococcal enterotoxins	--	x
Parasites		
Entamoeba histolytica	--	x
Giardia lamblia	--	x
Viruses		
Adenovirus	--	x
Astrovirus	--	x
Calicivirus	--	x
Coronavirus-like agents	--	x
Norovirus[a]	x (1-9)[b]	x (17)
Rotavirus (group A)	x (1)	x (431)

[a] Stool contained particles that were morphologically similar to norovirus.
[b] Multiple tests for viral enteropathogens were conducted on subsets of stool and serum samples, and the number of samples that tested positive for norovirus varied by test from 1 to 9 (Table 4.2).
SOURCE: Adapted with permission from Hyams et al. 1991.

Only 19 of the 432 soldiers in the study reported vomiting as a primary symptom. These cases were clustered temporally (in November and December) but not geographically. The testing of stool samples and paired serum samples suggested that norovirus was the principal etiologic agent in troops with vomiting (Table 4.2). Various investigators later conducted studies specifically on norovirus in the Gulf War context, as discussed below.

TABLE 4.2 Summary of Test Results for Viral Enteropathogens and Enterotoxins in Stool or Serum from Subsets[a] of US Military Personnel with Gastroenteritis During Operation Desert Shield

Enteropathogen	Identified	
	Yes (No. patients)	No (No. patients)
In stool samples from 19 patients with vomiting as a primary symptom, November-December 1990		
Enzyme immunoassay results:		
Adenovirus	--	x
Norovirus	x (3)	x (16)
Rotavirus (group A)	--	x
Immune electron microscopy results (in 13 of 19 specimens):		
Adenovirus	--	x
Astrovirus	--	x
Calicivirus	--	x
Coronavirus-like agents	--	x

Enteropathogen	Identified	
	Yes (No. patients)	No (No. patients)
Norovirus[b]	x (3)	x (10)
Rotavirus	--	x
In stool samples from 68 patients with diarrhea but no vomiting, November-December 1990		
Enzyme immunoassay results:		
Adenovirus	--	x
Norovirus	--	x
Rotavirus	--	x
Immune electron microscopy results (in 18 of 68 specimens):		
Adenovirus	--	x
Astrovirus	--	x
Calicivirus	--	x
Coronavirus-like agents	--	x
Norovirus[b]	x (1)	x (17)
Rotavirus	--	x
Paired serum samples from 11 patients with vomiting alone or vomiting and diarrhea		
Evaluated for a 4-fold or greater increase in serum antibody titer to:		
Adenovirus	--	x
Circulating *Clostridium perfringens* enterotoxins	--	x
Circulating staphylococcal enterotoxins	--	x
Norovirus	x (9)	x (2)
Rotavirus (group A)	--	x

[a] These groups of patients were part of a cohort of 432 troops.
[b] Stool contained particles that were morphologically similar to norovirus.
SOURCE: Adapted from Hyams et al. 1991.

Characterization of ETEC. The high prevalence of ETEC and *Shigella* isolates led investigators to characterize these organisms further (Table 4.3). Shigella isolates were identified by species; additional studies about the occurrence of *Shigella* among Gulf War troops are discussed below.

TABLE 4.3 Bacterial Enteropathogens Identified in Stool Specimens from 214[a] U.S. Military Personnel with Gastroenteritis

Enteropathogen	No. (%)[b] of Patients
Enterotoxigenic *E. coli*	
Heat-labile	15 (3.5)
Heat-stabile	44 (10.2)
Heat-labile and heat-stabile	64 (14.8)
Mixed[c] heat-labile and heat-stabile	2 (0.5)
Enteroinvasive *E. coli*	3 (0.7)
Shigella	
S. dysenteriae	4 (0.9)
S. flexneri	12 (2.8)
S. boydii	8 (1.9)
S. sonnei	89 (20.6)

Enteropathogen	No. (%)[b] of Patients
Salmonella (not *S. typhi*)	7 (1.6)
Campylobacter	2 (0.5)

[a] Bacterial enteropathogens were identified in 214 (49.5%) of the 432 stool samples collected.
[b] The total percentage of isolates is higher than the percentage of patients with an identified enteropathogen because 36 patients had mixed infections.
[c] Two patients had mixed heat-labile and heat-stabile enterotoxigenic *E. coli* infections, with individual colonies producing either heat-labile or heat-stable toxin alone.
SOURCE: Reprinted with permission from Hyams et al. 1991.

Hyams and colleagues tested *E. coli*-like organisms for heat-labile and heat-stabile toxin by using alkaline phosphate-conjugated oligonucleotide DNA probes and Y-1 adrenal cell and suckling-mouse assays (Hyams et al. 1991). Later, Wolf and colleagues further analyzed the Hyams et al. ETEC isolates for their toxin distribution, and other factors (Wolf et al. 1993). A given strain of ETEC may produce heat-labile enterotoxin (LT), heat-stabile enterotoxin (ST), or both. LT is nearly identical with the toxin that causes cholera. Some 85% of 132 ETEC isolates from 124 symptomatic Gulf War troops produced LT (Table 4.4).

TABLE 4.4 Toxin distribution Among 132 ETEC Isolates from 124 US Troops with Gastroenteritis during Operation Desert Storm

Toxin	No. (percentage) of isolates
LT and ST	59 (45)
LT	53 (40)
ST	20 (15)

SOURCE: Adapted with permission from Wolf et al. 1993.

Antimicrobial susceptibility. Using the disk-diffusion method, Hyams and colleagues determined which of five antibiotics would most effectively treat the strains of ETEC and *Shigella* identified in the stool cultures. Up to 63% of the ETEC and up to 85% of the *Shigella* specimens were resistant to several of the antibiotics most accessible to clinicians in the field (Table 4.5), including trimethoprim-sulfamethoxazole, the antibiotic most frequently used to treat diarrhea during the early stages of ODSh deployment. In contrast, the scientists found, ETEC and *Shigella* were 100% susceptible to ciprofloxacin and norfloxacin. Hyams and colleagues reported that empiric results of antibiotic treatment for diarrheal disease in the field led military clinicians to gravitate toward ciprofloxacin and norfloxacin over time. Clinicians also reportedly administered quinolone drugs to affected critical combat troops to shorten the duration of gastroenteric symptoms.

TABLE 4.5 Antimicrobial Resistance of Enterotoxigenic *E. coli* and *Shigella* Specimens

	Proportion of Resistant Specimens, %	
Antibiotic	Enterotoxigenic E. coli (N = 125)	Shigella (N = 113)
Trimethoprim-sulfamethoxazole	39	85
Tetracycline	63	68
Ampicillin	48	21
Ciprofloxacin	0	0
Norfloxacin	0	0

SOURCE: Adapted with permission from Hyams et al. 1991.

Epidemiologic Analysis

To learn the prevalence of and risk factors for diarrheal disease among US troops stationed in northeastern Saudi Arabia during ODSh, Hyams and colleagues administered an epidemiologic survey to 2,022 personnel from all branches of the military in October-December 1990 (Hyams et al. 1991). After an average of 2 months in Saudi Arabia, 57% of those surveyed had suffered at least one episode of diarrhea. The symptoms of diarrheal disease had led 22% of all respondents to seek medical care, and had prevented 20% of all respondents from performing their duties. Thirty-two percent of those surveyed had experienced two or more separate episodes of diarrhea. In some units, the attack rate was 5-10% per week.

A univariate analysis of potential risk factors for the transmission of diarrheal disease during ODSh suggested an association between an episode of diarrhea and eating salad, dining in a mess hall, and drinking from a canteen. (A laboratory study of 12 heads of lettuce obtained from food-distribution facilities in September 1990 found coliform bacteria in all 12; ETEC was identified in two (Hyams et al. 1991).) No association was found between an episode of diarrhea and obtaining food from local vendors, eating in a local restaurant, or drinking bottled water. A multivariate analysis of these risk factors and an evaluation of published research on the transmission of *Shigella* indicated that flies and relatively poor personal hygiene probably accounted for the spread of ETEC and *Shigella*.

The disabling effect of repeated outbreaks of diarrheal disease in US forces during ODSh despite the best available preventive measures led Hyams and colleagues to call for the development of a vaccine to protect troops (Hyams et al. 1991). DOD is supporting development of such vaccines (Stephens and Nataro 2004).

Shigella

The presence of immunoglobulin A (IgA) and immunoglobulin G (IgG) anti-*Shigella* lipopolysaccharide (LPS) in predeployment serum did not offer protective immunity to infection by *Shigella* spp. among US ground troops who participated in the Persian Gulf War, Hyams and colleagues reported (Hyams et al. 1995b). The investigators reached that conclusion by studying a cohort of 883 combat troops and support personnel in three Marine Corps units who were flown directly to Saudi Arabia in late December 1990 and directly back to the United States in May 1991. Initially stationed in Saudi Arabia, and then relocated to Kuwait, the subjects lived in remote, rugged, desert camps. US military personnel prepared most of their food, which came from the United States except for local fresh produce. The subjects drank both locally produced bottled water and water purified by reverse-osmosis (Hyams et al. 1993).

The investigators obtained serum samples from all members of the three units who were accessible during the week before their deployment and the 2 two days after their return (827 subjects). Paired serum samples were tested for antibodies to both *S. sonnei* and *S. flexneri*. Epidemiologic questionnaires were also administered to this cohort before and after deployment.

Among the 827 subjects, 18% seroconverted during ODSh and ODSt; that underscored earlier findings that troops deployed to ODSh and ODSt faced a considerable risk of *Shigella* infection. The study revealed the absence of an association between seroconversion and the occurrence of diarrheal symptoms. Overall, 60% of the cohort reported one or more episodes of diarrhea, and 18% reported diarrhea with fever. In contrast, many troops who seroconverted were asymptomatic.

Because *S. sonnei* LPS cross-reacts with the LPS of *Plesiomonas shigelloides*, some of the high concentrations of serum antibodies observed in samples from the 827 marines might not have been the result of exposure to *Shigella* spp. To determine whether exposure to *Shigella* led to persistently high antibody concentrations in some subjects and seroconversions in others, Mikhail and colleagues examined how a subset of the paired serum samples reacted to four *Shigella* invasion plasmids, which cross-react with just one enteroinvasive strain of *E. coli* (Mikhail et al. 1996). They also used ELISA to detect antibodies to *S. sonnei* LPS. In their report, the authors noted that antibodies to LPS and invasion plasmid antigens in serum increase and decrease within 4 months during naturally acquired *Shigella* infections.

Only 12 sets of serum samples were large enough to use for this experiment (six from seroconverters and six with persistently high concentrations of antibodies to *S. sonnei* LPS). By using Western blot, the investigators observed antibody reactions to numerous invasion plasmid antigens both before and after deployment in serum from troops with persistently high concentrations of antibodies to *S. sonnei* LPS, which suggest that they had been exposed to *S. sonnei* before deployment and were repeatedly exposed to it during deployment. In the postdeployment serum from troops who seroconverted, the scientists observed IgA and IgG recognition of additional invasion plasmid antigens and increased concentrations of antibodies to *S. sonnei* LPS—even in two soldiers who were asymptomatic for diarrheal illness throughout the war. The authors interpreted those results as an indication that troops who seroconverted had been exposed repeatedly to *S. sonnei* in the field.

Norovirus

Norovirus (NV) and Norwalk-like viruses caused both sporadic cases and outbreaks of acute gastroenteritis among ground troops and shipboard personnel throughout the Gulf War. Brief and debilitating, NV gastroenteritis usually causes acute vomiting, diarrhea, nausea, and abdominal cramps that last 1-2 days. Some people never develop symptoms even after direct challenge, but others are repeatedly susceptible to symptomatic infection. All infected people shed highly contagious NV in stools from as early as 15 hours after exposure to as late as 14 days after. Studies of NV infections among military personnel indicate that crowding is the most important risk factor for transmission (McCarthy et al. 2000).

After the Gulf War, Hyams and colleagues demonstrated the incidence of NV infection among troops deployed to Saudi Arabia and Kuwait from late December 1990 through May 1991 (Hyams et al. 1993). Using the paired serum samples from the 883-troop cohort described above, the investigators used ELISA to measure antibody activity to recombinant NV particles. The investigators defined evidence of infection as a 4-fold or greater increase in titer of anti-NV antibodies from predeployment serum to postdeployment serum.

Matching the ELISA results with the subjects' clinical symptoms, as reported in the aforementioned postdeployment epidemiologic questionnaire, the investigators obtained the results displayed in Table 4.6. After adjusting for oversampling of subjects with vomiting, the investigators estimated that NV infected 6% of the study population. The scientists could not determine the specific sources of infection, although they enumerated the probable opportunities for person-to-person spread of NV: rapid deployment of massive numbers of soldiers, overcrowding, and rugged desert living conditions that included communal temporary latrines and bathing facilities.

To aid the development of a vaccine against NV and Norwalk-like virus for the US military, Lew and colleagues compared the published genetic sequence of NV with sequences of NV strains extracted from three stool specimens from US troops who developed gastroenteritis while deployed to Saudi Arabia for ODSh (Lew et al. 1994).

TABLE 4.6 Number of Subjects with Various Clinical Manifestations of Enteric Disease and Serologic Evidence of Norovirus Infection

Clinical Manifestation	No. (%) with Complaint: Entire Cohort (n = 883)	No. (%) with Complaint: Subjects Tested for Norovirus Infection (n = 404)	No. (%) with ≥ 4-fold Increase in Norovirus Antibody (n = 32)
Vomiting alone	17 (1.9)	17 (4.2)	4 (23.5)
Vomiting and diarrhea	117 (13.3)	117 (29.0)	14 (12.0)
Diarrhea alone	406 (46.0)	170 (42.1)	11 (6.5)
No vomiting or diarrhea	343 (38.8)	100 (24.8)	3 (3.0)

SOURCE: Reprinted with Permission from Hyams et al. 1993.

Enteric Parasitic Infections

Enteric parasites may have infected a small percentage of troops deployed to the Persian Gulf region in 1990 and 1991 (Malone et al. 1991). Malone and colleagues studied the risk of enteric parasitic disease in a cohort of 422 marines returning from Saudi Arabia and Kuwait after 5 months of service on the front lines of ODSt. Like the marines described above, this cohort had little contact with local populations. The investigators collected stool samples from the troops within 2 days of their arrival in the United States. The specimens were analyzed for evidence of helminthic and protozoan infections according to the thimerisol (Merthiolate)-iodine-formalin concentration technique.

The only evidence of enteric parasitic infection found in the cohort was *Giardia lamblia* cysts in specimens from nine marines, or 2% of the subjects. Four of the nine troops had experienced an episode of diarrhea while deployed to the Middle East, and seven of the nine had previously been deployed aboard a ship that made port calls in the Mediterranean. None of the nine marines had diarrhea when their stool samples were obtained.

Oster and Sanford make passing reference to "a few" cases of amebiasis among troops deployed to the Persian Gulf War (Oster and Sanford 1992); however, the report lacks supporting epidemiologic, clinical, and microbiologic data. The committee is unaware of other reports of amebiasis among Gulf War troops.

Shipboard Military Personnel

About 46% of the 870 military personnel deployed to the Persian Gulf aboard the hospital ship USNS *Mercy* T-AH 19 had at least one episode of diarrhea in the period August 1990-January 1991 (Paparello et al. 1993). That finding is derived from the results of an epidemiologic survey designed to assess the prevalence and effects of diarrheal illness among shipboard personnel deployed to the Middle East during ODSh.

The USNS *Mercy* was a referral hospital for patients from other ships in the Persian Gulf and ground-based medical facilities during ODSh. From December 13, 1990, to January 7, 1991, investigators distributed a voluntary questionnaire to all Navy personnel aboard the ship; about 83% (N = 722) completed it (Table 4.6). The questions covered demographics; history of eating off the ship; job description; location of spaces where subjects worked, ate, and slept; and gastrointestinal symptoms. In contrast with the populations of most other studies described in this chapter, 32% of the subjects were female.

In addition to the results listed in Table 4.7, the investigators found that officers were more likely to report an episode of diarrhea and more often unable to perform routine duties due to diarrhea than enlisted personnel. One explanation, the authors speculated, is that officers tended to eat in a wide variety of local restaurants during visits to foreign ports, whereas enlisted personnel did not. The investigators also found independent associations between lower age (range, 17 to 31 years) and an episode of diarrhea with vomiting and between female sex and an episode of diarrhea with vomiting. The authors speculated about many explanations for the latter finding: that women were more likely to report symptoms to sick call, that a greater percentage of women than men were officers, and that women worked more closely with patients and thus were more often exposed to diarrheal pathogens.

TABLE 4.7 Morbidity Due to Diarrheal Disease Among 722 US Navy Shipboard Personnel Deployed to the Persian Gulf During ODSh

Symptoms and Outcomes	Fraction of Troops (N = 722), %
Diarrhea	46.3
Diarrhea and fever	11.6
Diarrhea and vomiting	6.2
Sick-call visit	7.6
Inability to work	6.0

SOURCE: Adapted with permission from Paparello et al. 1993.

Most of the 8.3% of subjects who received medication responded to treatment with norfloxacin or ciprofloxacin. The investigators suspected but could not confirm an infectious etiology for most cases of diarrheal disease among the USNS *Mercy*'s crew on the basis of the acute onset and short duration of most cases and a frequent association with eating in foreign ports. The relatively small space for living, eating, and attending to patients aboard the USNS *Mercy* promoted close contact that may have facilitated the transmission and spread of enteric pathogens among the crew and between patients and crew.

Gastroenteritis in Operation Enduring Freedom and Operation Iraqi Freedom

Epidemiologic Investigations of Gastroenteritis

An epidemiologic survey of 15,459 deployed troops conducted in January-March 2004 revealed that 74.5% of military personnel had experienced at least one episode of diarrhea while serving in OEF, OIF, or both (Sanders et al. 2005a). Sanders and colleagues of the Navy's Enteric Disease Research Program reached that finding and others through a survey designed to assess the incidence and effect of the most common illnesses and noncombat injuries among deployed US troops participating in OEF and OIF. The investigators' findings related to diarrheal disease are discussed here, and findings pertinent to respiratory disease and leishmaniasis are presented later.

The survey posed 199 questions that covered demographics, clinical information, general health, and health-risk behaviors and attitudes. The questions were dispersed among 20 unique single-page forms, each containing 19-21 questions (some questions appeared on multiple forms). That enabled the researchers to obtain a representative distribution of responses. The investigators verified the accuracy, integrity, and internal validity of the data obtained from each form.

The troops who completed the questionnaire represented about 11% of the US military force in OEF and OIF during the study period. The study subjects either were participating in the military's rest and recuperation (R&R) program in Doha, Qatar, or had stopped at an American air base en route to the United States for a 2-week break after an initial tour of duty in Afghanistan or Iraq.

Analysis of the survey data revealed that self-reported symptoms of diarrheal disease were moderately severe and multiple episodes common. Gastroenteritis occurred more frequently among troops deployed to Iraq (76.8%) than to Afghanistan (54.4%). The duration and severity of symptoms were greater for troops in Iraq than in Afghanistan. Table 4.8 contains additional salient data obtained through the survey about the occurrence of diarrheal illness among US forces during OEF and OIF.

TABLE 4.8 Impact of Diarrhea Among US Military Personnel Deployed to Iraq and Afghanistan, 2003-2004

Characteristics of illness	No. cases in Iraq (N, % or range[a])	No. cases in Afghanistan (N, % or range[a])	p
Experienced diarrhea	7,553 (76.8)	543 (54.4)	< 0.0001
Number of episodes	5 (2-8)	2 (2-5)	0.0003
Duration (days)	4 (1.5-4)	1.5 (1.5-4)	0.008
Maximal number loose stools per day	5 (2.5-5)	2.5 (2.5-5)	< 0.0001
Reported more than six stools per day	1,166 (20.8)	55 (14.0)	

Illness characteristics from Iraq and Afghanistan[b] combined	Percentage	95% CI
Sought care for diarrhea	40.2	38.0-42.5
Number of clinic visits[c]	2.0	1-2
Fever with diarrhea	25.8	22.3-29.2
Vomiting with diarrhea	18.0	15.0-21.1
Vomiting without diarrhea	16.5	14.0-19.1
Persistent diarrhea (>14 days)	9.8	7.5-12.1
Chronic diarrhea (>30 days)	3.3	1.9-4.7
Disposition		
Confined to quarters (bedrest)	14.2	11.5-16.9
Days in quarters[c]	2.0	1-2
Hospitalized	1.8	0.7-2.8

NOTE : CI = confidence interval.
[a] Ranges are from the 25th percentile to the 75th percentile (the interquartile range).
[b] No statistical differences in these characteristics were observed between sites.
[c] Values are median and interquartile range.
SOURCE: Adapted with permission from Sanders et al. 2005a.

Sanders and colleagues note that recall and selection bias may have influenced their results. They assert that the point estimates derived probably can be generalized to the entire population of US troops deployed to Iraq and Afghanistan for OEF and OIF.

The results presented above validate the findings of an earlier, smaller study in which Sanders and colleagues found that diarrheal illness among troops deployed to OEF and OIF occurred at a high rate and frequently manifested with severe symptoms (Sanders et al. 2005b; Sanders et al. 2004). They also found that diarrheal illness appeared to interfere with military operations more during OEF and OIF than during ODSh. They reached those conclusions by analyzing data collected from an anonymous questionnaire administered to 4,348 volunteers in the period October 27, 2003-January 27, 2004.

The epidemiologic questionnaire was designed to assess the incidence of diarrheal illness and its associated symptoms, treatment, and impact on military missions. Diarrhea was defined as three or more loose or liquid stools in 24 hours or two or more loose or liquid stools associated with other gastrointestinal symptoms or fever.

The respondents, who participated voluntarily, had been deployed for a median of 8 months to Iraq and 6.7 months to Afghanistan. Most were on R&R in Doha, Qatar; others were traveling through Incirlik Air Base, Turkey, after their deployment to Iraq had ended. Although Sanders and colleagues noted several sampling biases in their study, they concluded that it was unlikely that their results overestimated rates of diarrheal illness in the overall population of troops in Iraq and Afghanistan.

Sixty-four percent of respondents stationed in Afghanistan and 77% stationed in Iraq reported one or more episodes of diarrhea during their deployment. More than half the subjects reported multiple episodes. The amount of time spent off a military compound was associated with an increased risk of developing diarrhea. The investigators concluded that time spent off a base probably represented a surrogate measure of exposure to local food and drink.

The investigators found that diarrheal illness affected military operations in OEF and OIF more than it had during ODSh. Of the survey participants, 45% experienced an episode of diarrhea severe enough to decrease job performance for a median of 3 days; 62% of subjects sought medical care for diarrheal illness at least once, and 17% were consequently confined to bed rest for a median of 2 days. For nearly one-third of troops with diarrhea, treatment included intravenous rehydration. Personnel deployed to Iraq were more likely to experience diarrheal illness, to have multiple episodes, and to have severe diarrhea (more than 10 stools per day).

Sanders and colleagues did not attempt to identify the etiologic agents of diarrheal illness in their study population. Nevertheless, they speculated that ETEC and other enteropathogenic forms of *E. coli* probably caused most episodes of diarrhea that respondents described as watery (Table 4.9). They also speculated that norovirus caused many cases of diarrheal disease in troops who experienced vomiting as a primary symptom.

TABLE 4.9 Demographics and Diarrheal Illness Characteristics of US Military Personnel Deployed to Iraq and Afghanistan

Characterization[a] of Diarrhea	**Occurrence Among Troops Stationed in Iraq (N = 3915) [N (%)]**	**Occurrence Among Troops Stationed in Afghanistan (N = 255) [N (%)]**
Watery	2815 (72)	149 (58)
Vomiting (mainly)	317 (8)	6 (2)
Blood in diarrhea	128 (3)	5 (2)
Diarrhea with fever	471 (12)	23 (9)

[a] These characterizations reflect absolute responses that are not mutually exclusive and may include symptoms across multiple episodes.
SOURCE: Adapted with permission from Sanders et al. 2005b.

Laboratory Analysis of Gastroenteritis

More than any other type of infectious disease, gastroenteritis due to norovirus[1] and *Shigella* spp. plagued the population of 83,000 US marines deployed to Iraq in spring 2003 according to a study led by staff of a Navy preventive medicine laboratory that provided clinical

[1] Includes Norwalk-like viruses (Matson 2005).

and diagnostic support (Thornton et al. 2005). Located in a city about 175 km south of Baghdad, the laboratory collected and analyzed stool samples and other clinical specimens from 30 First Marine Expeditionary Force battalion aid stations and several other medical stations in the area. Thornton and colleagues published the results of their analysis of 129 stool specimens collected from April 24 to June 1, 2003, from 33 medical stations scattered across south-central Iraq.

The authors reported that large outbreaks of nausea, vomiting, and diarrhea lasting 24-48 hours occurred in the First Marine Expeditionary Force from early April though the middle of May, suggesting a viral etiology for most cases of gastroenteritis during that period. Febrile dysentery predominated in that population beginning in the middle of May.

Numerous factors placed the troops of the First Marine Expeditionary Force at risk for gastroenteritis, the authors wrote. The primitive nature of the camps, overcrowding, and filth flies in latrines and dining facilities characterized the troops' unsanitary living environment. Local ambient temperatures climbed to 40°C during the period of study. Some troops broke military rules to eat locally prepared food, particularly grilled chicken. Finally, a relatively small number of microorganisms are capable of causing shigellosis and norovirus gastroenteritis in humans. In an editorial commentary on Thornton's report, Matson postulates that robustly healthy people who become dehydrated during daily activity may face a greater risk of severe outcome when infected with norovirus (Matson 2005).

The investigators used plating, biochemical identification, antigen serologic testing, fluorescent antibody antigen detection, and enzyme immunoassay to evaluate stool specimens diagnostically for enteropathogens. Specifically, they tested specimens for pathogenic *E. coli*, *Campylobacter* spp., *Salmonella* spp., *Shigella* spp., *Giardia* spp., and *Cryptosporidium*. Suspect *E. coli* was tested for heat-labile and heat-stabile enterotoxins; additionally, investigators plated stool with gross blood or fecal leukocytes on sorbitol-MacConkey agar to detect enterohemorrhagic *E. coli.* The antimicrobial susceptibility of detected bacteria was evaluated with the disk-diffusion method.

Reverse-transcriptase polymerase chain reaction (PCR) was used to detect norovirus. In addition, the authors sequenced the RNA polymerase genes of detected norovirus to distinguish strains, compare the strains with each other and with known strains, and analyze the occurrence of norovirus strains by military unit and timing.

Table 4.10 illustrates the results of the laboratory-based diagnostic evaluation. One or more enteropathogens were detected in 57 of the 129 stool samples (44%). Norovirus was detected in 23% of the specimens; the investigators found 21 norovirus strains among 30 agent-positive patients. The most frequently detected bacterial enteropathogens were *Shigella sonnei* and *Shigella flexneri*; they were isolated from a total of 20% of the specimens. The presence of fecal leukocytes in 43 of 109 stool samples (39%) indicated inflammatory diarrhea, the investigators concluded.

Most of the bacterial isolates tested by Thornton and colleagues were doxycycline-resistant (Table 4.10), and several bacterial enteropathogens identified in prior studies of military populations were observed less frequently in this study population. For those reasons, both the authors and Matson (the editorial commentator) postulated that the mandatory dose of doxycycline (100 mg/day) taken by personnel in the First Marine Expeditionary Force for antimalarial prophylaxis may also have reduced the potential impact of bacterial enteric pathogens.

Extrapolating their results to the entire First Marine Expeditionary Force, Thornton and colleagues conservatively estimated that several thousand cases of norovirus illness occurred in

April and May 2003. They also postulated that norovirus is ubiquitous in Iraq, on the basis of their observations and reported outbreaks of viral gastroenteritis among other US and allied forces in different parts of the country.

TABLE 4.10 Major Findings from 129 Stool Specimens Obtained from Marines with Gastroenteritis During Operation Iraqi Freedom and Percentage of Bacterial Isolates Resistant to Antimicrobial Agents as Determined by Disk-Diffusion Assay

Agent	No. Agent-Positive Patients	No. Units with Agent-Positive Patients	Percentage of Drug-Resistant Isolates, by Drug					
			Doxycycline	Ciprofloxacin	TMP-SMZ	Cefoxitin	Cefazolin	Ceftriaxone
All bacteria	35	26	86	14	86	14	14	3
Shigella flexneri	13	8	92	0	77	0	0	0
Shigella sonnei	13	8	100	0	100	0	0	0
Campylobacter spp.[a]	5	5	40	100	100	100	100	20
Other bacteria[b]	4	4	75	0	50	0	0	0
Norovirus	30	14	NA	NA	NA	NA	NA	NA

NOTE: Doxycycline, 30μg in disk; ciprofloxacin, 5 μg; TMP-SMZ (trimethoprim-sulfamethoxazole), 1.25 μg of trimethoprim; cefoxitin, 30 μg; cefazolin, 30 μg; ceftriaxone, 30 μg.
NA = not applicable.
[a] Fifty-six stool samples were tested for Campylobacter spp.
[b] Putative enteroinvasive *Escherichia coli*: two cases; *Salmonella arizonae*: one case; *Plesiomonas shigelloides*: one case.
SOURCE: Reprinted with permission from Thornton et al. 2005.

Although the study by Thornton and colleagues was relatively robust in terms of methods, Matson noted three weaknesses in its design compared with similar studies in civilian populations: incomplete standardized clinical data collection, an unknown denominator from which the numerator of laboratory samples was derived, and lack of description of clinical illness and associated morbidity (Matson 2005). The investigators themselves acknowledged the lack of a solid denominator and attack rates in their report, attributing these limitations to the difficulty of gathering public health data and specimens during maneuver warfare.

RESPIRATORY DISEASE

Mild Acute Respiratory Disease in the Gulf War

Mild acute respiratory disease was one of the two leading infectious causes of morbidity among US troops who served in the Gulf War. Some investigators estimated that it accounted for about 7-12% of first-time outpatient visits to primary-care medical personnel in combat units (Wasserman et al. 1997). Crowded living conditions—and for some troops, residence in tightly constructed, air-conditioned buildings—probably facilitated the transmission of respiratory pathogens among US forces (Hyams et al. 1995a; Richards et al. 1993a). In one study, investigators identified *Streptococcus pyogenes*, *Neisseria meningitidis*, *Streptococcus pneumoniae*, *Haemophilus influenzae*, *Mycoplasma pneumoniae*, influenza virus types A and B, and adenovirus in clinical specimens obtained from soldiers who presented with respiratory symptoms (Richards et al. 1993a).

Crowding occurred frequently during ODSh because so many troops were deployed so quickly. Hyams and colleagues explain that, on arrival in Saudi Arabia, "combat troops were crowded together in warehouses and tents at initial staging areas and then moved to isolated desert locations" (Hyams et al. 1995a). Such conditions naturally facilitated the transmission of respiratory pathogens. That was dramatically illustrated by changes in the weekly rates of respiratory disease among of the 40,000 marines deployed to northeastern Saudi Arabia. Most of them were transported to the Persian Gulf in late August or late December 1990; the percentage of marines that received outpatient treatment for respiratory disease spiked during each deployment (Figure 4.1) (Hyams et al. 1995a).

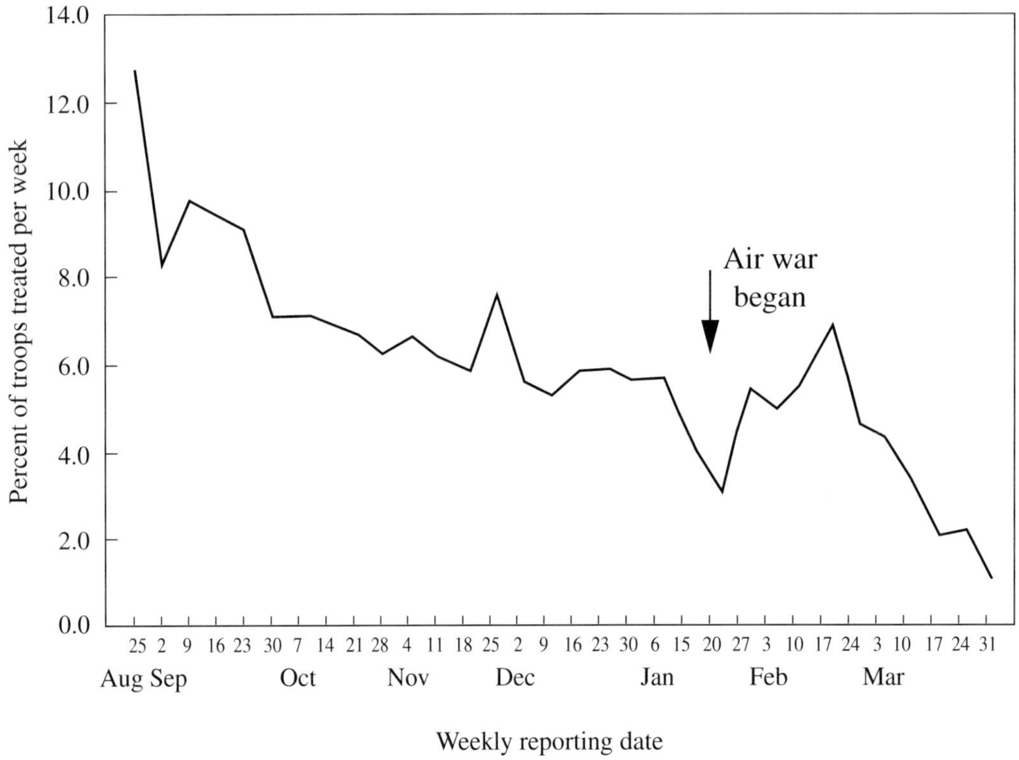

FIGURE 4.1 Weekly rates of total outpatient (sick call) visits among about 40,000 Marine Corps ground troops stationed in northeastern Saudi Arabia who participated in the US Navy's disease surveillance system.

SOURCE: Reprinted with permission from Hyams et al. 1995a.

Ground Troops

Richards and colleagues conducted epidemiologic, clinical, and environmental studies to determine the prevalence of risk factors for and severity of acute respiratory disease among US ground troops stationed in northeastern Saudi Arabia during ODSh (Richards et al. 1993a).

From November 1990 to January 1991, a voluntary questionnaire was administered to 2,598 men in four units selected to reflect diverse living conditions, geographic locations, and branches of the military (Army and Marine Corps). The rate of participation in the survey exceeded 95%. Respondents had been stationed in Saudi Arabia for a mean of 102 days.

When asked about symptoms of respiratory disease experienced at any time during their deployment, 34.4% of the survey respondents complained of sore throat, 43.1% of a cough, and 15.4% of chronic rhinorrhea. The symptoms of respiratory disease were severe enough to prevent 1.8% of respondents from performing their routine duties. The longer a soldier was deployed, the more likely he was to report respiratory problems. Having a history of respiratory disease (reported by 6% of respondents) or being a smoker (reported by 37% of respondents) significantly increased the likelihood of respiratory complaints.

The investigators asked survey participants where they slept—in tents, warehouses, non-air-conditioned buildings, or air-conditioned buildings—as a proxy measure of environmental exposure because troops often worked, relaxed, and slept in the same structure. Statistical analyses of the troops' responses revealed that the risk of developing a cough or sore throat increased as exposure to the outdoors decreased. Moreover, troops who slept in air-conditioned buildings were significantly more likely to develop both a sore throat and a cough. In contrast, exposure to the outdoors increased the risk of developing chronic rhinorrhea; troops who slept in tents were at highest risk. Controlling for smoking, time spent in the war theater, and a history of respiratory disease magnified those associations.

Blood and oropharyngeal-swab specimens were obtained from 68 military personnel who presented with acute respiratory symptoms at any of five medical facilities from October 1990 to January 1991. Using immunofluorescence, latex agglutination, and standard culture techniques, investigators identified bacterial and viral pathogens in 10 of the patients' specimens (Table 4.11).

Ground-surface samples of sand were collected from seven widely dispersed areas where US troops were stationed. No pathogenic bacterial or fungal organisms were isolated from the analyzed samples. The investigators did not collect or study airborne particles of sand.

TABLE 4.11 Pathogens Identified in Specimens from 68 Troops with Acute Respiratory Symptoms During Operation Desert Shield

Pathogen	No. Patients Infected (N = 14)[a]
Streptococcus pyogenes	3
Neisseria meningitidis	4
Streptococcus pneumoniae	1
Haemophilus influenzae	1
Mycoplasma pneumoniae	1
Influenza virus type A	1
Influenza virus type B	2
Adenovirus	1

[a] Etiologic agents were identified in specimens from only 14 of the 68 patients.
SOURCE: Richards et al. 1993a.

On the basis of the results of their epidemiologic, clinical, and environmental analyses, Richards and colleagues concluded that cases of cough and sore throat during ODSh probably had an infectious etiology, whereas environmental factors probably accounted for cases of chronic rhinorrhea. The investigators postulated that the recirculation of indoor air containing respiratory pathogens and the crowding of troops in air-conditioned buildings to escape the desert heat contributed to the high rate of mild acute respiratory disease observed during the Gulf War.

Shipboard Military Personnel

The reported risk of upper respiratory disease was lower among US ground troops than among Navy personnel who served aboard the 1,000-bed hospital ship USNS *Mercy* T-AH 19 during ODSh (Paparello et al. 1993). That was one conclusion of an epidemiologic study designed to assess the prevalence and impact of upper respiratory disease among shipboard personnel deployed to the Middle East during ODSh.

As described above, the USNS *Mercy* was a referral hospital for patients from other ships in the region and ground-based medical facilities during ODSh. From December 13, 1990-January 7, 1991, investigators distributed a voluntary questionnaire to all Navy personnel aboard the ship; about 83% (n = 722) completed it.

Among the surveyed population, 79% reported at least one upper respiratory complaint during their deployment. The respondents' symptoms generally were mild but persistent. Cold-like symptoms with fever were reported by 27.9%, cough by 53.2%, sore throat by 49.1%, and chronic rhinorrhea by 16.6%. The severity of such symptoms prevented 7.4% of respondents from performing their duties.

No significant association existed between smoking and respiratory complaints. Female sex and a history of respiratory disease were independently associated with cold-like symptoms plus fever and inability to perform duties. Investigators could not determine the reason for the sex-based association.

Pathogens probably caused the majority of respiratory disease aboard the USNS *Mercy* on the basis of the nature and short duration of reported symptoms, the investigators concluded. Moreover, they postulated that the relatively small total space for living, eating, and attending to patients promoted close contact that probably facilitated the transmission and spread of respiratory pathogens among the crew and between patients and crew.

Severe Acute Respiratory Disease in the Gulf War

More than 1,800 US military personnel deployed to the Persian Gulf region developed respiratory disease severe enough to require hospitalization of a day or more (Smith et al. 2004). Among those patients, 214 were diagnosed with pneumonia (etiologic agent unspecified), 90 with acute sinusitis, 102 with chronic sinusitis, and 81 with bronchitis; 678 cases were diagnosed as asthma, and the remaining cases of respiratory disease were not identified. The committee is unaware of published literature about the details of these cases other than what appears in this chapter.

Any of more than 50 viruses, bacteria, fungi, parasites, rickettsiae, chlamydiae, and mycoplasmas can cause pneumonia (Donowitz and Mandell 2000). A smaller array of viral, bacterial, and fungal organisms can cause acute sinusitis; however, such noninfectious agents as allergens and toxins may also instigate this disease. Acute bronchitis usually has a viral etiology, although it is also associated with *Bordetella pertussis*, *Mycoplasma pneumoniae*, and *Chlamydia pneumoniae* (strain TWAR) (Gwaltney 2000a). The pathogenesis of chronic sinus disease is poorly understood; at least six genera of bacteria have been cultured from patients with this diagnosis (Gwaltney 2000b).

Respiratory Disease in Operation Enduring Freedom and Operation Iraqi Freedom

About 70% of military personnel deployed to Iraq and Afghanistan in 2003 and the first quarter of 2004 contracted a respiratory infection during their tour of duty, according to the epidemiologic survey of 15,459 deployed troops described above (Sanders et al. 2005a). A cold or cough characterized nearly all self-reported cases of respiratory illness in that study (Table 4.12). A minority of subjects—2.6%—reported that they had been diagnosed with pneumonia; most of the cases were mild enough to obviate the need for hospitalization. A separate study found that more than 60 cases of pneumonia (severe and mild) occurred among US troops in Iraq from March 1, 2003 to August 20, 2003 (Anderson et al. 2005).

Nineteen deployed troops were hospitalized with acute bilateral pneumonitis with increased concentrations of eosinophils in March-August 2003 (CDC 2003a). All patients required intubation and mechanical ventilation; two ultimately died. The severity of this illness, its unknown cause, and its association with service in southwest and south-central Asia led the military to begin conducting special surveillance for severe acute pneumonia among troops deployed to OEF or OIF.

As of September 2003, laboratory evidence of infection with a pathogen had been identified in four of the 19 patients, as outlined in Table 4.13. In Chapter 6, the committee addresses idiopathic acute eosinophilic pneumonia (a syndrome whose etiology remains unknown).

TABLE 4.12 Impact of Respiratory Illness Among US Military Personnel Deployed to Iraq or Afghanistan, 2003-2004

	Percentage of Troops	**95% Confidence Interval**
No. of respiratory infections (cough or cold) during deployment		
None	30.9	27.6-34.4
1	19.1	16.4-22.2
2-3	35.6	32.3-39.2
>3	14.4	12.0-17.2
Sought medical care for respiratory infection	17.0	14.2-19.8
Received medicine from provider for respiratory infection	17.8	14.9-20.7
Self-medicated for respiratory infection	29.3	26.2-32.5
Experienced allergy attack	22.5	19.4-25.6
Experienced asthma attack	3.6	2.2-5.0
Developed pneumonia	2.6	1.4-3.8
Started or restarted smoking	47.6	41.7-53.6
No. of packs per day		
None	61.0	57.2-64.7
½	17.5	14.6-20.4
1	14.5	11.8-17.2
>1	7.0	5.1-9.0
Smoke Iraqi cigarettes	72.2	66.8-77.5

SOURCE: Adapted with permission from Sanders et al. 2005a.

Table 4.13 Four Cases of Severe Acute Pneumonitis with Evidence of Infectious Etiology

Case	Pathogen detected	Method of identification	Probable or suspect infection?
1	*Streptococcus pneumoniae*	Isolated from sputum culture	Probable
2	*S. pneumoniae*	Antigen detected in urine	Suspect
3	*Coxiella burnettii*	Serologic evidence	Suspect
4	*Acinetobacter baumanii*	Evidence in bronchoscopic culture	Suspect

SOURCE: CDC 2003a.

INSECT-BORNE DISEASES

Despite the endemicity of a number of insect-borne diseases in Saudi Arabia, Kuwait, and Iraq in 1990-1991, epidemiologic and laboratory surveillance for such diseases by military medical personnel identified very few cases among US troops who participated in the Gulf War (Richards et al. 1991; Richards et al. 1993b). A few dozen cases of leishmaniasis, malaria, and West Nile fever combined were diagnosed either in the field or after the war. In contrast, military medical facilities have reported more than 1050 cases of arthropod-borne disease—primarily cutaneous leishmaniasis—in troops who served in OEF and OIF. Several factors account for the difference. First, US troops serving in OEF and OIF have been present in southwest and south-central Asia year-round, including the warm seasons, when arthropods are most active. Second, many of the troops have served in or near settings where arthropods thrive, such as urban areas, areas where the infrastructure is dilapidated or destroyed, and estuaries. Finally, the Gulf War lasted only 10 months, whereas OIF and OEF are in their 4th and 5th years, respectively.

Leishmaniasis

Leishmaniasis is the umbrella term for a family of sand-fly-borne parasitic diseases that includes cutaneous leishmaniasis (CL), diffuse cutaneous leishmaniasis, mucocutaneous leishmaniasis (MCL), visceral leishmaniasis (VL, also called kala-azar), and viscerotropic leishmaniasis (VTL).

The signatures of CL are skin lesions that range in severity from small, dry, crusted areas to large, deep, mutilating ulcers. MCL is characterized by lesions that may lead to destruction of the nose, oral cavity, pharynx, and larynx. VL manifests as fever, enlargement of the liver and spleen, anemia, leukopenia, and hypergammaglobulinemia. VTL, a milder form of VL disease, may begin abruptly after infection or weeks to years later; alternatively, infected individuals may be asymptomatic. The acute syndrome is a febrile disorder that may include chronic fatigue and gastrointestinal symptoms; the chronic syndrome might consist of low-grade fever and malaise for several months.

Chapter 5 contains a detailed description of acute leishmaniasis and an analysis of its potential long-term adverse health outcomes. The following text summarizes what has been published about the cases of leishmaniasis contracted during the Gulf War, OEF, and OIF.

Leishmaniasis in the Gulf War

Clinicians at Walter Reed Army Medical Center (WRAMC) in Washington have identified 20 cases of CL and 12 cases of VTL among veterans of the Gulf War (Hyams et al. 1995a; Magill et al. 1993). Because VTL appeared to be clinically distinct from VL and had not previously been reported in the scientific literature, it has generated a substantial amount of attention and interest.

Viscerotropic Leishmaniasis

Twelve cases of VTL were identified in male US troops who had served in at least five military units in desert or urban locations in Kuwait, Iraq, and eastern Saudi Arabia (Hyams 1999; Magill et al. 1993; Magill et al. 1994). A cluster of these patients apparently became infected near the city of Dhahran along the Persian Gulf coast of Saudi Arabia about 200 miles south of the Saudi-Kuwaiti border (Magill et al. 1993).

From November 1990 to December 1993, 11 patients presented with unexplained fever, chronic fatigue, malaise, cough, intermittent diarrhea, or abdominal pain (Magill et al. 1993). Nine also had adenopathy or mild, transient enlargement of the liver and spleen. Serologic surveys conducted among troops in the same units as the first seven patients identified another infected person who was asymptomatic. Among the first seven cases, primary symptoms presented a median of 7 months after the soldiers had arrived in the Persian Gulf and within 5 months after they had departed. The ninth case became symptomatic, and the diagnosis was made 2 years after he left Saudi Arabia (Magill et al. 1994). The last three cases were identified and diagnosed in 1993 (Hyams 1999).

Leishmanial parasites were cultured from either bone-marrow aspirates or lymph-node biopsies from all 12 patients. With *Leishmania*-specific indirect immunofluorescent monoclonal antibody or direct fluorescent antibody, it was possible to visualize the parasites in smears of the aspirates or tissue from nine patients (such data were unavailable on three patients). *Leishmania tropica*, which usually causes CL, was identified through enzyme electrophoresis as the etiologic agent in at least 10 cases; however, none of the 12 patients displayed evidence of CL by either history or physical examination. While undergoing evaluation for leishmaniasis, three patients were found to have underlying conditions: acute retroviral syndrome and HIV seroconversion, renal-cell carcinoma, and acute Epstein-Barr viral infection (CDC 1992; Magill et al. 1993; Magill et al. 1994; Oster and Sanford 1992).

The published literature contains data on the treatment of nine of the 11 symptomatic patients for VTL. One of these patients' symptoms subsided without treatment; the other eight received parenteral sodium stibogluconate for up to 30 days. Clinicians aborted that treatment in two patients who developed severe thrombocytopenia after 8 and 18 days. The signs and symptoms of VTL resolved in five of the six patients who completed a 30-day course of sodium stibogluconate; after 10 months, the sixth patient underwent elective splenectomy to resolve his condition (CDC 1992; Magill et al. 1993; Magill et al. 1994; Oster and Sanford 1992).

Cutaneous Leishmaniasis

On the basis of the experience of allied forces stationed in Iraq and Iran during World War II, the US military anticipated that troops would be at risk for CL during the Gulf War (Hyams et al. 1995a; Martin et al. 1998). In fact, only 20 cases were recognized and diagnosed (Martin et al. 1998). The very low rate of infection has been attributed to several factors: use of insecticides and repellents; stationing of most combat troops in the open desert, as sand flies and their primary mammalian hosts (desert rodents) thrive in oases and urban areas; and deployment of the majority of ground troops during winter months, when sand flies are least active (Hyams et al. 1995a).

Few specifics about the 20 cases of CL have been published in scientific journals. Locations where patients became infected included from central Saudi Arabia, northeastern Saudi Arabia, and southern Iraq (Kreutzer et al. 1993). The first 17 cases presented with noduloulcerative disease typical of classic CL; the diagnosis was confirmed with examination of stained smears and cultures of aspirates or of biopsy specimens from the margin of an ulcer (Ohl et al. 1993). In specimens containing enough parasites for evaluation with isoenzyme analysis, *L. major* was identified as the etiologic agent (Kreutzer et al. 1993; Ohl et al. 1993). It was later determined that *L. major* caused all 20 cases (Magill 2005). It is unclear whether or how the 20 patients were treated for CL. Most skin lesions caused by *L. major* do not require treatment, because they heal spontaneously without persistent disfiguration, as described in Chapter 5 (Mandell et al. 2005).

Leishmaniasis in Operation Enduring Freedom and Operation Iraqi Freedom

Published reports and public presentations indicate that more than 1,000 US troops have had a diagnosis of leishmaniasis contracted during a tour of duty in OEF or OIF.

In the anonymous epidemiologic survey of nearly 15,500 troops conducted by Sanders and colleagues and described above, 2.1% of respondents reported receiving a diagnosis of leishmaniasis in 2003 or early 2004 (Sanders et al. 2005a). Extrapolating that finding to the entire force of 140,000 personnel deployed to Iraq and Afghanistan at that time suggests that 2,940 troops may have contracted the disease.

Cutaneous Leishmaniasis in Operation Enduring Freedom and Operation Iraqi Freedom

As of May 2005, military medical personnel had diagnosed and confirmed CL in more than 1,000 military personnel who served in OEF or OIF and were deployed to Afghanistan, Kuwait, or Iraq (Magill 2005; Willard et al. 2005; Zapor and Moran 2005). Each diagnosis was confirmed with light microscopy, culture, PCR assay, or a combination of these. Isoenzyme electrophoresis of cultured parasites from 176 patients consistently revealed *L. major* to be the etiologic agent in cases from Iraq (CDC 2004b; Magill 2005), and *L. tropica* caused CL in the cases from Afghanistan (Magill 2005).

Demographic data were collected from 361 patients treated for CL with sodium stibogluconate under an investigational new drug protocol administered at WRAMC (CDC 2004b). Sodium stibogluconate is a pentavalent antimony compound marketed as Pentostam® outside the United States. Although the patients came from multiple branches of the US military, most were in the Army's active force. It is believed that all but four of the 361 patients were infected in Iraq, particularly along the Iraqi border with Syria and Iran; two soldiers were infected in Kuwait and two in Afghanistan. Nearly 80% of the patients reported that their skin lesions first appeared in August-November 2003. Almost half first noted skin lesions characteristic of CL in September or October.

Staff at WRAMC reported successful treatment of the first 22 patients with 20 mg of sodium stibogluconate per kilogram (kg) of body weight per day by intravenous infusion for 20 days (CDC 2003b). Reversible side effects of the treatment protocol included fatigue, arthralgia, myalgia, headache, and chemical pancreatitis. In addition, a detailed report of 237 soldiers deployed from Fort Campbell, Kentucky, who acquired CL in OIF described diagnosis, clinical presentation, and response to therapy (Willard et al. 2005). It indicated that about 1% of Fort Campbell troops had a diagnosis of CL, that most were laboratory-confirmed, and that PCR was the most useful diagnostic technique. All cases responded to treatment. CL cases resulting from service in OIF are being managed with a variety of approaches, including oral fluconazole, sodium stibogluconate, cryotherapy, and ThermoMed (a device with FDA 510K clearance that delivers localized radiofrequency-generated heat directly to a lesion through a set of prongs placed onto the lesion).

US soldiers deployed to Iraq received dozens or even hundreds of insect bites beginning in April 2003 (Weina et al. 2004). DOD conducted surveillance from April to September 2003 to determine the prevalence of *Leishmania*-infected female phlebotomine sand flies—the vector for CL—in and near urban and periurban parts of Iraq where US soldiers have been stationed (CDC 2003b). Light traps facilitated the collection of about 65,000 of the flies, about half of them female. A fluorogenic PCR test revealed that 1.4% of the flies were infected with *Leishmania* spp.; the rate of infection ranged from zero in Diwaniya to 5% in An Nasiriya.

Visceral Leishmaniasis in Operation Enduring Freedom and Operation Iraqi Freedom

As of December 31, 2005, VL has been diagnosed and reported in two soldiers who were stationed in Iraq during OIF and three who participated in OEF (CDC 2004a; Magill 2005; Zapor and Moran 2005).

Case reports describing two of the three OEF soldiers affected by VL indicate that they were previously healthy men in their 30s who had served in the same Special Forces unit of the Army during distinct periods: March-September, 2003 (patient A) and May-October 2002 (patient B) (CDC 2004a). Both men presented with acute febrile illness in December 2003. On initial clinical evaluation, they displayed a few of the classic yet non-specific signs of advanced VL: fever, cachexia, enlarged liver and spleen, pancytopenia, and hypergammaglobulinemia with hypoalbuminemia. No leishmanial parasites were observed on light microscopic examination of bone-marrow and liver-biopsy specimens from patient A, nor were the parasites noted in cultured bone marrow. Genus-specific PCR analysis of the bone-marrow specimen also was negative. Clinicians then evaluated patient A for noninfectious diseases and evidence of infection by other etiologic agents. In February 2004, a combination of clinical and parasitologic criteria enabled clinicians to diagnose VL in patient A. By that time, he manifested all the classic signs of advanced VL. In addition, a re-examination of his liver-biopsy specimen with light microscopy revealed one definite and many probable *Leishmania* parasites. The etiologic species was not reported. After the first week of a 14-day course of treatment with liposomal amphotericin B (AmBisome®), the patient became afebrile and resumed physical training.

As in the case of patient A, light microscopic examination of a liver-biopsy specimen from patient B yielded positive results for *Leishmania* parasites. Genus-specific PCR analyses identified the etiologic agent as the *L. donovani-infantum* complex. A 15-day course of treatment with a lipid formulation of amphotericin B (Abelcet®) temporarily improved patient B's health, but he relapsed 2 weeks later. Thirty days after completing the first treatment protocol, he began a 28-day course of sodium stibogluconate (20 mg/kg of body weight per day) administered intravenously. The clinical outcome for patient B has not been reported.

The third reported case of VL from OEF was contracted during deployment to Seeb, Oman, in October 2001-March 2002 (Halsey et al. 2004). The patient, a 37-year-old male Air Force sergeant, became ill about 9 weeks after returning to the United States. His illness manifested as fever, chills, malaise, frontal headache, significant loss of weight, and enlarged liver and spleen. A bone-marrow biopsy was smear- and culture-negative for adult *Leishmania* protozoa (amastigotes) but PCR-positive. In addition, the patient's serum tested positive for *Leishmania*-specific immunoglobulin G in a novel enzyme-linked immunosorbent assay (ELISA). Clinicians determined the species to be *L. infantum-donovani* by using a second PCR assay that had species-specific primers and probes. The patient's symptoms quickly subsided after he began therapy with liposomal amphotericin B at 3 mg/kg per day on days 1-5, 14, and 21. Four months later, he remained free of symptoms, and his liver was functioning normally.

The two soldiers deployed to Baghdad who contracted VL presented with fever, enlarged liver and spleen, cytopenia, and hypergammaglobulinemia (Weina et al. 2004). On presentation, one had been deployed for 11 months, and the other had left Iraq 7 months earlier. Examination of bone-marrow biopsies from both patients revealed *Leishmania* parasites. The patients tested positive for *Leishmania* in an rK39 serologic test; and, their serum yielded titers of 1:1,024 or greater in a *Leishmania* immunofluorescent antibody test. Using a PCR assay with species-specific primers, clinicians were able to determine the species—*L. infantum-donovani*—in one case. The treatment protocols and their outcomes were not published.

Malaria

Very few cases of malaria have been reported in US veterans of the Gulf War, OEF, and OIF. That is not surprising because in 1990-1991, malaria had been eliminated from northeastern Saudi Arabia, where most US troops were stationed, and no indigenous malaria transmission occurred in Kuwait, Bahrain, or Qatar (Hyams et al. 1995a; Oldfield et al. 1991). Malaria due to *Plasmodium vivax* (vivax malaria) occurred in small numbers in northern Iraq during the late 1980s to 1991 (Oldfield et al. 1991). In the wake of the Gulf War, however, Iraq experienced a serious malaria epidemic; by 2000, vivax malaria had become a serious problem in that country (Schlagenhauf 2003). Moreover, the disease is endemic in many parts of Afghanistan.

Publications during the last 15 years about the threat of vivax malaria to US and allied forces in southwest and south-central Asia sound several consistent themes: the seriousness of the disease, shortcomings of chemical and personal countermeasures, and suboptimal rates of compliance with those countermeasures among troops of many nationalities. According to a 1995 report by the Army Medical Surveillance Activity, "after operations in highly endemic areas, sporadic cases [of malaria] may be expected despite compliance with all prevention guidelines" (MSMR 1995).

Malaria in the Gulf War

Vivax malaria existed in the Euphrates River valley of Iraq in 1990 and 1991 (Young et al. 1992). Seven cases of vivax malaria were reported among US troops who crossed into southern Iraq, where coalition forces operated briefly (Hyams et al. 1995a). No information was given on complications in those troops.

Malaria in Operation Enduring Freedom and Operation Iraqi Freedom

As of May 2005, 52 cases of vivax malaria had been reported in US troops who served either exclusively in Afghanistan or in both Afghanistan and Iraq (Kilpatrick 2005). It is believed that all 52 infections were contracted in Afghanistan, although *Plasmodium vivax* is endemic in areas of both countries (Wallace et al. 2002). None of the patients was diagnosed with malaria prior to leaving the war theater; this is not surprising, because vivax malaria is known to incubate in human hosts and may relapse up to 5 years after initial infection (Boecken and Bronnert 2005; Johnson 2004).

Thirty-eight of the 52 reported cases of vivax malaria occurred in a 725-man Army Ranger task force deployed to eastern Afghanistan in June-September 2002. Kotwal and colleagues, the primary-care clinicians for these rangers, collected and later analyzed data from the patients during their evaluation, treatment, and followup. In addition, a retrospective anonymous survey was administered to the whole task force in July 2003 to ascertain compliance with malarial countermeasures. Retrospective analysis led the authors to conclude that the 38 rangers became infected while working at two specific forward-operating bases during summer 2002 (Kotwal et al. 2005).

The antimalarial chemoprophylaxis prescribed for this Army Ranger task force consisted of 250-mg mefloquine tablets ingested weekly beginning 2 weeks before deployment and ending 4 weeks after deployment. To prevent the late onset of malaria, the troops also were instructed to ingest one 15-mg primaquine tablet daily for 2 weeks after deployment. In addition, it is expected that all US soldiers at risk of malaria are trained and supplied to minimize their exposure to mosquitoes by impregnating their uniforms and bed nets with permethrin, wearing the uniforms properly, using the bed nets, and frequently coating exposed skin with insect repellent that contains 33% DEET (Johnson 2004; Kotwal et al. 2005).

The first three rangers to become symptomatic had vivax malaria diagnosed in March and April 2003. Fifteen more rangers fell ill and had diagnoses in May; the remaining 20 cases came to light in June-November 2003 (Lay 2005). The attack rate for the 725-person task force was 52.4 cases per 1,000 soldiers.

P. vivax infection causes flu-like symptoms that are often severe and debilitating (Boecken and Bronnert 2005; Spudick et al. 2005). Most of the infected rangers presented with fever; many also complained of chills, headache, muscle aches, or nausea. A complete blood-cell count obtained for 31 of the patients demonstrated that most had mild to moderate anemia and thrombocytopenia. The attending physicians based their initial diagnoses on those clinical signs and symptoms. Each case was confirmed with microscopic visualization of malaria parasitemia in the patient's red blood cells on laboratory-prepared blood smears. A median of 233 days (range, 1-399 days) elapsed between these soldiers' return from the theater of war and confirmation of their diagnoses.

Two rangers relapsed after completing their first treatment regimen. One of those cases was complicated by life-threatening acute respiratory distress syndrome (ARDS) during the primary attack; the patient relapsed three times from June to December 2003. The multiple relapses indicated infection with primaquine-tolerant *P. vivax* (Spudick et al. 2005). Pulmonary complications, such as ARDS, might occur with vivax malaria more frequently than is generally recognized.

The results of the anonymous postdeployment survey reported by Kotwal and colleagues indicate that at least 72% of the 725-member task force complied poorly with most of the malarial countermeasures described above (Kotwal et al. 2005). Some 52% followed the US Army guidelines for mefloquine, 41% for primaquine, and 31% for both; 82% reportedly treated their uniforms with permethrin, but only 29% routinely applied DEET to exposed skin. Delayed presentation of vivax malaria is well described, primarily in people who fail to take primaquine as terminal prophylaxis after returning from malaria-endemic areas of the Middle East (Gasser et al. 1991).

Only 14 cases of malaria were reported in US troops in 2004, a 63% decrease from the year before (Lay 2005). All the cases were caused by *P. vivax* infection and were contracted in Afghanistan (Kilpatrick 2005), and they presented sporadically from February to November.

Kotwal and colleagues suggest that continuously educating field troops about the importance of countermeasures and having leaders monitor and enforce the use of chemoprophylaxis and personal protective measures might further reduce the occurrence of malaria among US forces (Kotwal et al. 2005). At the same time, they and others note several shortcomings of the countermeasures themselves (Boecken and Bronnert 2005; Kotwal et al.

2005; Spudick et al. 2005). Avoiding mosquito bites in the field is difficult and somewhat impractical. For example, nighttime patrols, use of night-vision devices, and vigilance during dusk and dawn place troops at higher risk of exposure to nocturnally active *Anopheles* mosquitoes, the vectors of malarial parasites, in endemic areas. Permethrin-impregnated bed nets have no utility for soldiers who are at work at night.

West Nile Fever

West Nile virus belongs to the Japanese encephalitis virus antigenic complex in the genus *Flavivirus* of the family Flaviviridae. Mosquitoes transmit West Nile virus, which was first isolated in 1937 from a febrile woman in the West Nile Province of Uganda. Although 80% of infected people are asymptomatic, those who develop clinical disease usually present with a nonspecific febrile illness lasting 3-6 days. Chapter 5 contains an in-depth discussion of this disease.

West Nile Fever in the Gulf War

Only one person who served in the Gulf War had a diagnosis of West Nile fever due to an infection contracted during the war (Richards et al. 1991). The patient was hospitalized with acute fever, debility, and arthralgias; these symptoms subsided without therapy after 4 days. Clinicians at the US Navy Forward Laboratory in Saudi Arabia tested the patient's serum with ELISA for immunoglobin M (IgM) and IgG antibodies to the etiologic agents of nine viral and rickettsial diseases: Congo-Crimean hemorrhagic fever, dengue fever, hantaviral disease (Hantaan virus), Q fever, Rift Valley fever, Sindbis, sand fly fever, typhus, and West Nile fever. The serum tested IgM-positive for West Nile virus, but IgM- and IgG-negative for the other arboviruses.

A separate study designed to determine the incidence of insect-borne infections among Gulf War troops identified 30 marines who had been infected with a flavivirus *before* deployment to Saudi Arabia (Richards et al. 1993b). In the study, an epidemiologic questionnaire was administered and a blood sample obtained from each of 865 marines just before deployment and immediately after. The serum samples were initially screened with ELISA for Crimean-Congo hemorrhagic fever, Rift Valley fever, sand fly fever, Sindbis, West Nile fever, and rickettsiae in the typhus and spotted-fever groups. Moderately increased titers of IgG to West Nile virus in the predeployment *and* postdeployment serum of 30 marines led investigators to test those blood samples for antibodies to other flaviviruses (for example, St. Louis encephalitis, dengue, and yellow fever viruses). Sera from those marines were reactive to the other flaviviruses.

West Nile Fever in Operation Enduring Freedom and Operation Iraqi Freedom

As of December 2005, there were no reported cases of West Nile fever in military personnel deployed to OEF or OIF.

BRUCELLOSIS

Brucellosis is a serious zoonotic disease endemic in many parts of the world including southwest and south-central Asia (Mandell et al. 2005). The etiologic agent, *Brucella* spp., has numerous mammalian reservoirs; infected animal hosts shed the bacteria in their milk and urine.

Humans can contract the disease by ingesting unpasteurized dairy products, by way of infected aerosols inhaled or inoculated into the conjunctival sac of the eyes, and through direct contact between animals or their secretions and cut or abraded skin.

Among all US soldiers who participated in the Gulf War, OEF, and OIF, only one case of brucellosis has been diagnosed (Andrews 2004). An Army helicopter pilot became ill in July 2004 about a week after he completed a 5-month tour of duty in Iraq and returned to his unit in Würzburg, Germany. His initial symptoms of malaise, intermittent chills and fevers as high as 103.9°F, and profuse sweating worsened during the next 5 days despite unspecified "symptomatic treatment" and a day of hospitalization. The patient was readmitted to Würzburg Army Hospital on day 5. Antibodies to *B. abortus* were identified through laboratory analysis of an unspecified tissue specimen. In addition, a *Brucella* isolate later identified as *B. melitensis* was isolated from the patient's blood. Medical personnel then diagnosed brucellosis. The case report on this patient lacks a description of the course of treatment administered, but the report notes that the patient completed a 14-day course of primaquine after redeploying (presumably to Iraq). The report also notes that the patient had taken chloroquine as malaria prophylaxis but missed his last weekly dose. Epidemiologic questioning of the patient identified only one possible source of the infection: observing the slaughter of a sheep in Iraq.

CHICKENPOX (VARICELLA)

Seventy-five US military personnel who served in ODSh or ODSt were hospitalized for chickenpox during their deployment (Smith et al. 2004). Although it is typically benign in children, chickenpox may cause a more severe disease in adults that might include pneumonitis, hepatitis, and encephalitis. Indeed, the disease kills one in 5,000 infected adults (Heymann 2004). A common complication is bacterial suprainfection, usually of the skin (Military Vaccine Agency 2005b). In 1995, the US Food and Drug Administration licensed a vaccine for this disease.

MENINGOCOCCAL DISEASE

Infectious diseases reportedly caused only one death among US troops deployed to ODSh or ODSt: a fatal case of meningococcal meningitis (Hyams et al. 2001a; Writer et al. 1996). No further information has been published about the death. The literature mentions a second, nonfatal case of meningococcal disease during ODSh or ODSt (Hyams et al. 1995a), but validating evidence is absent. The committee is unaware of other published literature on cases or outbreaks of meningococcal disease among US troops deployed to southwest and south-central Asia during the conflicts discussed in this report.

NOSOCOMIAL INFECTIONS

Gulf War

The committee is unaware of any reports of nosocomial infection among US troops deployed to the Persian Gulf region for ODSh or ODSt. About 470 military personnel who served in those operations suffered nonmortal wounds (Department of Defense 2005).

Operation Enduring Freedom and Operation Iraqi Freedom

More than 16,600 military personnel deployed to OEF and OIF have suffered nonmortal wounds (Defense Manpower Data Center 2006). Many of these troops lost limbs or parts of limbs as a result of explosions that caused traumatic or surgical amputation (Davis et al. 2005). Soil- and water-dwelling bacteria, including *Acinetobacter baumanii*, have colonized and infected many soldiers' amputation sites and other blast wounds (Zapor and Moran 2005). Indeed, orthopedic war wounds have become the most common reason for infectious-disease consultations since September 2001 at WRAMC (Zapor and Moran 2005). Cultured specimens from wounds have often implicated a multiple-drug-resistant strain of *A. baumanii* (Zapor and Moran 2005).

A. baumanii has long been a cause of nosocomial infections. Infected battle injuries from OEF and OIF, however, have increased the rate of bloodstream infections by *A. baumanii* by more than 2,000% at two major US military hospitals (Table 4.14) (CDC 2004c). Moreover, some strains of *A. baumanii* have demonstrated resistance to all but one antimicrobial agent in the present pharmacologic arsenal—colistin, a toxic drug (CDC 2004c).

The active-duty military personnel described below, who were generally young and healthy before sustaining war wounds, usually recovered from *A. baumanii* infection after receiving medical treatment.

TABLE 4.14 Increase in Incidence of *A. baumannii* Bloodstream Infections at Two Military Hospitals, 2000-2004

	No. Cases		
Hospital	pre-2003	January 2003-August 2004	**Percentage Increase in No. Cases**
Walter Reed Army Medical Center	2 (2001-2002)	45	2,150
Landstuhl Regional Medical Center	1 (2000-2002)	33	3,200

SOURCE: Scott et al. 2004.

Case Series 1: Brooke Army Medical Center

From March 1, 2003, to May 31, 2004, Brooke Army Medical Center (BAMC), in Houston, Texas admitted 151 injured active-duty soldiers who had been deployed to OEF or OIF (Davis et al. 2005). Davis and colleagues report that all patients but one had previously been admitted to Landstuhl Regional Medical Center (LRMC) in Landstuhl, Germany; three had also been admitted to a second US Army medical facility before BAMC.

Of the tissue samples obtained from 84 of those patients, 48 (32%) tested positive for *Acinetobacter calcoaceticus-baumanii* complex; 30 patients (63% of those colonized) were clinically infected, and 23 met the case definition for either *Acinetobacter* osteomyelitis or *Acinetobacter* wound infection (Table 4.15). None had been diagnosed with *Acinetobacter* spp. before evacuation from Iraq or Afghanistan.

All but one of the 23 patients with *Acinetobacter* osteomyelitis or *Acinetobacter* wound infection received parenteral antimicrobial drug treatment selected to match the susceptibility of the infecting *A. baumanii* strain (Table 4.16). The primary therapeutic challenge was antimicrobial resistance. Most patients with *Acinetobacter* osteomyelitis underwent a 6- to 8-week course of drug therapy complemented by multiple surgical debridements of necrotic bone; one patient was treated with surgical debridement alone. Drug therapy for 10 of the osteomyelitis patients involved two antimicrobials, usually imipenem and amikacin. In contrast, patients with

Acinetobacter wound infection received just one antimicrobial, generally for 10-16 days. All patients responded to therapy. Their followup had lasted a mean of 9 months (range, 1-23 months) at the time the report was published.

TABLE 4.15 Type of *Acinetobacter* Infection in 23 Wounded Soldiers Admitted to BAMC, March 2003-May 2004, and Therapies Received

Type of Infection	No. cases
Acinetobacter osteomyelitis	15
Acinetobacter osteomyelitis with bacteremia	3
Acinetobacter burn infection	2
Acinetobacter deep wound infection	3

SOURCE: Davis et al. 2005.

TABLE 4.16 Antimicrobial Drug Susceptibilities for 38 Isolates of *Acinteobacter calcoaceticu-baumannii* Complex Recovered from Wound or Blood Cultures

Antimicrobial Drug	Percentage of Susceptible Isolates
Amikacin	48
Amoxicillin/clavulanate	9
Ampicillin/sulbactam	50
Cefepime	14
Cefotetan	3
Ceftazidime	12
Ceftriaxone	6
Ciprofloxacin	11
Colistin[a]	100
Gentamicin	8
Imipenem	89
Tobramycin	14
Trimethoprim/sulfamethoxazole	29

[a] Colistin susceptibility evaluated in three multiple-drug-resistant isolates.
SOURCE: Davis et al. 2005.

Case Series 2: Walter Reed Army Medical Center and Landstuhl Regional Medical Center

Scott and colleagues report the identification of *A. baumannii* bloodstream infections in 102 patients at five military hospitals where active-duty military personnel injured in OEF or OIF received treatment (CDC 2004c). The cases were identified from January 1, 2002, to August 31, 2004. Table 4.17 displays the number of infected patients per hospital, their age range, and the subset who that been admitted with (mostly traumatic) injuries associated with OEF or OIF. At both WRAMC and LRMC, clinicians identified a significant percentage of *A. baumannii* bloodstream infections associated with activities in OEF or OIF within 48 hours of admission (62% at WRAMC and 67% at LRMC). The 78 *A. baumanii* isolates obtained from patients at WRAMC and LRMC manifested varied levels of resistance to antimicrobial agents commonly used to treat such infections (Table 4.18).

DOD has reportedly taken a number of actions to avert a widespread outbreak of *A. baumanii* nosocomial infections in military medical treatment facilities that serve troops deployed to OEF and OIF. The department has developed clinical management and wound-care guidelines to help clinicians prevent and mitigate *A. baumanii* infections in military treatment facilities and has launched an investigation into the sources of the pathogen. It is also conducting laboratory surveillance for *A. baumanii* at four major military hospitals in the United States and Germany and, to the extent possible, at US military medical treatment facilities on the ground in Iraq, Kuwait, and Afghanistan (CDC 2004c). Preliminary data have reportedly linked environmental isolates of *A. baumanii* obtained from field hospitals to patient isolates obtained during both surveillance and clinical evaluation (Zapor and Moran 2005).

TABLE 4.17 Cases of *A. baumanii* Infection Identified in Five Military Hospitals, January 2002-August 2004

Hospital	No. Cases	Median Age (Range) (years)	No. (%) Casualties Associated with OEF or OIF
Walter Reed Army Medical Center	45	30 (19-72)	29 (64)
Landstuhl Regional Medical Center	33	39 (6-86)	32 (97)
Brooke Army Medical Center	5	NP	5 (100)
National Naval Medical Center	8	NP	8 (100)
USNS Comfort	11	NP	11 (100)
TOTAL	102	---	85 ---

NOTE: NP = not published in the source article.
SOURCE: Scott et al. 2004.

TABLE 4.18 Pattern of Antimicrobial Susceptibility among Strains of *A. baumanii* Isolated from Patients with Bloodstream Infections at WRAMC and LRMC, January 2002-August 2004

Antimicrobial Drug	Percentage of Susceptible Isolates	
	WRAMC (N = 45)	LRMC (N = 33)
Imipenem	82	87
Amikacin	48	80
Ampicillin/sulbactam	35	8
Piperacillin/tazobactam	27	0
Cefepime	22	0
Ciprofloxacin	20	3

NOTE: WRAMC = Walter Reed Army Medical Center, LRMC = Landstuhl Regional Medical Center.
SOURCE: Scott et al. 2004.

Q FEVER

Q fever is a zoonotic disease endemic in southwest and south-central Asia (Wallace et al. 2002). The clinical syndrome may be acute or chronic. The acute illness usually manifests as a nonspecific febrile illness, pneumonia (sometimes atypical pneumonia), hepatitis, or a combination of the three; occasionally, it presents as acute meningitis or encephalitis. Chronic Q fever usually presents as endocarditis, granulomatous hepatitis, or vertebral osteomyelitis. Q fever frequently goes undiagnosed in humans; many cases are presumably subclinical or asymptomatic.

Cattle, sheep, and goats are the main reservoirs of the disease, which is caused by the bacterium *Coxiella burnetii*. A single organism can constitute an infectious dose. *C. burnetii* most frequently infects humans who inhale infected aerosolized body fluids of infected animals; the consumption of raw milk from *C. burnetii*-infected animals also has caused Q fever in humans.

Three cases of Q fever were reported in US troops who participated in the Gulf War (Hyams et al. 1995a), and 10 cases have been diagnosed in troops deployed to Iraq (Kilpatrick 2005).

Q Fever Contracted During the Gulf War

A case report about one of the three Gulf War troops who had a diagnosis of Q fever has been published (Ferrante and Dolan 1993). A 51-year-old man who had been involved in the ground war in ODSt presented with focal neurologic deficits suggestive of transient ischemic attacks in a crescendo pattern. Two weeks before the onset of symptoms, the patient had returned from Saudi Arabia, where he frequently worked around camels and had once driven a vehicle past a flock of sheep.

The first evaluation of the patient's cerebrospinal fluid (CSF) yielded an abnormal profile consistent with aseptic meningitis; however the sample was culture-negative for bacteria, fungi, and mycobacteria. Clinicians obtained two more CSF samples at 10 and 14 days; serology from the last puncture yielded a positive *C. burnetii* IgM indircct fluorescent antibody (IFA) titer consistent with recent Q fever infection. CDC confirmed that result, and Q fever meningoencephalitis was diagnosed. It is believed that the patient contracted the disease in Saudi Arabia through exposure to infected camels or sheep.

Clinicians treated the patient with a 21-day course of oral doxycyline (100 mg twice a day). Six weeks after the first lumbar puncture, serology for *C. burnetii* IgM IFA titer was negative. No further neurologic sequelae occurred during 12 months of followup.

Q Fever Contracted During Operation Enduring Freedom and Operation Iraqi Freedom

Ten cases of Q fever have been diagnosed in troops serving in OIF as of December 2005. All the patients became infected in northern Iraq (Kilpatrick 2005). We summarize here a report of about eight of the 10 cases; we are unaware of reports in the public literature about the other two patients.

During an investigation of a cluster of 19 cases of severe pneumonia in US troops serving in Iraq, extensive serologic testing for possible infectious etiologies revealed that three patients had positive antibody titers for *C. burnetii* by immunofluorescence assay (Anderson et al. 2005). The three patients' predeployment serum samples were negative in the same test. The results led investigators to examine whether *C. burnetii* accounted for other cases of pneumonia among military personnel deployed to Iraq during the same period (March 1-August 20, 2003).

Predeployment and postdeployment serum samples were available for 22 of 62 soldiers who had pneumonia diagnosed in Iraq. Serum was tested by immunofluorescence assay for phase I and phase II antibody to *C. burnetii*. Five of the 22 soldiers had seroconverted to *C. burnetii* before their postdeployment serum draws, leading the investigators to conclude that they also had contracted Q fever in the period March 1-August 20, 2003.

All eight patients in this study first sought medical care while stationed in northern Iraq. The first three patients were in northern Iraq when their symptoms of pneumonia began. The investigators postulated that humans may be at greater risk of contracting Q fever in northern Iraq owing to the larger concentrations of livestock that may exist there because the land is favorable for ruminants to graze. One of the first three patients reported drinking raw sheep's milk, two reported tick bites within 30 days of becoming ill, and all three reported contact with dogs, cats, sheep, goats, and camels (potential reservoirs of *C. burnetii*).

VIRAL HEPATITIS

Clinicians diagnosed a few cases of hepatitis A and B among deployed US troops during the Gulf War, according to Hyams and colleagues (Hyams et al. 1995a); the exact number of cases is unclear. The committee is unaware of published reports about those cases. The hospitalization rates for acute hepatitis among all active-duty military personnel in 1990 and 1991 were 187 per 100,000 and 168 per 100,000 respectively (Table 4.19) (Hyams et al. 2001b). The data do not indicate how many cases were associated with participation in ODSh or ODSt.

Staff at the Armed Forces Institute of Pathology diagnosed one case of hepatitis B and 15 cases of hepatitis C among Gulf War veterans from 1992 to 1997 (Specht et al. 2000). The investigators reportedly lacked the data to determine whether the patients had contracted hepatitis before, during, or after the war.

Hepatitis A and B vaccination policies differ among the services (IOM 1996). In the past, the Army, Navy, Marine Corps, and Coast Guard administered the hepatitis A vaccine as directed by the applicable surgeon general or the commandant of the Coast Guard; the Air Force vaccinated its personnel against hepatitis A when deploying them to a high-risk area. As of 1996, all services administered the hepatitis B vaccine to personnel in high-risk occupational groups or as directed by the applicable surgeon general or the commandant of the Coast Guard. More recently, DOD policy requires that all personnel be vaccinated for hepatitis A (Department of Defense 2006a; Military Vaccine Agency 2005a) and Army policy requires that all deployed personnel be vaccinated for hepatitis B (Department of the Army 2005a).

TABLE 4.19 Age- and Sex-Adjusted Hospitalization Rates per 100,000 Personnel for Acute Hepatitis Among Active Duty U.S. Military Forces, 1990 and 1991

	Acute Hepatitis A		Acute Hepatitis B		Acute Hepatitis C		Acute Unspecified Viral Hepatitis		Total	
Year	No.	Rate	No.	Rate	No.	Rate	No.	Rate	No.	Rate
1990	113	3.52	0	---	0	---	75	3.08	187	6.56
1991	74	2.87	25	0.96	1	0.05	72	3.07	168	6.75

SOURCE: Adapted with permission from Hyams et al. 2001a.

TUBERCULOSIS

No cases of active tuberculosis (TB) were recognized in military personnel who served in ODSt and ODSh (Hyams et al. 1995a). In many soldiers in some units, however, tuberculin skin tests (TSTs) were negative before the Gulf War and positive afterward (Oster and Sanford 1992). Among military personnel deployed to OEF and OIF, approximately 2.5 percent of those given pre- and post-deployment TSTs converted from negative to positive (Kilpatrick 2005). TST conversion is pathognomonic of acute infection with *Mycobacterium tuberculosis*; thus, transmission of *M. tuberculosis* occurred within some military units deployed to southwest and south-central Asia. Immunocompetent individuals who become infected with *M. tuberculosis* face a 10 percent lifetime risk for developing active TB in the absence of prophylactic treatment. The committee discusses TB at length in Chapter 5.

DEPARTMENT OF DEFENSE MEDICAL DATABASES

On January 10, 2006, IOM submitted a request to DOD to conduct a search of the Defense Medical Surveillance System (DMSS) database (described in Rubertone and Brundage (2002)) for numbers of cases of infectious diseases coded by the *International Classification of Diseases, Ninth Revision, Clinical Modification* (ICD-9-CM). The request included searching for infectious diseases diagnosed in military personnel deployed to the Gulf War, OIF, and OEF. DOD approved IOM's request on January 20. Because the DMSS database does not contain many data pertaining to in-theater morbidity during the Gulf War, DOD recommended that an additional search be conducted with a different DOD database on Gulf War in-theater hospitalization data.

On June 2, 2006, IOM received the results of the search of the Gulf War in-theater hospitalization database. Those results are presented in Table 4.20. DOD developed the database to investigate in-theater hospitalizations during the Gulf War (Smith et al. 2004). It contains records from almost 20,000 admissions occurring in the Kuwaiti theater of operations and evacuated admissions to hospitals in Europe. The committee reviewed the search results and determined that the results would not have changed the committee's approach to its charge or conclusions.

At the time of completion of this report, IOM had not received the results of the DMSS database search on infectious diseases diagnosed during OIF and OEF.

TABLE 4.20 Numbers of Cases of Infectious Diseases in the Gulf War In-Theater Hospitalization Database

ICD-9CM Category	Disease	No. Cases
003.0	Salmonella gastroenteritis	9
003.9	Salmonella infection, unspecified	2
004.9	Shigellosis, unspecified	3
005.0	Staphylococcal food poisoning	2
005.9	Food poisoning, unspecified	18
006.0	Acute amebic dysentery without mention of abscess	3
006.8	Amebic infection of other sites	3
006.9	Amebiasis, unspecified	14
008.5	Bacterial enteritis, unspecified	6
008.69	Other viral enteritis	2
008.8	Intestinal infection due to other organism, not elsewhere classified	86
009.0	Infectious colitis, enteritis, and gastroenteritis	23
009.1	Colitis, enteritis, gastroenteritis, presumed infectious origin	2
009.2	Infectious diarrhea	34
009.3	Diarrhea of presumed infectious origin	4
011.60	Tuberculous pneumonia (any form), unspecified examination	1
011.90	Unspecified pulmonary tuberculosis, unspecified examination	1
034.0	Streptococcal sore throat	19

ICD-9CM Category	Disease	No. Cases
035	Erysipelas	1
038.10	Staphylococcal septicemia, unspecified	1
038.9	Unspecified septicemia	2
040.0	Gas gangrene	1
041.10	Staphylococcus, unspecified, in condition classified elsewhere	1
041.4	Escherichia coli infection	1
042	Human immunodeficiency virus disease	2
047.9	Unspecified viral meningitis	3
048	Other enterovirus diseases of the central nervous system	1
052.1	Varicella (hemorrhagic) pneumonitis	1
052.7	Chickenpox with other specified complications	1
052.8	Chickenpox with unspecified complication	3
052.9	Varicella without mention of complication	64
053.8	Herpes zoster with unspecified complication	1
053.9	Herpes zoster without mention of complication	11
054.10	Genital herpes, unspecified	2
054.19	Other genital herpes	1
054.2	Herpetic gingivostomatitis	2
054.43	Herpes simplex disciform keratitis	3
054.79	Herpes simplex with other specified complications	1
054.9	Herpes simplex without mention of complication	1
055.9	Measles without mention of complication	1
057.8	Other specified viral exanthemata	1
057.9	Viral exanthem, unspecified	1
066.0	Phlebotomus fever	5
070.10	Viral hepatitis A without mention of a hepatic coma, lab test confirmed	4
070.30	Viral hepatitis B without coma, acute/ unspecified without hepatic delta, lab test confirmed	6
070.9	Unspecified viral hepatitis without hepatic coma	3
072.9	Mumps without mention of complication	1
074.1	Epidemic pleurodynia	1
075	Infectious mononucleosis	27
077.8	Other viral conjunctivitis	3
078.10	Other diseases due to viruses and chlamydiae, viral warts, unspecified	29
078.11	Other diseases due to viruses and chlamydiae, condyloma acuminatum	9
078.19	Other diseases due to viruses and chlamydiae, other specified viral warts	6
079.89	Other specified viral infections	5
079.98	Unspecified chlamydial	1
079.99	Unspecified viral infections	299
084.1	Vivax malaria (benign tertian)	7
084.6	Malaria, unspecified	4
085.0	Leishmaniasis visceral (kala-azar)	1
085.1	Cutaneous leishmaniasis, urban	1
085.9	Leishmaniasis, unspecified	2
091.3	Secondary syphilis of skin or mucous membranes	1
091.50	Syphilitic uveitis, unspecified	1
098.0	Acute gonococcal infection, lower genito-urinary tract	1
098.16	Acute gonococcal endometritis	1
099.3	Reiter's disease	6

ICD-9CM Category	Disease	No. Cases
099.40	Other nongonococcal urethritis unspecified	2
099.9	Venereal disease, unspecified	1
101	Vincents angina	1
110.3	Dermatophytosis of groin and perianal area	1
110.4	Dermatophytosis of foot	10
110.6	Deep seated dermatophytosis	1
111.0	Pityriasis versicolor	2
116.0	Blastomycosis	1
117.9	Other and unspecified mycoses	2
120.9	Schistosomiasis, unspecified	1
127.3	Trichuriasis	1
130.2	Chorioretinitis due to toxoplasmosis	3
130.7	Toxoplasmosis of other specified sites	1
133.0	Scabies	2
135	Sarcoidosis	16
136.1	Behcet's syndrome	1
136.9	Unspecified infectious and parasitic diseases	1
320.1	Pneumococcal meningitis	1
480.9	Pneumonia due to virus, unspecified	6
481	Pneumococcal pneumonia (streptococcus pneumoniae pneumonia)	1
482.30	Pneumonia due to streptococcus, unspecified	1
482.89	Pneumonia due to other specified bacteria	1
482.9	Pneumonia due to unspecified bacteria	3
483.0	Mycoplasma pneumoniae	5
485	Bronchopneumonia, organism unspecified	9
486	Pneumonia, organism unspecified	168
487.0	Influenza with pneumonia	1
487.1	Influenza with other respiratory manifestations	27
487.8	Influenza with other manifestations	2
711.06	Pyogenic arthritis involving lower leg	5
711.90	Unspecified infective arthritis, site unspecified	1
711.96	Unspecified infective arthritis involving lower leg	1
711.97	Unspecified infective arthritis involving ankle and foot	1

NOTE: ICD-9CM = International Classification of Diseases, Ninth Revision, Clinical Modification.
SOURCE: Smith 2006.

DEPARTMENT OF DEFENSE POLICY REGARDING PREDEPLOYMENT AND POSTDEPLOYMENT SERUM COLLECTION

DOD policy specifies that "predeployment serum specimens for medical examinations will routinely be collected within one year of deployment" and that "postdeployment serum specimens for medical examinations will be collected no later than 30 days after arrival at the demobilization site, home station, or in-patient medical treatment facility" (Department of Defense 2006b). Predeployment and postdeployment serum samples are required for all deployments outside the continental United States that are longer than 30 days and to areas without fixed US medical treatment facilities (Kilpatrick 2006). The serum samples are stored indefinitely at the DOD Serum Repository.

Routine testing of the serum samples is not conducted except testing for HIV (Kilpatrick 2006). However, the serum samples have been used for research studies (for example, on Lyme disease, *Helicobacter pylori* infection, and leishmaniasis), and for operational studies (for example, on severe acute pneumonia cases during OIF, malaria among Marines in Liberia, and WNV).

The committee agrees with DOD's overall policy regarding collection and use of serum specimens. However, for banked serum specimens to be most useful for determining whether infectious exposures occurred during deployment, the predeployment specimens need to be collected before travel. Current policy allows for collection of predeployment serum specimens up to a year after deployment. If specimens are not collected until after deployment, it would be difficult to ascertain whether any signs of infection found in the "predeployment" specimens are due to exposure during the current deployment or before it.

REFERENCES

Anderson AD, Smoak B, Shuping E, Ockenhouse C, Petruccelli B. 2005. Q fever and the US military. *Emerging Infectious Diseases* 11(8):1320-1322.

Andrews RB. 2004. Brucellosis in a soldier who recently returned from Iraq. *Medical Surveillance Monthly Report* 10(4):30.

Boecken GH, Bronnert J. 2005. Pathogenesis and management of a late manifestation of vivax malaria after deployment to Afghanistan: Conclusions for NATO Armed Forces Medical Services. *Military Medicine* 170(6):488-491.

CDC (Centers for Disease Control and Prevention). 1992. Viscerotropic leishmaniasis in persons returning from Operation Desert Storm—1990-1991. *Morbidity and Mortality Weekly Report* 41(8):131-134.

CDC. 2003a. Severe Acute Pneumonitis Among Deployed US Military Personnel—Southwest Asia, March—August 2003. *Morbidity and Mortality Weekly Report* 52(36):857-859.

CDC. 2003b. Cutaneous leishmaniasis in US military personnel—Southwest/Central Asia, 2002-2003. *Morbidity and Mortality Weekly Report* 52(42):1009-1012.

CDC. 2004a. Two cases of visceral leishmaniasis in US military personnel—Afghanistan, 2002-2004. *Morbidity and Mortality Weekly Report* 53(12):265-268.

CDC. 2004b. Update: Cutaneous leishmaniasis in US military personnel—Southwest/Central Asia, 2002-2004. *Morbidity and Mortality Weekly Report* 53(12):264-265.

CDC. 2004c. Acinetobacter baumannii infections among patients at military medical facilities treating injured US service members, 2002-2004. *Morbidity and Mortality Weekly Report* 53(45):1063-1066.

Davis KA, Moran KA, McAllister CK, Gray PJ. 2005. Multidrug-resistant Acinetobacter extremity infections in soldiers. *Emerging Infectious Diseases* 11(8):1218-1224.

Defense Manpower Data Center. *Military Casualty Information*. [Online]. Available: http://www.dior.whs.mil/mmid/casualty/castop.htm [accessed March 2006].

Department of the Army. 2005a. *Medical Screening of Personnel Mobilized for Deployment or Deployed in Support of Contingency Operations (Predeployment Screening Requirements)*. Falls Church, VA: Office of the Surgeon General.

Department of the Army. 2005b. *Release of Actionable Medical Information Policy Memorandum*. Fort Sam Houston, TX: Headquarters, United States Army Medical Command.

DOD (Department of Defense). 2005. *Principal Wars in Which the United States Participated US Military Personnel Serving and Casualties A*. [Online]. Available: http://www.dior.whs.mil/mmid/casualty/WCPRINCIPAL.pdf [accessed March 2006].

DOD. 2006a. *Individual Medical Readiness*. *Department of Defense Instruction*. Washington, DC.

DOD. 2006b. *Policy for Pre- and Post-Deployment Serum Collection*. Washington, DC: Assistant Secretary of Defense.

Donowitz GR, Mandell GL. 2000. Acute pneumonia. In: Mandell GL, Bennett JE, Dolin R, Editors. *Principles and Practice of Infectious Diseases*. 5th ed. New York: Churchill Livingstone. Pp. 717-743.

Ferrante MA, Dolan MJ. 1993. Q fever meningoencephalitis in a soldier returning from the Persian Gulf War. *Clinical Infectious Diseases* 16(4):489-496.

Gasser RA Jr, Magill AJ, Oster CN, Tramont EC. 1991. The threat of infectious disease in Americans returning from Operation Desert Storm. *New England Journal of Medicine* 324(12):859-864.

Gwaltney JM, Jr. 2000a. Acute Bronchitis. In: Mandell GL, Bennett JE, Dolin R, Editors. *Principles and Practice of Infectious Diseases*. 5th ed. New York: Churchill Livingstone. Pp. 703-706.

Gwaltney JM, Jr. 2000b. Sinusitis. In: Mandell GL, Bennett JE, Dolin R, Editors. *Principles and Practice of Infectious Diseases*. 5th ed. New York: Churchill Livingstone. Pp. 676-686.

Haberberger RL, Scott DA, Thornton SA, Hyams KC. 1994. Diarrheal disease aboard a US Navy ship after a brief port visit to a high risk area. *Military Medicine* 159(6):445-448.

Halsey ES, Bryce LM, Wortmann GW, Weina PJ, Ryan JR, DeWitt CC. 2004. Visceral leishmaniasis in a soldier returning from Operation Enduring Freedom. *Military Medicine* 169(9):699-701.

Heymann DL. 2004. *Control of Communicable Diseases Manual*. Washington, DC: American Public Health Association.

Hyams KC. 1999. Gulf War Syndrome: Potential role of infectious diseases. *Current Opinion in Infectious Diseases* 12(5):439-443.

Hyams KC, Bourgeois AL, Merrell BR, Rozmajzl P, Escamilla J, Thornton SA, Wasserman GM, Burke A, Echeverria P, Green KY, et al. 1991. Diarrheal disease during Operation Desert Shield. *New England Journal of Medicine* 325(20):1423-1428.

Hyams KC, Malone JD, Kapikian AZ, Estes MK, Xi J, Bourgeois AL, Paparello S, Hawkins RE, Green KY. 1993. Norwalk virus infection among Desert Storm troops. *Journal of Infectious Diseases* 167(4):986-987.

Hyams KC, Hanson K, Wignall FS, Escamilla J, Oldfield EC, 3rd. 1995a. The impact of infectious diseases on the health of US troops deployed to the Persian Gulf during operations Desert Shield and Desert Storm. *Clinical Infectious Diseases* 20(6):1497-1504.

Hyams KC, Malone JD, Bourgeois AL, Hawkins R, Hale TL, Murphy JR. 1995b. Serum antibody to lipopolysaccharide antigens of Shigella species among US military peronnel deployed to Saudi Arabia and Kuwait during Operation Desert Storm. *Clinical and Diagnostic Laboratory Immunology* 2(6):700-703.

Hyams KC, Riddle J, Trump DH, Graham JT. 2001a. Endemic infectious diseases and biological warfare during the Gulf War: A decade of analysis and final concerns. *American Journal of Tropical Medicine and Hygiene* 65(5):664-670.

Hyams KC, Smith TC, Riddle J, Trump DH, Gray G. 2001b. Viral hepatitis in the US military: A study of hospitalization records from 1974 to 1999. *Military Medicine* 166(10):862-865.

IOM (Institute of Medicine). 1996. *Interaction of Drugs, Biologics, and Chemicals in US Military Forces: Current and Future Issues*. Washington, DC: National Academy Press.

Johnson KE. 2004. Malaria, US Army, 2003. *Medical Surveillance Monthly Report* 10(1):6-8.

Kelly MT, Brenner DJ, Farmer JJIII. 1985. Enterobacteriaceae. In: Lennette EH, Balows A, Hausler WJ, Jr., Shadomy HJ, Editors. *Manual of Clinical Microbiology*. 4th ed. Washington, DC: American Society for Microbiology. Pp. 263-277.

Kilpatrick ME. 2005. *Presentation to IOM Committee on Gulf War and Health: Infectious Diseases*. Washington, DC.

Kilpatrick ME. 2006. Deployment Health Support Office of the Assistant Secretary of Defense, Health Affairs. Personal Communication.

Kotwal RS, Wenzel RB, Sterling RA, Porter WD, Jordan NN, Petruccelli BP. 2005. An outbreak of malaria in US Army Rangers returning from Afghanistan. *Journal of the American Medical Association* 293(2):212-216.

Kreutzer RD, Grogl M, Neva FA, Fryauff DJ, Magill AJ, Aleman-Munoz MM. 1993. Identification and genetic comparison of leishmanial parasites causing viscerotropic and cutaneous disease in soldiers returning from Operation Desert Storm. *American Journal of Tropical Medicine and Hygiene* 49(3):357-363.

Lay JC. 2005. Malaria, US Army, 2004. *Medical Surveillance Monthly Report* 11(1):7-10.

Lew JF, Kapikian AZ, Jiang X, Estes MK, Green KY. 1994. Molecular characterization and expression of the capsid protein of a Norwalk-like virus recovered from a Desert Shield troop with gastroenteritis. *Virology* 200(1):319-325.

Magill AJ. 2005. Leishmaniasis in Veterans of Desert Storm and Iraqi Freedom. *Presentation to IOM Committee on Gulf War and Health: Infectious Diseases*. Washington, DC.

Magill AJ, Grogl M, Gasser RA Jr, Sun W, Oster CN. 1993. Visceral infection caused by Leishmania tropica in veterans of Operation Desert Storm. *New England Journal of Medicine* 328(19):1383-1387.

Magill AJ, Grogl M, Johnson SC, Gasser RA Jr. 1994. Visceral infection due to Leishmania tropica in a veteran of Operation Desert Storm who presented 2 years after leaving Saudi Arabia. *Clinical Infectious Diseases* 19(4):805-806.

Malone JD, Paparello S, Thornton S, Mapes T, Haberberger R, Hyams KC. 1991. Parasitic infections in troops returning from Operation Desert Storm. *New England Journal of Medicine* 325(20):1448-1449.

Mandell GL, Bennett JE, Dolin R. 2005. *Principles and Practice of Infectious Diseases*. 6th ed. Philadelphia, PA: Elsevier Churchill Livingstone.

Martin S, Gambel J, Jackson J, Aronson N, Gupta R, Rowton E, Perich M, McEvoy P, Berman J, Magill A, Hoke C. 1998. Leishmaniasis in the United States military. *Military Medicine* 163(12):801-807.

Matson DO. 2005. Norovirus gastroenteritis in US Marines in Iraq. *Clinical Infectious Diseases* 40(4):526-527.

McCarthy M, Estes MK, Hyams KC. 2000. Norwalk-like virus infection in military forces: Epidemic potential, sporadic disease, and the future direction of prevention and control efforts. *Journal of Infectious Diseases* 181(2 Suppl):S387-S391.

Mikhail MM, Mansour MM, Oyofo BA, Malone JD. 1996. Immune response to Shigella sonnei in US Marines. *Infection and Immunity* 64(9):3942-3945.

Military Vaccine Agency. 2005a. *Hepatitis A Infection and Hepatitis A Vaccine*. Military Vaccine (MILVAX) Agency, Office of The Army Surgeon General, US Army.

Military Vaccine Agency. 2005b. *Chickenpox Vaccination Program: Questions and Answers*. Military Vaccine (MILVAX) Agency, Office of The Army Surgeon General, US Army.

MSMR (Medical Surveillance Monthly Report). 1995. Malaria in active duty soldiers. *Medical Surveillance Monthly Report* 1(4):9.

Ohl CA, Hyams KC, Malone JD, Oldfield E 3rd. 1993. Leishmaniasis among Desert Storm veterans: A diagnostic and therapeutic dilemma. *Military Medicine* 158(11):726-729.

Oldfield EC 3rd, Wallace MR, Hyams KC, Yousif AA, Lewis DE, Bourgeois AL. 1991. Endemic infectious diseases of the Middle East. *Reviews of Infectious Diseases* 13(3 Suppl)S199-S217.

Oster CN, Sanford JP. 1992. Febrile illness in a Desert Storm veteran. *Hospital Practice (Office Edition)* 27(11):145-148, 151, 155-160.

Paparello SF, Garst P, Bourgeois AL, Hyams KC. 1993. Diarrheal and respiratory disease aboard the hospital ship, USNS-Mercy T-AH 19, during Operation Desert Shield. *Military Medicine* 158(6):392-395.

Richards AL, Hyams KC, Merrell BR, Dasch GA, Woody JN, Ksiazek TG, LeDuc JW, Watts DM. 1991. Medical aspects of Operation Desert Storm. *New England Journal of Medicine* 325(13):970-971.

Richards AL, Hyams KC, Watts DM, Rozmajzl PJ, Woody JN, Merrell BR. 1993a. Respiratory disease among military personnel in Saudi Arabia during Operation Desert Shield. *American Journal of Public Health* 83(9):1326-1329.

Richards AL, Malone JD, Sheris S, Weddle JR, Rossi CA, Ksiazek TG, LeDuc JW, Dasch GA, Hyams KC. 1993b. Arbovirus and rickettsial infections among combat troops during Operation Desert Shield/Desert Storm. *Journal of Infectious Diseases* 168(4):1080-1081.

Rubertone MV, Brundage JF. 2002. The Defense Medical Surveillance System and the Department of Defense serum repository: Glimpses of the future of public health surveillance. *American Journal of Public Health* 92(12):1900-1904.

Sanders JW, Putnam SD, Riddle MS, Tribble DR, Jobanputra NK, Jones JJ, Scott DA, Frenck RW. 2004. The epidemiology of self-reported diarrhea in operations Iraqi freedom and enduring freedom. *Diagnostic Microbiology and Infectious Disease* 50(2):89-93.

Sanders JW, Putnam SD, Frankart C, Frenck RW, Monteville MR, Riddle MS, Rockabrand DM, Sharp TW, Tribble DR. 2005a. Impact of illness and non-combat injury during operations iraqi freedom and enduring freedom (Afghanistan). *American Journal of Tropical Medicine and Hygiene* 73(4):713-719.

Sanders JW, Putnam SD, Riddle MS, Tribble DR. 2005b. Military importance of diarrhea: Lessons from the Middle East. *Current Opinion in Gastroenterology* 21(1):9-14.

Schlagenhauf P. 2003. Malaria in Iraq—the pitfalls of Plasmodium vivax prophylaxis. *Lancet Infectious Diseases* 3(8):460.

Scott P, Artis D, Uzonna J, Zaph C. 2004. The development of effector and memory T cells in cutaneous leishmaniasis: The implications for vaccine development. *Immunological Reviews* 201:318-338.

Smith TC. 2006. *Results of IOM Requested Database Search for Infectious Disease Cases During the Gulf War*. San Diego, CA: Department of Defense Center for Deployment Health Research, Naval Health Research Center.

Smith TC, Corbeil TE, Ryan MA, Heller JM, Gray GC. 2004. In-theater hospitalizations of US and allied personnel during the 1991 Gulf War. *American Journal of Epidemiology* 159(11):1064-1076.

Specht CS, Lewin-Smith MR, Kalasinsky VF, Peterson MR, Mullick FG. 2000. The surgical pathology and cytopathology of US Persian Gulf War military veterans: Identification of diseases endemic to the theater of operations. *Archives of Pathology and Laboratory Medicine* 124(9):1299-1301.

Spudick JM, Garcia LS, Graham DM, Haake DA. 2005. Diagnostic and therapeutic pitfalls associated with primaquine-tolerant Plasmodium vivax. *Journal of Clinical Microbiology* 43(2):978-981.

Stephens I, Nataro JP. 2004. Prevention of enteric diseases. *Advances in Experimental Medicine and Biology* 549:71-82.

Thornton SA, Sherman SS, Farkas T, Zhong W, Torres P, Jiang X. 2005. Gastroenteritis in US Marines during Operation Iraqi Freedom. *Clinical Infectious Diseases* 40(4):519-525.

Wallace MR, Hale BR, Utz GC, Olson PE, Earhart KC, Thornton SA, Hyams KC. 2002. Endemic infectious diseases of Afghanistan. *Clinical Infectious Diseases* 34(5 Suppl):S171-S207.

Wasserman GM, Martin BL, Hyams KC, Merrill BR, Oaks HG, McAdoo HA. 1997. A survey of outpatient visits in a United States Army forward unit during Operation Desert Shield. *Military Medicine* 162(6):374-379.

Weina PJ, Neafie RC, Wortmann G, Polhemus M, Aronson NE. 2004. Old world leishmaniasis: An emerging infection among deployed US military and civilian workers. *Clinical Infectious Diseases* 39(11):1674-1680.

Willard RJ, Jeffcoat AM, Benson PM, Walsh DS. 2005. Cutaneous leishmaniasis in soldiers from Fort Campbell, Kentucky returning from Operation Iraqi Freedom highlights diagnostic and therapeutic options. *Journal of the American Academy of Dermatology* 52(6):977-987.

Wolf MK, Taylor DN, Boedeker EC, Hyams KC, Maneval DR, Levine MM, Tamura K, Wilson RA , Echeverria P. 1993. Characterization of enterotoxigenic Escherichia coli isolated from US troops deployed to the Middle East. *Journal of Clinical Microbiology* 31(4):851-856.

Writer JV, DeFraites RF, Brundage JF. 1996. Comparative mortality among US military personnel in the Persian Gulf region and worldwide during Operations Desert Shield and Desert Storm. *Journal of the American Medical Association* 275(2):118-121.

Young RC Jr, Rachal RE, Huguley JW 3rd. 1992. Environmental health concerns of the Persian Gulf War. *Journal of the National Medical Association* 84(5):417-424.

Zapor MJ, Moran KA. 2005. Infectious diseases during wartime. *Current Opinion in Infectious Diseases* 18(5):395-399.

5

LEVELS OF ASSOCIATION BETWEEN SELECT DISEASES AND LONG-TERM ADVERSE HEALTH OUTCOMES

Only 10% of the roughly 90 infectious diseases endemic in southwest and south-central Asia are likely to pose a long-term health risk to exposed US military personnel. As noted in Chapter 3, the long-term adverse health outcomes of most diseases endemic in the region would usually become apparent during or immediately after the acute illness, and many of the health outcomes are rare. However, nine of the infectious diseases meet the inclusion criteria outlined in Box 5.1 and discussed in Chapter 2. Those nine diseases and their associated long-term adverse health outcomes are the subject of this chapter (Table 5.1).

Following the paradigm of past Institute of Medicine Committees on Gulf War and Health, the committee determined the strength of association between each infection[1] and specific long-term adverse health outcomes in humans. For every health outcome discussed in this chapter, there is limited or suggestive evidence of an association, sufficient evidence of an association, or sufficient evidence of a causal relationship with the infectious disease. Several delayed long-term adverse health outcomes of the nine diseases are listed in Chapter 3 but not reviewed here; the committee determined that there is inadequate or insufficient evidence of an association between these health outcomes and the infectious diseases. To reach its conclusions, the committee assessed the available evidence published in the biomedical literature about the long-term adverse outcomes of the diseases on human health.

BOX 5.1 Inclusion Criteria

The committee used these questions to evaluate the dozens of infectious diseases endemic in southwest and south-central Asia or commonly found among troops in wartime (Table 2.1). If the answer to every question was yes, a disease met the criteria for in-depth evaluation in this chapter.

1. Was the infection or disease diagnosed in US troops in appropriate temporal relationship to deployment to the Gulf War, Operation Enduring Freedom, or Operation Iraqi Freedom, given the natural history of the disease?
2. Is the risk of contracting the disease during deployment in southwest or south-central Asia equal to or greater than the risk of contracting it in the United States?
3. Does the disease have a known or suspected long-term adverse health outcome?
4. Would there be a delay between the infection or the end of the acute illness and the onset of the long-term adverse health outcome?

[1] In this context, the term *infection* refers to a primary infection that leads to disease.

TABLE 5.1 The Nine Infectious Diseases Studied for Strength of Association with Specific Long-Term Adverse Health Outcomes

Infectious Disease	Long-Term Adverse Health Outcomes Evaluated for Strength of Association
Brucellosis	Arthritis Cardiovascular system infections Ophthalmologic manifestations Genito-urinary tract manifestations Hepatic abnormalities Neurologic manifestations Respiratory system infections Other symptoms (fatigue, inattention, amnesia, depression)
Campylobacter infection	Guillain-Barré syndrome Reactive arthritis Uveitis
Leishmaniasis	Delayed presentation of visceral leishmaniasis (VL)[a] Reactivation of VL in the context of future immunosuppression Post-kala-azar dermal leishmaniasis
Malaria	Clinical relapse Late presentation or recrudescence of disease Hematologic manifestations Ophthalmologic manifestations Nephrologic disease Neurologic and neuropsychiatric disease
Coxiella burnetii infection (Q fever)	Chronic hepatitis Endocarditis Osteomyelitis Post-Q fever fatigue syndrome Vascular infection
Salmonella (nontyphoid) infection	Reactive arthritis
Shigella infection	Hemolytic uremic syndrome Reactive arthritis
Tuberculosis[b]	Activation of latent tuberculosis infection Late manifestations of pulmonary and extrapulmonary tuberculosis
West Nile virus infection[c]	Persistent deficits in cognition, movement, and daily functioning

[a] Viscerotropic leishmaniasis is considered a subset of VL for the purposes of this discussion.
[b] Tuberculosis (TB) does not meet inclusion criterion 1 (Box 5.1), because there have been no published reports of military personnel who developed active TB while deployed to the Gulf War, Operation Enduring Freedom (OEF), or Operation Iraqi Freedom (OIF). However, in a presentation to the committee, Kilpatrick (2005) indicated that 2.5% of military personnel deployed to OEF and OIF and given predeployment and postdeployment skin tests for TB seroconverted during their deployment; that is, they acquired new TB infections. Immunocompetent people who are infected with TB have a 10% lifetime risk of developing active TB; this risk increases dramatically in people who become immunosuppressed. Therefore, the committee decided to evaluate TB in depth.
[c] West Nile virus infection does not meet inclusion criterion 4 (Box 5.1), because its health outcomes usually are manifested at the time of the acute illness. However, dramatic changes in the epidemiology of West Nile virus infection since the middle 1990s led the committee to decide to review it in depth.

This chapter contains nine sections, with similar formats: one for each disease. Each begins with an introduction to the disease and its etiologic agent, which is followed by a brief description of the acute illness. Then, a summary of diagnostic criteria and methods and of treatment protocols is presented. Each section ends with an evidence-based discussion of the infection's known long-term adverse health outcomes and their pathogenesis; this discussion is the basis of the committee's conclusions about the strength of association between the primary infection and each long-term adverse health outcome.

DIARRHEAL DISEASES: *CAMPYLOBACTER*, NON-TYPHOID *SALMONELLA*, AND *SHIGELLA* INFECTIONS

Among the many pathogens known to have caused diarrheal disease among US troops deployed to the Gulf War, Operation Enduring Freedom (OEF), or Operation Iraqi Freedom (OIF), three merit an examination of their potential long-term, adverse outcomes to veterans' health: *Campylobacter, Shigella,* and *Salmonella.*

Campylobacter Infection

Campylobacter infections are common causes of acute diarrheal illnesses in humans globally (Blaser 2005). The committee examined three potential long-term adverse health outcomes of *Campylobacter* infection: Guillain-Barré syndrome, reactive arthritis, and uveitis.

The most common pathogenic *Campylobacter* species is *C. jejuni*, but disease may also be caused by other species, especially *C. coli, C. upsaliensis*, *C. lari*, and *C. fetus*. The typical illness is acute diarrheal disease lasting 2-5 days accompanied by abdominal pain and fever. The illness responds well to antibiotic treatment but often is self-limited. *Campylobacter* occasionally causes an acute systemic infection.

Transmission of *Campylobacter*

Campylobacter species (spp.) infect humans most often through contaminated food or water. Drinking untreated water is a major risk factor for both sporadic and epidemic campylobacteriosis (Allos 2001; Blaser 2005). Foodborne infections occur chiefly after the consumption of improperly heated foods of animal origin; common vehicles include unpasteurized milk and undercooked chicken. Among wild and domesticated animals, *Campylobacter* spp. may be normal flora or pathogens (Blaser 2005). Rarely, the bacteria are transmitted by person-to-person contact; this occurs chiefly from the handling of feces of incontinent people, such as infants, who are infected.

People suffering from an enteric illness may be infected with two or more bacterial, viral, protozoan, or helminthic pathogens. Some laboratory analyses of stool specimens from deployed troops who had a diagnosis of diarrheal illness found dual infections in a subset of patients, as described in Chapter 4.

Endemicity in Southwest and South-Central Asia

Campylobacter is a common cause of acute diarrhea in southwest and south-central Asia (Wilson 1991). In the United States, the bacteria frequently instigate both sporadic diarrhea and outbreaks (Wilson 1991).

Acute Illness

Patients with *Campylobacter* infections often present with a short prodrome of symptoms consisting chiefly of headache, myalgias, back pain, and fever. Within 24 hours, the illness centers on the gastrointestinal tract, producing abdominal pain and diarrhea (either may come first). Common characteristics of the abdominal pain are unlocalized cramping that may be so severe as to mimic acute appendicitis; however, diarrhea predominates over abdominal pain in most patients.

On the first day of diarrheal illness, the patient usually has four to 20 loose stools, and 25% of them may contain visible blood. Laboratory examination of stool specimens usually reveals gross or microscopic blood in all and leukocytes in 70%. Fever continues from the prodrome and persists for 24-48 hours.

Symptoms usually begin to recede after 48 hours and resolve during the next few days. In rare cases, the illness may last longer. In the absence of antibiotic treatment, relapse occurs in about 20% of cases; relapses are usually milder than the initial episodes.

Some people with *Campylobacter* infections are bacteremic (Mandell et al. 2005); this condition represents either a primary bacteremia or, rarely, the seeding of a distant organ (Blaser et al. 1986).

Diagnosis During and After Acute Illness

Diagnosis of the acute illness is based on culture of feces and, rarely, of blood. Culture-based tests even in the acute phase can have false-negative results, especially in infection by non-*jejuni* species, because *Campylobacter* spp. are difficult to grow in culture. Alternatively, the bacteria can be detected with polymerase-chain-reaction (PCR) assay of genetic material from stool specimens. Antibody testing, which is not commercially available, is less reliable because of the diversity of *Campylobacter* strains, the time required for a response to occur, and differences in magnitudes of responses among hosts.

Infected people shed *Campylobacter* in stool for a mean of 2-3 weeks after the onset of symptoms; virtually no immunocompetent hosts are still shedding the organism after 8 weeks (Karmali and Fleming 1979; Svedhem and Kaijser 1980; Taylor et al. 1988). Thus, a culture or PCR test conducted more than 2 months after an acute episode of *Campylobacter* enteric disease would rarely be positive. After 2 months have elapsed, there is no reliable diagnostic test for exposure to *Campylobacter* in people who manifest diseases that could be late adverse health outcomes of a *Campylobacter* infection.

Treatment of Acute Illness

Fluid and electrolyte replacement is the treatment of choice for diarrheal illnesses. In patients who are still symptomatic at the time of diagnosis, antimicrobial treatment is recommended, particularly with fluoroquinolones and macrolides. Clinicians should be cognizant of *Campylobacter*'s growing resistance to those antimicrobials; the degree of resistance will reflect the use of antimicrobials in animal farming and in the local human population.

Long-Term Adverse Health Outcomes of *Campylobacter* Infection

On occasion, infection by *Campylobacter* spp. leads to long-term adverse health outcomes. The most serious health outcome associated with campylobacteriosis is Guillain-Barré syndrome (GBS). Reactive arthritis appears to occur after campylobacteriosis at a frequency greater than the background frequency. There is some evidence that uveitis is associated with *Campylobacter* infection.

Guillain-Barré Syndrome

The first report of an association between *Campylobacter jejuni* infection and GBS was published in 1982 (Rhodes and Tattersfield 1982). Numerous scientists have since investigated the relationship between the two diseases and have published more than 200 reports in peer-reviewed journals. By the year 2000, those investigations had established that infection by *C. jejuni* causes about 30% of all cases of GBS (Allos 1997; Dingle et al. 2001; McCarthy and Giesecke 2001; Nachamkin 2002; Nachamkin et al. 1998; Nachamkin et al. 2001; Sinha et al. 2004; Tam et al. 2003). A number of other infectious diseases are also associated with GBS.

GBS is a severe acute neurologic disease characterized by ascending paralysis with involvement of motor neurons and sometimes sensory neurons (Rhodes and Tattersfield 1982). Developing over a period of days, the symptoms of GBS may lead to paralysis of the respiratory muscles and death; however, with rapid supportive care, the fatality rate has been reduced from more than 10% to less than 5%. Between 10 and 20% of affected persons have permanent neurologic deficits, such as persistent muscle weakness and contractures. Most patients with GBS require hospitalization, and more than 20% require ventilatory support at some time during their illness. Recommended treatment should be started immediately and may include plasmapheresis and intravenous administration of immunoglobulins.

Approximately 0.01-0.03% of US patients who suffer acute gastrointestinal disease due to *C. jejuni* will develop GBS (Allos 1997; Tauxe and Blake 1992). The risk of developing GBS during the 2 months after a symptomatic episode of *C. jejuni* infection is about 100 times greater than the risk in the general population (McCarthy and Giesecke 2001). The symptoms of GBS usually are manifested 7-28 days after the onset of gastrointestinal symptoms (Allos 1997; McCarthy and Giesecke 2001). There is no association between the severity of *C. jejuni*-induced gastrointestinal illness and the risk of developing GBS (Allos 2001).

Rigorous serologic and culture studies have found and validated evidence of recent infection by *C. jejuni* in high percentages of patients with GBS. Several studies, including at least two case-control studies, showed that GBS patients were more likely than controls to have increased titers of antibodies to *C. jejuni* (Liu et al. 2003; Mishu et al. 1993). They demonstrated important trends and associations in populations but are neither standardized nor sufficiently accurate to be used for conclusive diagnosis in an individual patient. In another line of inquiry, seven independent studies found that 8-50% (mean, 30%) of stool specimens obtained from patients with GBS at the onset of symptoms were culture-positive for *C. jejuni* (Enders et al. 1993; Gruenewald et al. 1991; Hariharan et al. 1996; Kuroki et al. 1993; Rees et al. 1995; Ropper 1988; Speed et al. 1984). A positive culture is sufficient for diagnosis of *Campylobacter*-induced GBS but may be falsely negative, depending on the accuracy of the cultural procedures used, timing after symptom onset, clinical status, and antibiotic use.

There are several types of GBS, including acute inflammatory demyelinating polyneuropathy (AIDP), acute motor axonal neuropathy (AMAN), and Miller-Fisher syndrome (MFS). Antecedent *Campylobacter* infections have been linked with AMAN and MFS (Dingle et al. 2001; Kuwabara et al. 2004; Nachamkin et al. 1998); their association with AIDP is controversial (Kuwabara et al. 2004; Nachamkin et al. 1998).

Molecular mimicry is believed to play a role in the nerve damage that occurs in *Campylobacter*-associated GBS (Nachamkin et al. 1998). Although the mechanism is unknown, some molecular structures on the surface of particular strains of *Campylobacter* appear to mimic either the glycolipids of peripheral nerves or specific proteins found in myelin (Allos 2001).

The committee concludes that there is sufficient evidence of an association between *Campylobacter jejuni* infection and GBS, if the GBS is manifested within 2 months of the infection.

Reactive Arthritis

Reactive arthritis (ReA), an acute nonpurulent form of arthritis, is a complication of many infectious diseases that affect parts of the body distinct from those involved in the acute illness (Yu and Kuipers 2003). The disease chiefly follows urogenital or diarrheal infections by multiple etiologic agents, including *Campylobacter*. ReA that occurs after an episode of campylobacteriosis usually is manifested within several weeks of the acute gastrointestinal illness (Blaser 2000).

The clinical manifestations ReA range from isolated transient monoarthritis to severe multisystem disease. Although it can be highly inflammatory and severe, ReA usually is moderate in intensity. Patients often manifest such constitutional symptoms as fatigue, malaise, fever, and weight loss. The arthritis typically is asymmetric and additive, with new joints becoming involved over days or weeks. Joints of the lower extremities suffer most. Tendinitis is common, as are urogenital, ocular, and mucocutaneous lesions. Rarely, ReA is associated with aortic insufficiency and cardiac conduction abnormalities. Reiter's syndrome—the triad of arthritis, urethritis, and conjunctivitis—makes up just one portion of the ReA spectrum and is more closely associated with *Shigella* and *Chlamydia trachomatis* infections than with *Campylobacter*.

ReA following infections by various agents occurs most often, although not exclusively, in people who have the gene that encodes a histocompatibility antigen called HLA-B27. Between 30% and 85% of ReA patients have the HLA-B27 gene. However, only 8% of healthy people have the HLA-B27 gene, and only about 20% of them will develop ReA if they contract the triggering infections (NIH 2002). People who are 18-40 years old are at greatest risk for ReA. Men and women are equally likely to contract ReA from enterically-acquired infections; in contrast, ReA from sexually-acquired infections predominantly affects men.

Long-term followup studies of patients who have ReA suggest that some joint symptoms persist for months in 10-60% of cases and that acute symptoms commonly recur (Hannu et al. 2004a; Hannu et al. 2002; Rees et al. 2004). Up to 25% of affected people must change or curtail their work because of joint symptoms. The symptoms of ReA usually last 1-21 weeks and occasionally up to a year (Skirrow and Blaser 2002). Symptoms that persist beyond a year tend to be mild and nondeforming.

ReA is a clinical diagnosis, but the finding of HLA-B27 positivity is helpful. Treatment is symptomatic and uses primarily anti-inflammatory agents, including nonsteriodal anti-inflammatory agents, especially indomethacin.

Population-based studies have provided the most convincing evidence of an association between *Campylobacter* infection and ReA. Two such studies found that 7% and 1.8% of patients with laboratory-confirmed *Campylobacter* infection later developed ReA (Hannu et al. 2002; Rees et al. 2004). They validated the results of three independently conducted rheumatologic surveys administered after distinct outbreaks of *Campylobacter* infection (Bremell et al. 1991; Eastmond et al. 1983; Hannu et al. 2004a). The surveys found that 0.7-2.6% of adults infected with *Campylobacter* later developed ReA. The scientific literature also contains reports of at least 40 sporadic cases of ReA associated with *Campylobacter* infection (Hannu et al. 2002). The disparate geographic locations of the studies—including Finland and California—indicate that the association of *Campylobacter* with ReA is a general, not local, phenomenon.

The pathogenesis of bacteria-induced ReA is poorly understood. *Campylobacter* organisms invade such host cells as monocytes and dendritic cells, which transport the bacteria through the bloodstream to multiple locations, including joints (Yu and Kuipers 2003). How *Campylobacter* and other ReA-causing bacteria survive persistently in joint cells remains unknown, as does the viability of *Campylobacter* organisms in those cells. Yu and Kuipers (2003) present a plausible hypothesis for the mechanism by which *Campylobacter* organisms induce joint-specific inflammation: that macrophages present antigenic peptides to $CD8^+$ T lymphocytes through histocompatibility antigen HLA-B27. The T-cell receptor of $CD8^+$ T lymphocytes is specific for both foreign and self peptides carried by HLA-B27. The process may activate $CD8^+$ T lymphocytes and produce the initial inflammatory response. The mechanism of sustained inflammatory response is unknown.

Despite the ambiguous pathogenesis of postinfection ReA, the weight of epidemiologic evidence convincingly illustrates that a small percentage of people infected by *Campylobacter* spp. later develop ReA.

The committee concludes that there is sufficient evidence of an association between *Campylobacter* infection and reactive arthritis (ReA), if the ReA is manifested within 3 months of the infection. Most cases of ReA are manifested within a month of the infection.

Uveitis

Uveitis is an inflammation inside the eye that affects the uvea. Known causes of uveitis include autoimmune disorders, infection, and exposure to toxins (MedlinePlus Medical Encyclopedia 2006). In many cases, the cause is unknown.

Three case reports describe uveitis after *C. jejuni* infection (Hannu et al. 2004b; Howard et al. 1987; Lever et al. 1984). The first report involves one of 350 patients who contracted *C. jejuni* infection in an outbreak in Finland in August 2000 (Hannu et al. 2004b). The subject of the report, a 72-year-old woman who had gastritis, developed pain and mucopurulent exudation in her left eye without marked redness after the *C. jejuni* outbreak. Although *C. jejuni* infection was not confirmed with a stool culture, it was "epidemiologically highly probable" that her prior gastrointestinal symptoms were caused by *C. jejuni* (Hannu et al. 2004b). About 3 weeks after the acute illness, the woman sought medical attention for the eye symptoms, and mild acute anterior uveitis was diagnosed. An HLA-B27 antigen test was negative. She was treated with local corticosteroid drops and corticosteroid-antibiotic ointment. The condition resolved about 2 months after the acute illness. In a second case report, a previously healthy 39-year-old woman with a culture-confirmed *C. jejuni* infection developed redness and pain in her eyes about 4 weeks after the gastritis resolved (Howard et al. 1987). The eye condition was diagnosed as nonspecific anterior uveitis. The eye inflammation was treated and resolved over a period of 2 weeks. An HLA-B27 antigen test was negative. In the third case report, acute anterior uveitis was reported in a 34-year-old woman who had a culture-confirmed *C. jejuni* infection (Lever et al. 1984). She also had hypogammaglobulinemia and chronic diarrhea. No information was given on how the uveitis was treated, how long after onset of the infection the uveitis developed, or how long it took the condition to resolve.

The committee concludes that there is limited or suggestive evidence of an association between *C. jejuni* infection and uveitis, if the uveitis is manifested within a month of the infection.

Nontyphoidal *Salmonella* Infection

The genus *Salmonella* comprises commensal and pathogenic bacteria found in humans, mammals, reptiles, birds, and insects worldwide. These gram-negative, largely motile bacilli are highly adaptable facultative anaerobes 2-3 μm long that reside mainly in the intestines of their hosts. Salmonellae are classified in two species, *S. enterica* and *S. bongori*; the former is divided into six subspecies and more than 2,500 serotypes (or serovars) according to their somatic, surface, and flagellar antigens and their habitats (Box 5.1) (Center for Infectious Disease Research and Policy 2006; Pegues et al. 2005).

BOX 5.1 Classification of *Salmonella*

Salmonella enterica
- subspecies *enterica* (I)
- subspecies *salmae* (II)
- subspecies *arizonae* (IIIa)
- subspecies *diarizonae* (IIIb)
- subspecies *houtenae* (IV)
- subspecies *indica* (VI)

Salmonella bongori

SOURCE: Pegues et al. 2005.

Salmonella enterica serotypes Typhi and Paratyphi cause life-threatening typhoid fever and paratyphoid fever (typhoidal salmonellosis), respectively. Those diseases' severity, short incubation period, and other salient characteristics would lead to rapid detection, diagnosis, and treatment in deployed US military personnel (CDC 2005b; Olsen et al. 2003). In contrast, uncomplicated infection with nontyphoidal salmonellae causes an array of generally milder illnesses that appear similar to other diarrheal diseases and usually resolve without medical attention. Therefore, the committee devotes attention exclusively to infection with nontyphoidal salmonellae in this chapter.

Transmission of Nontyphoidal Salmonellae

Nontyphoidal salmonellae are most commonly transmitted by the ingestion of contaminated food, especially food of animal origin. Food derived from infected animals that is uncooked, inadequately cooked, unpasteurized, or inadequately pasteurized may transmit the bacteria to humans. Alternatively, such products may cross-contaminate other food that then becomes a vehicle for transmission. Outbreaks of salmonellosis also have arisen from the consumption of fresh produce contaminated with human or animal feces containing salmonellae (Pegues et al. 2005).

Drinking contaminated water infrequently leads to transmission of nontyphoidal salmonellae to humans (Pegues et al. 2005). Exposure to salmonella-infected pets, especially reptiles, can lead to transmission to humans. Rarely, transmission occurs through the transfusion of tainted blood products (Wilson 1991).

Endemicity in Southwest and South-Central Asia

Salmonella spp. is present in all countries (Wilson 1991). The centralized production and wide distribution of manufactured foods in developed nations periodically facilitates large outbreaks of salmonellosis (Pegues et al. 2005).

Acute Illness

Salmonella Gastroenteritis

Gastroenteritis is the most common syndrome of infection with nontyphoidal *Salmonella*. Some 60-80% of cases occur sporadically. After an incubation period of 6-72 hours, patients experience sudden onset of diarrhea, nausea, and sometimes vomiting. Those symptoms are frequently accompanied by fever, headache, abdominal pain, and chills. Myalgia is sometimes reported. Rarely, patients manifest pseudoappendicitis or mimicry of the intestinal changes of inflammatory bowel disease (Heymann 2004; Pegues et al. 2005).

Microscopic examination of stool specimens during the acute phase reveals neutrophils and sometimes red blood cells.

Salmonella gastroenteritis is usually self-limited. Fever commonly resolves within 48-72 hours after onset. Diarrhea usually resolves within 3-7 days, after 10 days at most; however, patients continue to shed the agent in stool for 4-5 weeks, depending on the serotype of *Salmonella*. Patients who receive antimicrobial therapy may shed for longer periods (Pegues et al. 2005).

Severe *Salmonella* gastroenteritis leads to dehydration and hospitalization in 2.2 cases per million in the US population. The disease causes about 580 deaths per year in the United States, primarily in elderly or immunocompromised people (Pegues et al. 2005).

Salmonella Bacteremia

Bacteremia occurs in 1-4% of immunocompetent patients who have *Salmonella* gastroenteritis. Any serotype of the agent may be responsible. Among adults, the risk of bacteremia is greater for *Salmonella*-infected people who are immunocompromised (Pegues et al. 2005).

Diagnosis of Acute Illness

Salmonella infection may be microbiologically confirmed by plating freshly passed stool samples onto a primary culture medium. Selenate-based enrichment broths can facilitate the recovery of low numbers of organisms. Rapid immunoglobulin M (IgM) antibody-based serologic tests may supplement stool culture (Pegues et al. 2005).

Treatment of Acute Illness

Uncomplicated gastroenteritis may be treated simply with ingestion of oral rehydration solution to replace water and electrolytes. Antibiotics are indicated in adults who are debilitated; who have HIV infection, continued fever, or high fever; or who manifest extraintestinal infection. Ciprofloxacin, ampicillin, or amoxicillin may be administered to adults. Trimethoprim-sulfamethoxazole and chloramphenicol may be effective for treating people who have microbial-resistant strains (Heymann 2004).

Coinfection with Nontyphoidal Salmonellae and Human Immunodeficiency Virus

Salmonellosis is sometimes the first manifestation of HIV infection. People with HIV are at much higher risk than the general population for salmonellosis, and the risk of *Salmonella* bacteremia is 20-100 times greater. *Salmonella* bacteremia often recurs in HIV-infected people; indeed, such recurrence is a criterion for the classification of AIDS by the Centers for Disease Control and Prevention (CDC) (CDC 1992; Heymann 2004; Kim et al. 2004; Pegues et al. 2005).

Long-Term Adverse Health Outcome of Nontyphoidal *Salmonella* Infection

As discussed above, ReA is an acute nonpurulent form of arthritis that complicates infections at other sites of the body. The most commonly affected joints are the knees and ankles (Locht et al. 2002). If ReA follows an acute episode of nontyphoidal S*almonella* infection, it is manifested 1-2 weeks after the gastrointestinal illness. The reported incidence of ReA among cases of acute nontyphoidal *Salmonella* infection ranges from only 1% to as high as 29% (Buxton et al. 2002; Dworkin et al. 2001; Hannu and Leirisalo-Repo 1988; Lee et al. 2005; Leirisalo-Repo et al. 1997; Locht et al. 1993; Locht et al. 2002; Maki-Ikola and Granfors 1992; Maki-Ikola et al. 1991; Maki-Ikola et al. 1992; Mattila et al. 1994; Mattila et al. 1998; Nikkari et al. 1999; Sinha et al. 2003; Thomas and Hedayati 1986; Thomson et al. 1994; Thomson et al. 1992; Thomson et al. 1995). Factors that influence the incidence include older age, longer duration of diarrhea, and the presence of HLA-B27.

The duration of symptoms is variable, ranging from months to years (Lee et al. 2005; Leirisalo-Repo et al. 1997; Mattila et al. 1994; Thomson et al. 1995). Antibiotic treatment for the diarrheal illness does not affect the severity of ReA or its duration (Locht et al. 1993; Mattila et al. 1998). Ankylosing spondylitis occasionally follows ReA.

ReA is a clinical diagnosis, but the presence of HLA-B27 is helpful. Symptom-based treatment involves primarily the administration of anti-inflammatory agents.

> **The committee concludes that there is sufficient evidence of an association between nontyphoidal *Salmonella* infection and reactive arthritis (ReA) if the ReA is manifested within 3 months of the infection.**

Shigella Infection

Like *Campylobacter* and nontyphoidal *Salmonella* infections, *Shigella* infections are common causes of acute diarrheal illnesses in humans globally (Halpern et al. 1989; Shears 1996; Taylor et al. 1991) and have been diagnosed in US troops during the Gulf War, OEF, and OIF. Occasionally, *Shigella* infections lead to long-term adverse health outcomes, notably ReA and hemolytic uremic syndrome. Each adverse health outcome appears to occur after an episode of shigellosis at frequencies greater than background rates.

Transmission of *Shigella* Infection

Humans are the reservoir for the four known species of *Shigella*: *S. dysenteriae*, *S. flexneri*, *S. boydii*, and *S. sonnei*. They are transmitted by the fecal-oral route and through fecal contamination of unpurified water, or uncooked or undercooked food. Person-to-person transmission is common and is facilitated by lack of hand-washing facilities and inadequate supply of potable water. In military camps, where sewerage is not regular, shigellosis may become epidemic. Although *Shigella* spp. occasionally infects other primates, such infections have little impact on transmission among humans.

Endemicity in Southwest and South-Central Asia

Shigella is endemic, hyperendemic, or epidemic in locales with minimal sanitation. Shigellosis is well recognized in southwest and south-central Asia. *S. flexneri* and *S. dysenteriae* are more common in southwest and south-central Asia than in the United States, where *S. sonnei* dominates.

Acute Illness

Shigella infection causes an acute diarrheal illness. Symptoms are constitutional; they frequently include malaise and fever, and they immediately involve abdominal bloating, cramping, and diarrhea.

During shigellosis, diarrhea may be nonbloody and watery or bloody; the latter condition is generally termed dysentery. Laboratory examination of stool specimens usually reveals numerous leukocytes. The number of loose stools can range from several per day to more than 20 on the worst day of the illness. Fever and constitutional symptoms typically peak during the period of most severe diarrheal symptoms. The diarrhea may be accompanied by tenesmus, or painful straining while defecating. The illness usually is self-limiting, and patients recover within a week. In the absence of antibiotic treatment, however, shigellosis can be severe or even, rarely, fatal (Bennish 1991).

Diagnosis of Acute Illness

Diagnosis is based on culture of fecal specimens and very rarely blood. When PCR methods are available, they can be equally valuable. People with acute shigellosis remain culture-positive for up to 4 weeks. Beyond that timeframe, culture is inadequate to confirm or refute any relationship of symptoms with *Shigella.*

Treatment of Acute Illness

Treatment of all acute gastrointestinal infections must be based first on fluid replacement. The use of antibiotics is recommended because it shortens the duration of shigellosis and the likelihood of transmission to other hosts (Bhattacharya and Sur 2003). Resistance to sulfonamides, chloramphenicol, and tetracyclines is nearly universal, and resistance to ampicillin and trimethoprim-sulfamethoxazole is frequent. Treatment with fluoroquinolines or azithromycin is successful, even in short courses (1-3 days). The use of antimotility agents may induce more severe disease and is contraindicated.

Long-Term Adverse Health Outcomes of *Shigella* Infection

Reactive Arthritis

As discussed above, ReA is an acute nonpurulent form of arthritis that complicates infections at other sites of the body. If ReA follows an acute episode of shigellosis, it is usually manifested 2-3 weeks after the gastrointestinal illness (Calin and Fries 1976; Chen et al. 2002; Finch et al. 1986; Good 1979; Noer 1966; Sieper et al. 1993; Simon et al. 1981). It is most common after *S. flexneri* infection; it also follows infection by *S. dysenteriae* (Good 1979) but rarely *S. sonnei* (Good 1979; Kaslow RA 1979; Lewis 1982; Simon et al. 1981). Ankylosing spondylitis occasionally follows ReA and may be considered as a consequence of *Shigella*-induced ReA. The symptoms of ReA cause up to 25% of affected people to change or curtail their work. Followup studies suggest that some joint symptoms persist in 30-60% of patients for up to a year, but most patients recover within a few months (Calin and Fries 1976; Rongnoparat and Panpanit 1987). ReA after shigellosis is rare: in studies of Israeli soldiers with acute diarrheal illnesses, 336 cases of shigellosis were documented from 1993 to 1997 in the field units under surveillance, and none of the subjects developed ReA or ankylosing spondylitis (Bloom et al. 1994).

The most conclusive evidence regarding the incidence of ReA due to *Shigella* infection comes from the recent population-based study of Hannu et al. (2005). Of 278 patients with *Shigella*-positive stool cultures, 7% had ReA, and an additional 2% developed other reactive musculoskeletal symptoms; one of the 597 controls had ReA. In the *Shigella*-positive patients, the odds ratio for developing ReA was 16.2 (95% CI, 2.1-123.9). Some 36% of the ReA patients were HLA-B27-positive. Several additional studies and case reports support the findings of Hannu et al. (Chen et al. 2002; Davies et al. 1969; Finch et al. 1986; Lauhio et al. 1988; Neithercut et al. 1984; Noer 1966; Sieper et al. 1993; Simon et al. 1981).

The committee concludes that there is sufficient evidence of an association between *Shigella* infection and reactive arthritis (ReA), if the ReA is manifested within 3 months of the infection. Most cases of ReA will be manifested within 1 month of the infection.

Hemolytic Uremic Syndrome

Acute shigellosis may lead to hemolytic uremic syndrome (HUS), a life-threatening disease that afflicts primarily young children and the elderly (Ilnyckyj et al. 2003; Okhuysen et al. 2004). HUS is defined as a clinical triad of hemolysis, thrombocytopenia, and renal dysfunction. It is usually manifested within 6-10 days of the onset of shigellosis; more rarely, people with shigellosis-associated HUS can come to clinical attention as late as 30 days after the onset of enteritis (Nathoo et al. 1995; Parsonnet and Griffin 1993).

Shiga toxins produced by some *Shigella* strains (particularly *S. dysenteriae*) cause HUS by damaging endothelial cells, especially in the kidneys. The damage leads to microangiopathy, which results in microangiopathic hemolytic anemia, renal failure, and systemic illness.

There have been many published cases of HUS that occurred after shigellosis. For example, HUS occurred after *Shigella* infection in two of 42 US tourists to Mexico in 1988 (Parsonnet et al. 1989), 40 of 320 (12%) patients in Bangladesh admitted to a hospital (Rahaman et al. 1975), nine of 241 (4%) patients in Bangladesh (Koster et al. 1978), and seven of 36 (19%) patients in South Africa (Bloom et al. 1994).

The committee concludes that there is sufficient evidence of an association between *Shigella* infection and hemolytic uremic syndrome (HUS), if HUS is manifested within 1 month of the infection. Most cases of HUS will be manifested within 10 days of the infection.

BRUCELLOSIS

Human brucellosis is a chronic intracellular infectious process that involves *Brucella* spp. and the human reticuloendothelial system. The process may harm any organ in the human body. Up to 10% of people infected with brucellae may develop chronic disease, which is often due to relapses after partial therapy or to disease progression after undiagnosed and untreated acute disease. Although brucellosis occurs sporadically in many countries, it is endemic in areas of southwest and south-central Asia. The committee discusses below the clinical spectrum of chronic brucellosis and determines criteria for linking long-term adverse health outcomes to infection during military service in the Gulf War, OEF, or OIF.

Brucellae are small, gram-negative coccobacilli that are facultative intracellular pathogens with the ability to survive and multiply in mononuclear phagocytic cells of infected hosts. Eight *Brucella* species have been identified, but only a subgroup is associated with human disease (Table 5.2). At present, all *Brucella* species are considered biovars of *B. melitensis*.

B. melitensis contains two circular replicons of 1.1 and 1.2 Mb. Its genome contains 3,197 open reading frames. *B. melitensis*, *B. abortus* biotypes 1 and 4, and *B. suis* biotype 1 are very similar. In contrast, *B. suis* biotypes 2 and 4 contain two replicons of 1.35 and 1.85 Mb, and *B. suis* biotype 3 contains a single circular replicon of 3.3 Mb (Pappas et al. 2005).

TABLE 5.2 Nomenclature and Characteristics of *Brucella* spp.

Species	Biotype	Animal Hosts	Human Virulence[a]
B. melitensis	1-3	Goats, sheep, camels	++++
B. abortus	1-6, 9	Cows, camels, yaks, buffalo	++ to +++
B. suis	1-5	Pigs (biotypes 1-3), wild hares (biotype 2), caribou (biotype 4), reindeer (biotype 4), wild rodents (biotype 5)	+
B. canis		Canines	+
B. ovis		Sheep	-
B. neotomae		Rodents	-
B. pinnipediae and *B. cetaceae*		Minke whales, dolphins, porpoises, seals	+

[a] Virulence is graded on a scale from no virulence (-) to the highest degree of virulence (++++).
SOURCE: Adapted with permission from Pappas et al. 2005.

Transmission and Endemicity of Brucellosis

Human brucellosis is a zoonosis; almost all infections are derived directly or indirectly from exposure to animals. Humans may be infected through direct contact of abraded skin or cuts with infected animals, their tissues or fluids, inhalation, inoculation of mucosal or conjunctival membranes, or ingestion of infective animal products (most often unpasteurized dairy products) (Lulu et al. 1988).

Human brucellosis occurs sporadically in many developed or industrialized countries, including the United States, but most cases occur in three distinct endemic zones: the Near East and Middle East, including Iran, Iraq, Kuwait, Saudi Arabia, Israel, Jordan, and Turkey; the Mediterranean region, including Spain, Portugal, Italy, and Greece; and Latin American countries, including Peru, Argentina, and Mexico (Abo-Shehada et al. 1996; Bodur et al. 2003; Geyik et al. 2002; Gottesman et al. 1996; Gungor et al. 2002; Gur et al. 2003; Hasanjani Roushan et al. 2004; Khateeb et al. 1990; Lubani et al. 1989b; Lulu et al. 1988; McLean et al. 1992; Memish and Venkatesh 2001; Mousa et al. 1987; Norton 1984; Tasova et al. 1999; Trujillo et al. 1994; Zaks et al. 1995). Endemic disease in those regions is usually associated with *B. melitensis* infection.

In the endemic zones, infections are acquired typically through consumption of dairy products, especially unpasteurized goat cheese and untreated milk. Human-to-human transmission of brucellosis species is rare but has been associated with transplantation of infected bone marrow, blood transfusion, and possibly sexual transmission of the organism in semen

(Goossens et al. 1983; Ruben et al. 1991). Brucellosis probably is endemic in Afghanistan, but data on its occurrence there are sparse.

Between 100 and 200 US cases of human brucellosis were reported annually to CDC during the 1990s. Brucellosis cases in the United States have begun to shift from people who are occupationally exposed to animals and animal products (such as butchers, abattoir workers, veterinarians, and farmers) to people who ingest unpasteurized goat-milk products imported from Latin America (Chomel et al. 1994; Taylor and Perdue 1989). The disease is 8 times more prevalent at the US-Mexico border than elsewhere in the United States (Doyle and Bryan 2000; Fosgate et al. 2002). In the United States, cattle-associated *B. abortus* has been the etiologic agent of human brucellosis acquired directly from animals, and *B. melitensis* the agent of human brucellosis acquired from dairy products (CDC 1986; Spink 1954).

Acute Brucellosis

The acute form of human brucellosis is usually manifested 2-4 weeks after infection as a nonspecific febrile illness accompanied by profuse sweating, headache, malaise, arthralgia, arthritis, myalgia, back pain, or a combination of these. Hematologic abnormalities may include anemia, leukopenia, thrombocytopenia, and clotting disorders that are usually mild and resolve with therapy (Crosby et al. 1984; Pappas et al. 2004). Severe thrombocytopenia is rare (Young et al. 2000). Brucellosis in animals (especially that caused by *B. abortus*) is associated with spontaneous abortion. Although brucellosis may result in human abortion, it may be no more common than abortion that occurs during any infectious process (Khan et al. 2001; Makhseed et al. 1998).

Diagnosis of Acute Brucellosis

The diagnosis of brucellosis should be considered in the appropriate clinical setting with appropriate demographic risk factors. Laboratory analysis may disclose mild leukopenia, thrombocytopenia, and anemia with minimally to moderately abnormal liver-function tests. Definitive diagnosis involves recovering organisms, usually from blood or bone marrow. Culturing of bone marrow is the most sensitive method of diagnosis (Gotuzzo et al. 1986). In rare cases, brucellae may also be recovered from synovial fluid, cerebral spinal fluid, urine, or biopsy samples (Gotuzzo et al. 1986). Rapid automated bacterial identification systems may occasionally misidentify brucellae, for instance, as *Moraxella phenylpyruvica* (Roiz et al. 1998). PCR and other molecular techniques may be used, but they are not yet used widely in clinical settings (Colmenero et al. 2002; Fox et al. 1998; Morata et al. 2001; Queipo-Ortuno et al. 1997). If microbiologic cultures are negative, diagnosis of human brucellosis usually involves serologic analysis.

A number of serologic tests for diagnosing brucellosis exist (Al Dahouk et al. 2003; Young 1991). The most widely used is a serum agglutination test (SAT), which measures IgM and immunoglobulin G (IgG) brucella antibody titers. SAT titers above 1:160 are diagnostic for brucellosis in the appropriate clinical setting (Young 1991). A 2-merceptoethanol assay can increase the specificity of the SAT by distinguishing IgG from IgM responses (Baldi et al. 1996). Drawbacks of the SAT include cross-reactivity and inability to diagnose *B. canis* infection. In some people with brucellosis, an SAT response will not occur. Blocking antibodies may be present, or a Coombs test may be positive (Pascual et al. 1988). An enzyme-linked immunosorbent assay (ELISA) specific for brucella has higher sensitivity and specificity than the

SAT (Almuneef and Memish 2003; Ariza et al. 1992; Khateeb et al. 1990; Lulu et al. 1988) and may be positive when other tests are negative. In evaluating people for neurobrucellosis when the SAT is negative, an ELISA should be performed (Araj et al. 1988). If neurobrucellosis is considered and serum antibody tests and microbiologic cultures are negative, cerebral spinal fluid can be evaluated for the presence of antibrucella antibodies (Kochar et al. 2000a; McLean et al. 1992).

Treatments for Brucellosis and Related Long-Term Toxicity

Treatment of people for brucellosis usually involves administration of tetracyclines (usually doxycycline) with rifampin for 6 weeks (WHO 1986). However, a regimen of oral doxycycline for 6 weeks and streptomycin for 2-3 weeks is more effective (Solera et al. 1995). Streptomycin may be replaced with gentamicin. Administration of aminoglycoside antibiotics is associated with renal and cranial VIIIth nerve toxicity, although if aminoglycosides are appropriately administered during short-course therapy, such complications are rare and often transient.

Coinfection

Although *Brucella* spp. are intracellular pathogens, there has been no apparent increase in morbidity and mortality during coinfection with brucellae and other intracellular pathogens or infections that disrupt the cellular immune system, such as HIV infection.

Long-Term Adverse Health Outcomes of Brucellosis

Acute brucellosis may be a nonspecific flu-like illness, so a specific diagnosis might not be made. People with untreated brucellosis are at risk for the relapsing and chronic health outcomes described below. In addition, antimicrobial therapy is not 100% effective, and even treated people are at risk for relapse and chronic disease. Clinical manifestations due to relapsing or chronic brucellosis usually are evident within 2-6 months of acute illness and if untreated can persist for years or decades (Spink 1951). Manifestations may be protean and nonspecific. Focal infections have also been reported up to 30 years after probable acute disease (Ariza et al. 2001; Colmenero et al. 2002; Martin et al. 1961; Mousa et al. 1986; Norton 1984; Williams and Crossley 1982; Zinneman et al. 1961).

Diagnosis of Chronic Brucellosis

Diagnosis during chronic brucellosis is similar to that during acute disease. During chronic brucellosis, bacteriologic confirmation may include detecting the organism in a bone marrow sample or in a focal infectious process or abscess. Serologic evaluation is usually positive. Isolated involvement of the central nervous system is rare and is usually diagnosed with serologic analysis or antibody analysis of cerebral spinal fluid.

Major Manifestations of Chronic Brucellosis

The major manifestations of relapsing or chronic brucellosis include the following conditions and organ systems.

Arthritis

Bone and joint complications are the most common manifestation of chronic and relapsing brucellosis, occurring in 10-80% of cases in various studies (Mousa et al. 1987; Tasova et al. 1999; Zaks et al. 1995). Arthritis is usually peripheral and monoarticular and often involves the knee or hip; however, some patients develop polyarthritis (Geyik et al. 2002; Gotuzzo et al. 1982; Gotuzzo et al. 1987; Hasanjani Roushan et al. 2004). Peripheral arthritis may be infectious (in which case it is usually monoarticular, and the organism may be recovered from the joint) or reactive (in which case involvement is often polyarticular or pauciarticular, and the organism will not be recovered from the joint) (Bravo et al. 2003). Sacroiliitis is the second-most frequent articular lesion (Alarcon et al. 1981; Ariza et al. 1993; Khateeb et al. 1990); it is usually unilateral. Spondylitis may affect 5-10% of patients with *Brucella* arthritis (Ariza et al. 1985; Gotuzzo et al. 1982; Namiduru et al. 2004; Solera et al. 1999). Radiographic features may include the presence of lytic and blastic lesions, erosion of the anterior superior part of the vertebral body (a "parrot peak" sign) (Ibero et al. 1997), and spondylodiscitis. Postinfection spondyloarthritis, bursitis, tenosynovitis, and infection of joint prostheses have also been reported (Weil et al. 2003). Although any joint might be involved during brucellosis, arthritis of the hips and knees is most common during acute disease and is usually manifested within 12 months of infection; involvement of the axial skeletal system and spondylitis are most common during chronic disease; and sacroiliitis might occur during either acute disease or chronic disease (Akritidis and Pappas 2001; Ariza et al. 1985; Colmenero et al. 1996; Doganay et al. 1993; Gotuzzo et al. 1987; Mousa et al. 1987; Namiduru et al. 2004; Norton 1984).

The committee concludes that there is sufficient evidence of an association between brucellosis and arthritis and spondylitis. Arthritis is usually manifested within 12 months of the acute illness; spondylitis might be manifested later.

Hepatic Involvement

Human brucellosis is often associated with changes in liver function and has been associated with granulomatous hepatitis (Harrington et al. 1982; Lulu et al. 1988; Williams and Crossley 1982). Hepatomegaly may be present (Lulu et al. 1988), but cirrhosis has not been reported. Chronic abscesses of the liver and spleen may occur (Ariza et al. 2001; Colmenero et al. 2002; Vallejo et al. 1996).

The committee concludes that there is sufficient evidence of an association between brucellosis and hepatic abnormalities, including granulomatous hepatitis.

Neurologic Involvement

Neurobrucellosis has been reported in 1-5% of adults who have *Brucella* infections (al Deeb et al. 1989; Bashir et al. 1985; Bouza et al. 1987; Young 1983). It usually involves meningitis or meningoencephalitis that is often chronic (al Deeb et al. 1989; Bashir et al. 1985; Bodur et al. 2003; Bouza et al. 1987; McLean et al. 1992; Mousa et al. 1986; Pascual et al. 1988). Fever, headache, nuchal rigidity, and altered consciousness may occur (Bodur et al. 2003; Gokul et al. 2000). Evaluation of cerebrospinal fluid usually reveals lymphocytic pleocytosis, increased protein concentration, and normal or moderately decreased glucose (Pascual et al. 1988). Microbiologic cultures of cerebrospinal fluid are positive for brucellae in 10-20% of cases. Rare brain or epidural abscesses, myelitis-radiculoneuritis, demyelinating meningovascular syndromes, deafness, sensorineural hearing loss, and GBS have been reported (Dalrymple-Champneys 1950; Kochar et al. 2000a; Lubani et al. 1989a; McLean et al. 1992;

Mousa et al. 1986; Oliveri et al. 1996; Riestra-Castaneda et al. 1996; Thomas et al. 1993). The diagnosis of neurobrucellosis may be made even in the setting of negative microbiologic cultures of cerebrospinal fluid and negative serologic assays if specific antibodies are found in the cerebrospinal fluid (Kochar et al. 2000a; Sanchez-Sousa et al. 1990).

The committee concludes that there is sufficient evidence of an association between brucellosis and chronic meningitis and meningoencephalitis and between brucellosis and infection of the nervous system.

The committee concludes that there is limited or suggestive evidence of an association between brucellosis and myelitis-radiculoneuritis, demyelinating meningovascular syndromes, deafness, sensorineural hearing loss, and Guillain-Barré syndrome

Ophthalmologic Involvement

Anterior-posterior uveitis is the most common ocular manifestation of brucellosis (al-Kaff 1995; Gungor et al. 2002; Rolando et al. 1985a; Rolando et al. 1985b; Rolando et al. 1987; Tabbara 1990). Papilledema, optic neuritis, episcleritis, nummular keratitis, and multifocal choroiditis have also been reported (Gungor et al. 2002; Lyall 1973; McLean et al. 1992; Rabinowitz et al. 2005; Rolando et al. 1985b; Rolando et al. 1987; Walker et al. 1992). Without proper treatment, secondary glaucoma, cataracts, and retinal detachment may occur (Rabinowitz et al. 2005; Rolando et al. 1985a).

The committee concludes that there is sufficient evidence of an association between brucellosis and uveitis.

The committee concludes that there is limited or suggestive evidence of an association between brucellosis and papilledema, optic neuritis, episcleritis, nummular keratitis, and multifocal choroiditis.

Genitourinary Tract Manifestations

Orchioepididymitis may occur in up to 20% of men with brucellosis (Ibrahim et al. 1988; Memish and Venkatesh 2001; Navarro-Martinez et al. 2001; Papatsoris et al. 2002). It is most often unilateral and accompanied by normal urine sediment (Navarro-Martinez et al. 2001). Pyelonephritis and chronic renal abscesses have been reported in association with brucellosis (Zinneman et al. 1961).

The committee concludes that there is sufficient evidence of an association between brucellosis and orchioepididymitis and between brucellosis and local infections of the genitourinary system (for example, pyelonephritis or renal abscesses).

Cardiovascular System Infections

Endocarditis causes the majority of *Brucella*-related deaths even though it occurs in less than 2% of chronic cases (al-Harthi 1989). Involvement of the aortic valve is most common, and pericarditis and mycotic aneurysms of blood vessels may occur (McLean et al. 1992).

The committee concludes that there is sufficient evidence of an association between brucellosis and cardiovascular system infections.

Respiratory System Infections

Respiratory tract involvement with brucellosis may include pneumonia, pleural effusion, lung nodules or abscesses, miliary lesions, and thoracic lymphadenopathy (Pappas et al. 2003; Wortmann 2004).

The committee concludes that there is sufficient evidence of an association between brucellosis and respiratory system infections.

Other Symptoms

People who have chronic brucellosis often report fatigue, inattention, amnesia, and depression (Gokul et al. 2000; Imboden et al. 1959; Khateeb et al. 1990; Martin et al. 1961; Sacks and Van Rensburg 1976; Spink 1951).

The committee concludes that there is limited or suggestive evidence of an association between brucellosis and fatigue, inattention, amnesia, and depression.

LEISHMANIASIS

Leishmaniasis is an intracellular infection caused by a diverse group of protozoa in the genus *Leishmania*. It affects an estimated 12 million people worldwide; there are 1-1.5 million new infections each year.

Leishmaniasis presents as one of three major clinical syndromes: visceral leishmaniasis (VL, also known as kala-azar), cutaneous leishmaniasis (CL) and (infrequently) mucocutaneous leishmaniasis (MCL). About 90% of VL cases occur in India, Bangladesh, Sudan, and Brazil; 90% of CL cases in Afghanistan, Brazil, Iran, Peru, Saudi Arabia, and Syria; and 90% of MCL cases, in Bolivia, Brazil, and Peru (Desjeux 2004; Murray et al. 2005). The three syndromes have been divided into a complex taxonomic and etiologic scheme that is explained briefly here (Table 5.3).

CL is divided into Old World CL (referring to occurrences in southern Europe, the Middle East, and parts of southwest Asia and Africa) and New World CL (southern United States and Latin America). *L. tropica, L. major* and *L. aethiopica* occasionally disseminate to cause diffuse cutaneous leishmaniasis (DCL). *L. braziliensis* can cause mucosal leishmaniasis.

TABLE 5.3 Clinical Syndromes Caused by *Leishmania* Species and Their Geographic Distribution

Clinical Syndromes	*Leishmania* species	Location
Visceral leishmaniasis:		
Kala-azar; generalized involvement of reticuloendothelial system (spleen, bone marrow, liver)	*L. donovani*	Indian subcontinent, northern and eastern China, Pakistan, Nepal
	L. infantum	Middle East, Mediterranean littoral, Balkans, central and southwestern Asia, northern and northwestern China, northern and sub-Saharan Africa
	L. donovani (archiba)	Sudan, Kenya, Ethiopia
	L. chagasi	Latin America
	L. amazonensis	Brazil (Bahia state)
	L. tropica	Israel, India; viscerotropic form of disease in Saudi Arabia (US troops)

	L. spp.	Kenya, Ethiopia, Somalia
Post-kala-azar dermal leishmaniasis	*L. donovani*	Indian subcontinent, East Africa
	L. spp.	Kenya, Ethiopia, Somalia
Old World cutaneous leishmaniasis:		
Single or few skin lesions	*L. major*	Middle East, northwestern China, northwestern India, Pakistan, Africa
	L. tropica	Mediterranean littoral, Middle East, western Asia, Indian subcontinent
	L. aethiopica	Ethiopian highlands, Kenya, Yemen
	L. infantum	Mediterranean basin
	L. donovani (archibaldi)	Sudan, east Africa
	L. spp.	Kenya, Ethiopia, Somalia
Diffuse cutaneous leishmaniasis	*L. aethiopica*	Ethiopian highlands, Kenya, Yemen
New World cutaneous leishmaniasis:		
Single or few skin lesions	*L. mexicana* (chiclero ulcer)	Central America, Mexico, Texas
	L. amazonensis	Amazon basin and neighboring areas, Bahia, other states in Brazil
	L. (V.) braziliensis	Multiple areas of Central America and South America
	L. (V.) guyanensis (forest yaws)	Guyana, Suriname, northern Amazon basin
	L. (V.) peruviana (uta)	Peru (western Andes), Argentine highlands
	L. (V.) panamensis	Panama, Costa Rica, Colombia
	L. (V.) pifanoi	Venezuela
	L. (V.) garnhami	Venezuela
	L. (V.) venexuelensis	Venezuela
	L. (V.) colombiensis	Colombia, Panama
	L. chagasi	Central America, South America
Diffuse cutaneous leishmaniasis	*L. amazonensis*	Amazon basin and neighboring areas, Bahia and other states in Brazil
	L. (V.) pifanoi	Venezuela
	L. mexicana	Mexico, Central America
	L. spp.	Dominican Republic
Mucosal leishmaniasis	*L .(V.) braziliensis* (espundia)	Multiple areas in Latin America

NOTE: *V.* denotes subgenus *Vianna*. All others subgenus *Leishmania*.
SOURCE: Adapted with permission from Guerrant et al. 1999.

Parasites in the *L. donovani* complex cause VL cases globally. Historically, *L. tropica* was rarely reported to cause VL; a few cases were reported in east Africa (Kenya) and southwest Asia. However, a handful of US soldiers deployed to the Gulf War developed a mild visceral form of leishmaniasis caused by *L. tropica* (termed viscerotropic disease). Those cases are described in Chapter 4.

Transmission of Leishmaniasis

The *Leishmania* organisms have two forms: the promastigote (which is flagellated) and the amastigote. The sand fly is the vector and carries the promastigote form. Sand flies inject the promastigote form of the parasite into humans. Infection is then established with the amastigote form, which is harbored in human macrophages.

Two transmission cycles have been described. In the zoonotic cycle, dogs are the primary animal reservoir, and humans are an occasional host when they are infected by the bite of the sand fly. In south-central Asia (Afghanistan), great gerbils *(Rhombomys opimus)* are the vertebrate hosts of *L. major* and thus determine the clinical distribution of associated CL. In the anthroponotic cycle, humans are the sole reservoir, and sand flies remain the critical vector. *Phlebotomus papatasi* is the sand fly species that transmits *L. major* throughout most of the Middle East and is present in south-central Asia. *Phlebotomus sergenti* was recently identified as the species responsible for transmission of *L. tropica* in Afghanistan (Wallace et al. 2002).

Sand fly bites are exceedingly common in the Middle East. In August 1943, sand fly fever (caused by a phlebovirus) occurred at a peak rate of 235 per 1,000 military personnel deployed to the Persian Gulf (Hertig and Sabin 1964). Because sand flies are most active during warm months, however, there is seasonal variation in the risk of infection. Only 31 cases of leishmaniasis were diagnosed among 697,000 troops deployed during the Gulf War, and deployment to the open desert during cooler weather was thought to be a partial reason for the low incidence of the disease (Cope et al. 1996). Even in areas that are important foci of *Leishmania* infection, the prevalence of sand fly-caused infection with *Leishmania* spp. is unpredictable (Fryauff et al. 1993).

Finally, humans have acquired leishmaniasis through parenteral exposure (because of contaminated injection equipment and blood products) and through sexual contact, but those cases are rare.

Endemicity in Southwest and South-Central Asia

Southwest Asia and south-central Asia are home to Old World CL and VL (Oldfield et al. 1991). The potential for anthroponotic acquisition of CL is especially high in Kabul, Afghanistan, where 270,000 persons (in a population of 2 million) were estimated to be infected in 1996 (World Health Organization as cited in Hewitt et al. 1998). Some 4,700 cases of CL were reported in northern Syria in 1999, an increase from the 3,900 cases reported in 1998 (WHO 2002); most CL in the Middle East is caused by *L. major*.

Acute Leishmaniasis

Old World CL has an incubation period of 2 weeks to 2 months. The most common etiologic agent is *L. major,* which causes papular lesions that can ulcerate (Wallace et al. 2002). Most (90-95%) CL lesions heal spontaneously, and they rarely cause persistent disfiguration. *L. recidivans* can cause a chronic cutaneous ("ring") lesion.

VL has an incubation period of 2-4 months, although it has been reported to be as long as 2 years. Most infected persons remain asymptomatic during the acute phase. When VL evolves to the clinically evident form, classic symptoms include fever, weight loss, weakness, diarrhea, dysentery, and abdominal swelling. The typical triad of diagnostic findings consists of anemia, fever, and hepatosplenomegaly. Complications of the acute infection arise typically from superimposed bacterial infection, sometimes exacerbated by the neutropenia that can result from bone marrow infiltration. Cytokine disruption is probably critical in determining the clinical presentation and in mediating the outcome of infection, even with treatment (Murray et al. 2005). The predominant cell-mediated immune response is characterized by activity of Th1-type CD4+

cells and associated interferon-γ-induced macrophage activation. That response sets the stage for control, but probably not uniform eradication, of the parasite. Macrophage defenses required to kill *Leishmania* have been extensively studied, as have the pathogen's antiphagocytic defenses (Cunningham 2002; Teixeira et al. 2006).

Of the twelve people who had viscerotropic leishmaniasis caused by *L. tropica* in the Gulf War, one was asymptomatic, and the remainder had a mixed picture involving many of the classic features of VL (Hyams et al. 1995; Magill et al. 1994). Those presentations were distinguished from typical VL in that anemia was typically the sole hematologic sign, and most patients had modest increases in liver enzymes. Three of the patients had an underlying disease of relevance: HIV, acute infection with Epstein-Barr virus, and renal-cell cancer (Hyams et al. 1995).

Diagnosis of Leishmaniasis

Several methods have been used to diagnose the various forms of leishmaniasis. Most CL is diagnosed on the basis of its classic clinical appearance, although if the lesion is atypical, prolonged, or not responsive to therapy, biopsy may be performed at the margin of the lesion. PCR is increasingly used in this setting, especially because misdiagnosis may occur (many lesions clinically diagnosed as CL are bacterial in origin). PCR was the mainstay of diagnosis in a recent description of 237 cases of CL acquired in OIF (Willard et al. 2005). Skin testing based on antigens of *L. major* demonstrates prior infection with *Leishmania* spp. and is usually positive in active CL caused by *L. major.*

VL is often diagnosed on the basis of histopathologic detection of amastigotes in biopsy or aspirate of bone marrow, spleen, or lymph nodes. Indirect immunofluorescent monoclonal antibody can also be applied to those tissues. Biopsy samples can be directly cultured, and isoenzyme analysis used for further speciation. Serum antibody testing, often used in assessment of persons with suspected VL, is most commonly performed with the direct agglutination test. However, the performance of this test is highly variable; in fact, serology was negative in a number of the viscerotropic cases identified in Gulf War soldiers. Available serologic tests are based on *L. major* antigens, so the relevance to viscerotropic leishmaniasis (caused by *L. tropica*) is unclear. Finally, some investigators have reported that urine-based assays that detect either *Leishmania* antigen (Sundar et al. 2005) or *Leishmania*-specific IgG (Islam et al. 2002) were valuable in diagnosing VL.

Treatments for Leishmaniasis and Related Long-Term Toxicity

Most cases of CL will resolve without specific medical therapy. Oral azoles (fluconazole and ketoconazole), cryotherapy, or paromomycin ointment may hasten resolution. Under study is a device called ThermoMed that delivers radiofrequency-generated heat directly to a lesion through a set of prongs placed on the lesion; the device has Food and Drug Administration 510K clearance as of this writing.

Systemic treatment is always indicated for VL. The mainstay of therapy has been pentavalent antimonials, including sodium stibogluconate and meglumine antimonite (Aronson et al. 1998; Murray 2000; Murray 2004). Liposomal amphotericin B was traditionally reserved for antimony-treatment failures, but it is increasingly used as first-line therapy and has been the regimen of choice for soldiers who acquired VL in OEF. Antimonials are not well tolerated in the acute treatment period. Gastrointestinal intolerance, bone marrow suppression, and hepatotoxicity occur in up to 50% of patients (and are usually reversible). Pancreatitis and abnormalities of cardiac repolarization also occur; the latter is generally unassociated with arrhythmia and resolves within two months after completion of treatment. At least one case of laryngeal edema has been reported to be associated with antimony therapy. Oral miltefosine has also been used for treatment for VL and CL. None of these drugs appears to be associated with long-term toxicity.

Coinfection by Leishmania Parasite and Human Immunodeficiency Virus

VL is estimated to be the third-most common opportunistic infection in HIV-infected persons in southern Europe (Choi and Lerner 2002). The association emphasizes immune control of the organism and reactivation of quiescent infection in the setting of reduced cell-mediated immune response. Indeed, *Leishmania* infection might reactivate in patients with CD4 counts below 200/μL (Choi and Lerner 2002). The World Health Organization (WHO) estimates that 25-70% of adult VL cases in southern Europe now occur in HIV-infected patients and that AIDS increases the risk of VL by a factor of 100-1,000 (Choi and Lerner 2002). Clinically, leishmaniasis in HIV-infected persons is characterized by atypical presentations (including pulmonary disease, lingual and esophageal ulcerations, and fever of unknown origin), reduced rates of treatment response, progression from cutaneous to visceral disease, higher rates of death, and reduced sensitivity of serologic tests.

Long-Term Adverse Health Outcomes of Leishmaniasis

Cutaneous Leishmaniasis

Infections with *L. major* have not led to viscerotropic infection, parenteral or vertical transmission, or presentation as an opportunistic infection associated with HIV. Old World CL as a rule resolves spontaneously and rarely causes chronic scarring. All of the numerous cases of CL that have occurred in soldiers involved in OIF (CDC 2003b; CDC 2004b) have reportedly responded to relatively short courses of sodium stibogluconate (Weina et al. 2004; Willard et al. 2005). However, some cases have been associated with large lesions and long duration. Given the difficulty in diagnosis, unrecognized CL has the potential to cause substantial cosmetic problems.

DCL is not as responsive to therapy as CL and can cause progressive disfiguration and destruction of skin and soft tissue.

Visceral Leishmaniasis

The organisms responsible for VL also infect monocytes and macrophages; however, in contrast with *L. major*, they may establish latency in these cells. This phenomenon results in a demonstrable risk of recurrence in the setting of immunosuppression induced by chemotherapy, transplantation-related processes, or HIV infection (Basset et al. 2005). As discussed above, immune control of VL involves primarily CD4+ T-cell activity (Th1-type response). Conversely, VL promotes formation of Th2-type cytokines, which can inhibit control of the disease. VL is itself an immunosuppressive disease, partly because of infiltration of reticuloendothelium of liver, spleen, and bone marrow and because it has been associated with polyclonal B-cell activation and increased production of numerous autoantibodies. One case report of GBS that predated the clinical appearance of VL by about a month has been reported;

the authors postulated that the parasite could mediate autoimmune damage to peripheral nerve myelin (Fasanaro et al. 1991).

Because *L. infantum* has been responsible for most cases of HIV-related VL (Russo et al. 2003), it might be particularly likely to persist in macrophages and monocytes. This organism was identified in one of the two cases of VL acquired in Afghanistan (CDC 2004a) but has not been identified in veterans of other conflicts. Of those two cases, one was diagnosed 14 months after deployment ended in Afghanistan, and the patient had symptoms of clinical recurrence. In addition, VL is estimated to be the third-most common opportunistic infection in HIV-infected persons in southern Europe, as detailed above (Russo et al. 2003).

Because the period of latent infection with VL organisms can be long (10 years is commonly cited), immune suppression can allow reactivation of a latent infection. In the description of the viscerotropic cases that occurred in the Gulf War, the authors stated that "if *L. tropica* is also capable of surviving in a latent state, visceral leishmaniasis will need to be included in the differential diagnoses of illness in veterans of Operation Desert Storm for years to come" (Magill et al. 1993). Although chronic infection is clearly plausible, no systematic studies have investigated the possibility prospectively, in part because there is no accurate and noninvasive screening test for the infection (Ohl et al. 1993). However, intensive evaluation among 150 Gulf War veterans with complaints was unable to identify prior or current infection with *Leishmania* spp. (Hyams et al. 1995).

Post-kala-azar dermal leishmaniasis (PKDL) is a well-documented long-term adverse health outcome of VL that occurs on the Indian subcontinent and in east Africa (Zijlstra et al. 2003). On the basis of the Indian experience, this health outcome may develop in 5-10% of patients several years after apparently successful treatment for VL (Zijlstra et al. 2003). PKDL has been mistaken for leprosy, and patients with this presentation remain infectious (Zijlstra et al. 2003). Nerve involvement (as is seen in leprosy) has been reported rarely with PKDL (El Hassan et al. 1992; Khandpur et al. 2004).

The committee concludes that

- **There is sufficient evidence of an association between infection with an etiologic agent of visceral leishmaniasis (VL) and delayed presentation of the acute clinical syndrome.**
- **There is sufficient evidence of an association between infection with an etiologic agent of VL and the reactivation of VL in the context of future immunosuppression.**
- **There is sufficient evidence of an association between VL and development of post-kala-azar dermal leishmaniasis (PKDL) if PKDL occurs generally within 2 years of the initial infection.**

MALARIA

Human malaria is caused by infection with one or more of four species in the genus *Plasmodium*: *P. falciparum, P. vivax, P. ovale,* and *P. malariae*. Although estimates vary, there are probably 350-500 million clinical episodes of malaria each year and 0.7-2.7 million deaths (Breman 2001; WHO 2003). Malaria occurs worldwide in tropical and subtropical regions, typically affecting poor and developing areas most severely. *P. falciparum* predominates in tropical areas; *P. vivax*, in temperate regions. The two other species are less frequently encountered: *P. malariae* is found worldwide, and the geographic range of *P. ovale* is limited mostly to tropical Africa, the Middle East, southeast Asia, and the western Pacific.

Transmission of Malaria

Malaria infection occurs when a *Plasmodium*-infected *Anopheles* mosquito feeds on a susceptible human host, delivering sporozoites that initially invade hepatocytes and mature into merozoites that then invade erythrocytes. The cycle is completed when a competent female *Anopheles* mosquito feeds on a parasitemic human, obtaining gametocytes that then initiate infection in the mosquito. Many *Anopheles* species are potential vectors of malaria in different parts of the world, so mosquito species-specific behaviors, including host feeding preference and daily activity patterns, tend to result in varied regional transmission patterns. Often, several mosquito species will combine to constitute an overall vector profile for a region. In tropical areas, transmission intensity is often linked to rainy seasons—typically one major and another less severe. In temperate or seasonally arid regions, a single transmission period is evident (Guerrant et al. 1999).

Endemicity in Southwest and South-Central Asia

The best recent estimates of overall malaria morbidity and mortality in southwest and south-central Asia are about 6 million cases and 59,000 deaths per year (RBM 2005a). Afghanistan and Yemen alone account for an estimated 5.5 million of all cases, on the basis of 2004 data (RBM 2005b). In the malaria-endemic countries of Tajikistan, Azerbaijan, Armenia, Georgia, Kyrgyzstan, and Uzbekistan, malaria occurred at a rate of 0.11 case per 1,000 population in 1990-2003 (RBM 2005h). In contrast, the case rate was about three per 1,000 during the same period in southwest Asia, Afghanistan, and Pakistan combined (RBM 2005h).

About 70% of all infections are caused by *P. vivax*, but this varies regionally. *P. malariae* is *not* reported to be endemic in most parts of southwest or south-central Asia and is rare in areas where it has been reported. Diagnosis and reporting in some areas, such as Iraq and Afghanistan, have been hindered in recent years because of war-related interruptions to the public-health infrastructure. Transmission is highly seasonal and peaks in late July to September.

In Iraq, malaria is endemic in Duhok, Erbil, Ninawa, Sulaimaniya, Tamim, and Basrah provinces. Some 362 cases were recorded in Iraq in 2003. The disease is due exclusively to *P. vivax*; peak transmission takes place in May-November. The main vectors are *A. sacharovi*, *A. superpictus*, *A. maculipennis*, *A. stephensi*, and *A. pulcherrimus*. Most of the cases occur in the northern governorates, mainly in the Zakho district in Dohuk, where four of the five vector species reside (RBM 2005e).

Malaria is endemic in Afghanistan in all areas below 2,000 m in altitude. Afghanistan reported about 600,000 cases in 2003, 93% of which were caused by *P. vivax* and 7% by *P. falciparum* (Kolaczinski et al. 2005). Estimates of the rates of feeding of infective vectors on humans in eastern Afghanistan indicated that *A. stephensi* would contribute 76% of infective bites and *A. fluviatilis* and *A. culicifacies* 7% and 3%, respectively. Because of chloroquine resistance, numbers of *P. falciparum* infections in eastern Afghanistan have increased from 1% of all infections in 1970 to 20% in 2002 (Kolaczinski et al. 2005; RBM 2005c).

Saudi Arabia tends to have equal percentages of infection with *P. vivax* and *P. falciparum* but low case totals (1,700 cases in 2003). The primary vector in Saudi Arabia is *A. arabiensis* (RBM 2005g).

Pakistan reported more than 125,000 laboratory-confirmed cases in 2003, 4 million probable cases, and 14 deaths. Of the laboratory-confirmed cases, almost 70% were caused by *P. vivax*. The primary mosquito vectors of malaria in Pakistan are *A. culicifacies* and *A. stephensi* (RBM 2005f).

In Iran, three provinces in the southeastern corner account for most of the 23,000 cases reported in 2003, 21% of which were caused by *P. falciparum*. Primary mosquito vectors include *A. fluviatilis*, *A. stephensi*, and *A. culicifacies* (RBM 2005d).

Acute Malaria

All four *Plasmodium* species can cause cyclic fevers, particularly in naïve populations. Known as malarial paroxysms, the cycles are characterized by rapid onset of high fever with chills followed by rapid resolution, often with intense diaphoresis. The cycles are associated with erythrocyte lysis that occurs at the end of the erythrocytic cycle of infection. The classical (but infrequently observed) periodic attacks occur every second day with the "tertian" parasites (*P. falciparum*, *P. vivax*, and *P. ovale*) and every third day with the "quartan" parasite (*P. malariae*).

Among populations in endemic areas, the development of partial immunity leads to milder illness and even asymptomatic infections. However, the immune response does not block repeated infections or infections with multiple strains or species. In temperate climates, the long latent phase with *P. vivax* and *P. ovale* appears to provide the opportunity for the resumption of transmission when the mosquito season returns in the next year (Guerrant et al. 1999).

Malaria is diagnosed with microscopic examination of blood smears stained with Giemsa or Wright's stain. An experienced technician can diagnose most cases with examination of routine blood smears (thin smears), but examination of thick smears is more sensitive in detecting those with less severe parasitemia. The key to diagnosis is recognizing the potential for malaria in a potentially exposed person who has fever, anemia, and thrombocytopenia. Deaths from malaria in travelers returning to the United States, most notably with *P. falciparum*, continue to occur, often in association with delays in diagnosis and in effective therapy (Newman et al. 2004). Other diagnostic techniques have been developed, including fluorescence microscopy, immunologic diagnosis of falciparum malaria with antibodies to the protein HRP2, DNA probes specifically for *P. falciparum*, and PCR methods (Amino et al. 2005; Berry et al. 2005; Wilson et al. 2005).

Treatments for Malaria and Related Long-Term Toxicity

Resistance to chloroquine and multiple-drug resistance are major problems with *P. falciparum* in most of Africa, Asia, and South America. Drug-resistant *P. falciparum* has also been found in the Middle East and southwest Asia, including Iraq (Guerrant et al. 1999). Resistance to chloroquine is an emergent problem with *P. vivax* in some parts of Asia, Oceania, and South America (Kurcer et al. 2006).

Antimalarial drugs have well-documented acute adverse effects on the skin, gastrointestinal tract, central nervous system, and other organ systems, but evidence of long-term adverse health outcomes is sparse (Taylor and White 2004). Moderate to severe neuropsychiatric complications have been reported in association with mefloquine, doxycycline, combined chloroquine and proguanil, and combined atovaquone and proguanil (Schlagenhauf et al. 2003; Taylor and White 2004). Although retinopathy associated with high-dose long-term chloroquine use has been described, it has rarely been associated with modern prophylaxis. Additional discussion on the health effects of antimalarial drugs can be found in the section on ophthalmologic complications below.

Coinfection with *Plasmodium* Spp. and Human Immunodeficiency Virus

There is clear evidence that HIV infection, particularly with lower CD4+ cell counts, is associated with an increased risk of malaria, higher levels of parasitemia, and higher mortality (Butcher 2005). Nevertheless, malaria and HIV coinfection in a soldier deployed to southwest or south-central Asia would be highly improbable, given the low rates of HIV in southwest and south-central Asia, segregation of US military troops from civilian populations, periodic HIV screening of troops and removal of soldiers testing HIV-positive from overseas service, and low malaria transmission rates.

Long-Term Adverse Health Outcomes of Infection with *Plasmodium* Spp.

Infection by *Plasmodium* potentially has long-term repercussions for human health. Long-term adverse health outcomes of infection can be manifested in neurologic, neuropsychiatric, ophthalmologic, hematologic, or renal disease. In addition, malaria itself can present after a latency of months to years or may break out anew because of undertreatment.

The epidemiology of malaria in Afghanistan and Iraq suggests that *P. vivax* is the principal threat to US troops deployed to OEF and OIF. *P. falciparum* was not known to circulate in Iraq in 1991-2005, and, although reported in Afghanistan, it is far less prevalent than *P. vivax*. Although *P. falciparum* predominates in Saudi Arabia, only seven cases of malaria were reported in US troops during the Persian Gulf War, as described in Chapter 4. *P. ovale* and *P. malariae* are rare in southwest and south-central Asia.

Hematologic Complications

Splenic rupture is a well-described complication of malaria, particularly that caused by *P. vivax*. It can occur weeks to months after the acute infection. Hyperreactive malaria syndrome or tropical splenomegaly can be noted months or years after malarial infection (Metha et al. 1996).

Anemia is a principal complication of malaria. It is expected as an acute event, but it may be detected months or even years after the infection. Only in cases of fulminant falciparum malaria is anemia so severe as to be debilitating or life-threatening. Repeated hemolysis, presumably due to subcurative treatments, is reported as a chronic complication (Metha et al. 1996).

> **The committee concludes that there is sufficient evidence of a causal relationship between malaria infection and hematologic manifestations weeks or months later, particularly splenic rupture after vivax malaria and anemia after falciparum malaria.**

Ophthalmologic Complications

A number of case reports describe the complication of retinal hemorrhage associated with severe cerebral malaria and following vivax malaria. Permanent visual loss may result from this complication (Choi et al. 2004). The capillary permeability associated most notably with falciparum malaria has been associated with retinal hemorrhage and edema, with occasional serious visual impairment, in adults and children (Beare et al. 2003; Hidayat et al. 1993; Kochar et al. 2000b; Lewallen 1998; Tripathi et al. 1995). Retinal manifestations may be noted months or years after the acute malaria infection (Biswas et al. 1996).

Malaria-associated chronic ophthalmologic disorders include side effects of the chronic prophylactic use of antimalarial drugs, such as hydroxychloroquine and chloroquine (Balo et al. 1996; Easterbrook 1999; Lozier and Friedlaender 1989; Niemeyer and Fruh 1989; Portnoy and Callen 1983; Ruiz and Saatci 1991; Tzekov 2005; Wei et al. 2001). The associations have been recognized for decades (Begue 1964; Bernstein 1967; Giles and Henderson 1965; Rubin 1968; Sugiyama et al. 1967). Chloroquine-based prophylaxis is not being used for US troops deployed to OEF and OIF. Oxidative stress has been cited as a possible contributing etiology (Toler 2004). Rynes and Bernstein (1993) highlight the relative rarity of the retinal complications and the need for long-term administration of the drugs.

> **The committee concludes that there is sufficient evidence of a causal relationship between malaria infection and ophthalmologic manifestations, particularly retinal hemorrhage and scarring, recognized for the first time months or years after the infection.**

Neurologic and Neuropsychiatric Complications

Neurologic complications, particularly cerebral malaria due to *P. falciparum*, are characterized by confusion, clouding of consciousness progressing to coma, and seizures. Cerebral malaria is due largely to sequestration of infected red blood cells in the cerebral circulation (Renia et al. 2006), but coma can also be caused by such other malaria complications as hypoglycemia, uremia, or hypoxia due to pulmonary edema (Idro et al. 2005). Cerebral malaria is fatal in 15-20% of cases, and residual neurologic deficits have been reported in 1-3% of adults and 10% of children (Bajiya and Kochar 1996). It is notable that over 97% of afflicted adults who survive the cerebral episode of falciparum malaria are left without detectable chronic sequelae.

A postmalaria neurologic syndrome has been described in people who were treated for malaria due to *P. falciparum* (Falchook et al. 2003). The manifestations include confusion, psychosis, seizures, and a fine tremor (Malviya et al. 2005; Meier et al. 2004). There may be an associated magnetic resonance imaging finding of enhancement of nonspecific white-matter lesions (Dey et al. 2001).

Two other postmalaria neurologic complications have been described in case reports and case series. Acute inflammatory demyelinating polyneuropathy and Guillain-Barré syndrome have been reported after falciparum malaria and less frequently after vivax malaria (Chakravarty et al. 2004; Shubhakaran and Sharma 2003). Onset of neurologic symptoms can occur during the acute stage of the illness or days to weeks after the end of the acute illness (Shubhakaran and Sharma 2003; Kanjalkar et al. 1999). Cerebellar ataxia, often with tremors, has also been described after falciparum malaria, possibly resulting from demyelinating lesions in the cerebellum (Metha et al. 1996; Senanayake and de Silva 1994). All reports of patients who experienced acute inflammatory demyelinating polyneuropathy and cerebellar ataxia described complete recovery within months of onset (Chakravarty et al. 2004; Kanjalkar et al. 1999), although the natural history of these disorders after other conditions has been associated with slow recovery and persistent neurologic deficits in some of those affected (Kanjalkar et al. 1999).

One report dealt with neurologic deficits among veterans who had experienced cerebral malaria from *P. falciparum* during the Vietnam War (Varney et al. 1997). Veterans with a self-reported history of cerebral malaria were found to have a greater frequency of neuropsychiatric symptoms than veterans who suffered combat wounds. The report raises questions about the potential for cerebral malaria to produce subtle, persistent neurologic deficits that may not have been apparent in examinations conducted during routine medical treatment and followup (Shamo 2001).

The committee concludes that there is limited or suggestive evidence of an association between *Plasmodium vivax* and *Plasmodium falciparum* infections and demyelinating polyneuropathy and Guillain-Barré syndrome.

The committee concludes that there is limited or suggestive evidence of an association between *Plasmodium falciparum* infection and neurologic disease, neuropsychiatric disease, or both, months to years after the acute infection.

Renal Complications

Chronic untreated *P. malariae* infection can be manifested with chronic glomerulonephritis even years after the onset of infection (Eiam-Ong 2003; Kibukamusoke 1986). In contrast, the nephrotic syndrome and acute glomerulonephritis are far more common near the onset of infection (days to weeks later), may be associated with any malaria infection, and would be manifested after months or years only very rarely.

The committee concludes that there is sufficient evidence of an association between *Plasmodium malariae* infection and the manifestation of immune-complex glomerulonephritis years to decades later.

The committee concludes that there is sufficient evidence of a causal relationship between malaria infection and renal disease, especially the nephrotic syndrome that may occur weeks to months after acute infection.

Relapse and Recrudescence of Malaria

Some *P. vivax* and *P. ovale* parasites remain dormant as hypnozoites in the liver for months after primary infection. The latent period is generally 6-11 months (Mandell et al. 2005), although one report found the latent period to be less than 4 months (Oh et al. 2001).

At the end of their dormancy, *P. vivax* or *P. ovale* hypnozoites initiate the same process that occurs during acute malaria, generating tissue schizonts that rupture and release merozoites into the bloodstream. When the merozoites invade and lyse red blood cells, the patient experiences a relapse with acute symptoms resembling de novo infection (Mandell et al. 2005). Such relapses have been described as occurring periodically but irregularly almost always within 2 years after primary infection (Eliades et al. 2005; Shute et al. 1977).

Thus, relapse of malaria may occur after either symptomatic or asymptomatic infection by *P. vivax* and *P. ovale*, particularly in people who are taking such prophylactic antimalarials as chloroquine that neither prevent *Plasmodium* spp. from infecting hepatocytes nor eliminate *Plasmodium* hypnozoites (Guerrant et al. 1999). In contrast, treatment with primaquine mitigates hepatic infection, reducing the risk of relapse after primary infection by *P. vivax* or *P. ovale* (Baird 2005; Shanks and Edstein 2005; Taylor and White 2004). The diagnosis of persistent hepatic infection by *P. vivax* or *P. ovale* can be made only if relapse occurs and blood smears or other suitable diagnostics are confirmatory.

The phenomenon of persistent latent hepatic infection does not occur with *P. falciparum* or *P. malariae*. However, there are other mechanisms whereby both these species can lead to hepatic disease months or years after the acute infection. Delayed recurrence or delay in onset several months after exposure may occur with *P. falciparum* if drug-resistant parasites are inadequately treated (Guerrant et al. 1999). That would be expected to occur weeks to months later, rather than years later. *P. malariae* may lead to chronic, low-level parasitemia that may be difficult to detect and may persist for many decades. The unusual cases of truly chronic malaria due to *P. malariae* may require immunodiagnostic techniques or repeated smears to detect the parasite because of low levels of parasitemia.

The committee concludes that there is sufficient evidence of a causal relationship between malaria infection and relapse of disease (*Plasmodium vivax* or *Plasmodium ovale*) or late presentation of disease (*Plasmodium malariae*) months to years after acute infection.

The committee concludes that there is sufficient evidence of an association between infection by *Plasmodium falciparum* and recrudescence weeks to months after the primary infection, but only in the case of inadequate therapy.

Q FEVER (INFECTION BY *COXIELLA BURNETII*)

Coxiella burnetii is the etiologic agent of the zoonosis Q fever, which was first described in abattoir workers in Australia in 1935 (Derrick 1937). The organism has since been demonstrated to have a worldwide distribution and has been isolated in a wide variety of animal and arthropod species. Remarkable for its heterogeneity, it is a highly pleomorphic gram-negative coccobacillus that uses multiple routes of transmission.

In vertebrate hosts, *C. burnetii* targets the host macrophage, where it survives as an obligate intracellular pathogen in the harsh acidic environment of the phagolysosome. The bacteria exhibits phase variation on passage through cell culture; from the phase I virulent stage observed in natural and animal infections, it can shift to an avirulent phase II stage after repeated passage through cell culture. Under adverse conditions, *C. burnetii* undergoes sporulation, yielding an atypical spore-like form that can survive extreme environmental conditions. It is highly infectious, producing disease after infection with a single organism.

C. burnetii infection causes a wide array of acute and chronic presentations in humans, as described below. Nonetheless, only about 40% of people infected with it report clinical symptoms. About 7% of the general US population is seropositive for *C. burnetii* (McQuiston and Childs 2002).

Transmission of *Coxiella burnetii*

Most human cases of Q fever result from the inhalation of aerosols contaminated with *C. burnetii* of animal origin (Raoult et al. 2005). Infected aerosols may be generated by domesticated farm animals—especially cattle, sheep, and goats—but can also arise from cats, dogs, and birds. Although the organism is not known to cause overt disease in animals, it is shed in milk, urine, feces, and especially amniotic fluid and products of conception. The placenta of an infected ewe may contain up to a billion infectious doses of *C. burnetii* per gram of tissue; thus, the parturition of livestock can generate highly infectious aerosols.

Most humans who become infected with *C. burnetii* are exposed through direct contact with farm animals, domesticated animals, or animals in abattoirs. However, several outbreaks of Q fever appear to have been caused by *C. burnetii* aerosols transported by wind (Tissot-Dupont et al. 2004) or through fomites, such as contaminated straw used in industrial packaging (van Woerden et al. 2004). For example, the largest outbreak of Q fever ever reported in the UK occurred in 1989 in large, metropolitan Birmingham (West Midlands) probably as a consequence of the windborne spread of *C. burnetii* spores from farms outside the city (Hawker et al. 1998; Smith et al. 1993).

Less common routes of *C. burnetii* transmission include the ingestion of infectious raw milk, direct inoculation with contaminated material, and tick bites. Even rarer are reports of transmission within households, through sexual contact, and through blood transfusion (Milazzo et al. 2001).

Endemicity in Southwest and South-Central Asia

Most countries have reported *C. burnetii* infections (Wilson 1991). Q fever is widespread in Iran, Afghanistan, and Pakistan and is common in the Arabian Peninsula and Syria (Wilson 1991). Studies conducted in Turkey and Oman have demonstrated that 8-12% of the adult populations of those countries have been exposed to the organism, and rates are higher among those who work with animals (Cetinkaya et al. 2000; Scrimgeour et al. 2003). Several clinical reports document the frequency of Q fever among Israelis; one study found that almost 6% of 346 patients who has a diagnosis of community-acquired pneumonia had laboratory evidence consistent with *C. burnetii* infection (Oren et al. 2005; Siegman-Igra et al. 1997).

Acute Q Fever

Acute Q fever occurs within 10-17 days after exposure to contaminated aerosols. Patients most frequently present with pneumonia, hepatitis, or a self-limited, influenza-like febrile illness. The clinical presentation of Q fever appears to vary geographically; for instance, *C. burnetii*-induced pneumonia is more common in eastern Canada, and *C. burnetii*-induced hepatitis predominates in Spain. The acute phase usually lasts 1-3 weeks and resolves without specific therapy or adverse health outcomes.

Coxiella burnetii Pneumonia

The symptoms of Q fever pneumonia include prominent headache, cough, pleuritic chest pain, and fever (Tissot-Dupont et al. 1992). Radiographic findings can vary widely, although nonsegmental and segmental pleural-based opacities are a common feature. Chest films of patients who have been exposed to parturient cats often show multiple rounded opacities (Gordon et al. 1984). Although some patients with Q fever pneumonia develop acute respiratory distress syndrome, the vast majority of patients' symptoms resolve without adverse health outcomes.

Coxiella burnetii Hepatitis

Q fever hepatitis is characterized by mildly increased transaminases, thrombocytopenia, and frequent autoantibodies. Liver biopsy often reveals a highly specific histology known as a doughnut granuloma (Travis et al. 1986).

Atypical Presentations of Acute Q Fever

Unusual presentations of acute Q fever include aseptic meningitis, meningoencephalitis, peripheral neuropathy, GBS, myocarditis, pericarditis, thyroiditis, bone marrow necrosis, erythema nodosum, glomerulonephritis, and orchitis. Q fever in pregnancy can lead to miscarriage and neonatal death (Raoult et al. 2002).

Treatment of Acute Q Fever and Related Long-Term Toxicity

Although acute Q fever usually resolves spontaneously, antibiotic treatment can reduce the duration of symptoms and may diminish the risk of complications. The treatment of choice is tetracycline or doxycycline given for 7-14 days. Alternative antibiotic regimens include chloramphenicol, quinolones, rifampin, and trimethoprim. In vitro efficacy of erythromycin is poor, but there is some evidence of clinical efficacy in vivo (Raoult 2003).

Possible long-term toxicity of tetracycline use includes nervous and sensory system effects. Benign intracranial hypertension has been described in children and adults on tetracycline and doxycycline (Digre 2003; Gardner et al. 1995; Lochhead and Elston 2003); this complication has resulted in visual-field loss (Digre and Corbett 2001; Gardner et al. 1995; Lochhead and Elston 2003).

Diagnosing Q Fever

The diagnosis of Q fever should be considered in patients who have an appropriate clinical presentation and substantial animal exposure. Nonspecific laboratory findings include increased erythrocyte sedimentation rate, low platelet counts, increased liver enzymes, and multiple transient autoantibodies.

Specific diagnosis of Q fever is complicated. Growth of *C. burnetii* in culture is not only difficult, but also fraught with biosafety hazards because of its high infectivity and tendency to aerosolize. Most cases of *C. burnetii* infection are diagnosed serologically. Acute infection is accompanied by a rise in IgM antibody to phase II antigens followed by an IgG response to phase II antigen. In contrast, chronic infection is characterized by high titers of IgA and IgM to phase I and II antigens. IgM antibodies can remain increased for long periods and are not indicative of recent infection (Fournier et al. 1998).

Current methods of antibody detection include indirect immunofluorescence assay (IFA), ELISA, and the less sensitive and less specific complement-fixation assay. Indirect immunofluorescence is now considered to be the reference for serologic diagnosis. Acute infection can be diagnosed on the basis of a 4-fold rise in titer in paired serum samples. Single IFA titers of 1:50 IgM and 1:200 IgG to phase II antigen are considered diagnostic of acute infection, and a titer of 1:800 IgG to phase I antigen is considered diagnostic of chronic infection. Probes that use DNA amplification with PCR are now available to identify *C. burnetii* in blood, urine, and tissue samples (Parker et al. 2006).

Coinfection with *Coxiella burnetii* and Human Immunodeficiency Virus

Relatively little is known about *C. burnetii* infection in HIV patients. In principle, as an intracellular pathogen with long-term persistence in human hosts, *C. burnetii* might be expected to cause more frequent and more severe infections in the immunocompromised state. Indeed, Raoult et al. (1993) noted a 10-fold increase in the incidence of Q fever among HIV-seropositive patients in France. Later studies have yielded conflicting results (Madariaga et al. 2004; Montes et al. 1995; Raoult et al. 1993).

Long-Term Adverse Health Outcomes of Q Fever

C. burnetii persists in circulating monoctyes and bone marrow of healthy people who had a diagnosis of Q fever and recovered from the acute illness.

Complications of Acute Q Fever

About 2% of patients with acute Q fever manifest neurologic involvement. Long-term neurologic deficits have been described in that population: motor weakness, blurred vision, residual paresthesia, sensory loss, peripheral neuropathy, and behavioral changes (Bernit et al. 2002; Drancourt et al. 1991; Ferrante and Dolan 1993; Raoult et al. 2005). There are case reports of other rare neurologic deficits. Although the neurologic deficits can be long-term, onset occurs during the acute syndrome. Thus, the association between acute Q fever with neurologic involvement and long-term neurologic deficits is self-evident.

Chronic Sequelae of *Coxiella burnetii* Infection

The scientific literature contains evidence of five chronic syndromes associated with *C. burnetii* infection: post-Q fever chronic fatigue syndrome, culture-negative endocarditis, vascular infection, chronic hepatitis, and osteomyelitis. In general, older age and immunosuppression appear to be risk factors for the development of chronic Q fever (Fenollar et al. 2001). There also appear to be risk factors specific to particular syndromes. Although infection with *C. burnetii* may be chronic, chronic Q fever itself is rarely reported and usually occurs among those with pre-existing abnormalities of cardiac valves or endovascular grafts.

The largest case series to date reviewed 74,202 suspect cases referred to the French National Reference Center for Rickettsial Diseases during a 14-year period (1985-1998) (Raoult et al. 2000). Serum samples were initially screened with the IFA assay for reactive IgM and IgA antibodies to *C. burnetii*. Samples that tested positive underwent a second IFA assay to determine antibody titers; a phase II IgG titer of at least 200:1 and a phase II IgM titer of at least 50:1 indicated recent Q fever. With that method, investigators identified 7,543 probable cases. To confirm them, the reference center collected, tested, and cultured additional serum, blood, or tissue samples from the patients. *C. burnetii* was detected with the IFA assay in the samples of 1,383 cases whose serum had IgG titers of at least 800:1. Clinical data on the confirmed cases indicated that 1,070 of the patients suffered acute Q fever and 313 chronic Q fever. Raoult and colleagues reported the clinical and epidemiologic characteristics of these cases (Raoult et al. 2000). The committee drew on their findings (Table 5.4) and others to reach conclusions about the strength of association between *C. burnetii* infection and the five long-term adverse health outcomes noted above.

TABLE 5.4 Prevalence of Various Forms of Chronic Q Fever Among 295 Cases from France

Condition	Identified Cases	
	No.	%
Endocarditis	229	73
Vascular infection	25	8
Abnormal Pregnancy (outcome)	13	6
Chronic hepatitis	8	3
Osteoarticular infection	7	2
Chronic pericarditis	3	1
Adenopathy	1	< 1
Splenic pseudotumor	1	< 1
Lung pseudotumor	1	< 1
Chronic neurofoci	1	< 1
No identified foci	6	2

SOURCE: Reprinted with permission from Raoult et al. 2000.

Endocarditis

The most common and well-studied form of chronic Q fever is endocarditis (Brouqui et al. 1993; Raoult et al. 2000; Saah 2000; Stein and Raoult 1995). Most patients have abnormal or prosthetic cardiac valves; however, any part of the vascular tree may become infected (Raoult et al. 1986; Saah 2000). Fenollar et al. (2001) found that 30-50% of patients who had a diagnosis of acute Q fever and underlying cardiac valvular lesions would develop endocarditis. The delay between infection and the onset of endocarditis remains undefined.

Acute Q fever is not a prerequisite of Q fever endocarditis. In the French study noted above, only one-third of the endocarditis patients reported a previous febrile syndrome of unknown etiology within the year preceding the onset of chronic symptoms (Raoult et al. 2000).

Q fever endocarditis differs from typical endocarditis caused by pyogenic bacteria in that fever is often absent and vegetation can be difficult to detect with echocardiography (Fenollar et al. 2001; Fenollar et al. 2006; Gami et al. 2004). Vegetation is distinct on microscopy, which reveals a chronic inflammatory infiltrate and large, foamy macrophages (Marrie 1990; Marrie 2000).

Untreated endocarditis usually leads to death. Even with treatment, mortality is high (23.5%) (Brouqui et al. 1993). Treatment for chronic Q fever endocarditis usually involves combination antibiotic therapy. Regimens may include doxycycline with quinolone alone or with rifampin. Hydroxycholoroquine has also been used in combination therapeutic regimens (Raoult et al. 1999). The optimal duration of treatment is unclear; some experts treat for 18-24 months, and others recommend lifelong therapy given the high rates of relapse after cessation of antibiotics (Maurin and Raoult 1999).

The committee concludes that there is sufficient evidence of an association between infection by *Coxiella burnetii* and endocarditis years after primary infection.

Vascular Infection

Vascular infections can occur in aneurysm and vascular grafts and are often accompanied by a nonspecific illness characterized by weight loss and fever. The authors of a recent case series suggest that the incidence of *C. burnetii* vascular infection is underestimated and recommend that *C. burnetii* serologic tests be routinely carried out in cases of unexplained illness in patients with a history of underlying vascular disease (Fournier et al. 1998).

The committee concludes that there is sufficient evidence of an association between infection by *Coxiella burnetii* and vascular infection years after primary infection.

Chronic Hepatitis

Several investigators have documented isolated chronic hepatitis as an infrequent manifestation of chronic Q fever (Raoult et al. 2000; Saah 2000; Turck et al. 1976; Yebra et al. 1988). It presents with mildly increased liver enzymes; granulomatous hepatitis is histologically typical when liver biopsy is performed. Patients whose acute Q fever is manifested as hepatitis or who have underlying alcoholic cirrhosis may be more likely to develop this health outcome (Raoult et al. 2000). The time between acute infection and diagnosis of chronic hepatitis may be as long as 2 years (Yebra et al. 1988). This health outcome appears to account for less than 5% of all chronic manifestations of *C. burnetii* infection.

The committee concludes that there is sufficient evidence of an association between infection by *Coxiella burnetii* and chronic hepatitis years after primary infection.

Osteomyelitis

Osteomyelitis is another rare manifestation of chronic Q fever. Of the 313 people with confirmed chronic Q fever as identified by Raoult et al., seven had osteomyelitis. Only one of those had an earlier documented acute infection with *C. burnettii*, although several reported a febrile illness within the previous year (Raoult et al. 2000). Nourse et al. identified three additional cases and described 11 previously reported cases; almost half the cases were in children, and nearly all the patients had contact with farm animals (Nourse et al. 2004). In summary, chronic Q fever sometimes is manifested as osteomyelitis, which may occur with a previously diagnosed Q fever illness or in the context of a known history of acute Q fever.

The committee concludes that there is sufficient evidence of a causal relationship between exposure to *Coxiella burnetii* and osteomyelitis.

Post-Q Fever Fatigue Syndrome

A post-Q fever chronic fatigue syndrome has been described in several populations of exposed patients (Ayres et al. 1998; Hatchette et al. 2003; Marmion et al. 1996; 2005; Wildman et al. 2002). Five years after the previously mentioned outbreak in the West Midlands, UK, 42.4% of those with diagnosed Q fever reported symptoms of chronic fatigue compared with only 26% of a control group (Ayres et al. 1998). A second study documented high levels of fatigue in exposed subjects 10 years after exposure (Wildman et al. 2002). Twenty-seven months after an outbreak of Q fever in Newfoundland, 52% of patients had persistent symptoms that hampered their activities to the same extent as type 2 diabetes mellitus and coronary arterial disease affected cohorts of Americans (Hatchette et al. 2003).

Those studies have limitations that prevent the scientific community—including the investigators themselves—from definitively confirming the existence of a post-Q fever fatigue syndrome. For instance, the outbreak of Q fever in Newfoundland led farms to close, leaving many people unemployed; this socioeconomic factor may have confounded the study results (Hatchette et al. 2003). Data on comorbidity were unavailable, followup serologic data were incomplete, and the study also may have been limited by participation bias: subjects who continued to have symptoms may have been more likely to participate in both questionnaire surveys.

Later studies have reported differences in immune-response genes among those who report post-Q fever fatigue compared with those who are unaffected (Helbig et al. 2005; Helbig et al. 2003). One hypothesis is that after C. *burnetii* infection, *Coxiella* may persist universally in the bone marrow and be regulated by the host's immune response. A subset of patients with subtle differences in their immune response may later develop post-Q fever fatigue. That and other hypotheses are under active investigation in Australia and the UK.

> **The committee concludes that there is limited or suggestive evidence of an association between infection by *Coxiella burnetii* and post-Q fever chronic fatigue syndrome years after primary infection.**

TUBERCULOSIS

The unique properties and history of tuberculosis (TB) led the committee to approach this section differently from the rest of the chapter in two ways. First, initial infection with *Mycobacterium tuberculosis* (TB infection) is usually asymptomatic, the onset of the disease (TB) is almost always delayed, and relapse of TB may occur years after successful treatment. Thus, TB infection has the potential for delayed long-term adverse health outcomes both because of the onset of clinically evident TB months to decades after initial infection and because of the long-term consequences of acute disease.

Second, TB has a long history of occurrence and transmission in military settings and remains a cause of potential delayed adverse health outcomes in US troops and veterans of the Gulf War, OEF, and OIF—especially those who are or were deployed to regions where TB is highly endemic. The committee discusses TB in the military at the end of this section.

TB is a chronic necrotizing granulomatous infection caused primarily by the acid-fast bacillus *Mycobacterium tuberculosis*. An obligate aerobe, *M. tuberculosis* grows best in such tissues with high oxygen tension as the apices of the lung and the renal cortex; this explains why most infections are manifested as pulmonary disease. *M. bovis,* a related organism, causes a substantial number of TB cases in regions where milk is not routinely pasteurized and where *M. bovis*-infected cattle are not identified and destroyed.

Transmission of Tuberculosis

TB is transmitted primarily through exposure to airborne *M. tuberculosis*. When an infected person coughs, sneezes, yells, or sings, microscopic droplets containing *M. tuberculosis* are expelled into the air. Heavier particles quickly settle out of the air, and lighter ones remain suspended, often for several hours. Inhaled droplets of 1-5 μm in diameter are small enough to reach the alveoli, where the mycobacteria colonize and infect the lung tissue of their new hosts (IOM 2000).

Detection of Tuberculosis Transmission

The human immune system usually does not recognize *M. tuberculosis* as a foreign body until 2-6 weeks after inoculation. During that lag time, the organisms proliferate, spreading from the lungs to the lymphatics and disseminating in the bloodstream. Once the human immune system mounts its primary response to *M. tuberculosis*, further growth and proliferation of the pathogen are usually suppressed; most people maintain a latent TB infection (LTBI) that is believed to persist as a benign condition for life unless progression to active TB develops. The initial infection with *M. tuberculosis* in adults is usually asymptomatic and results in long-lasting cell-mediated immunity to purified protein derivative (PPD) of *M. tuberculosis*. Only 1-2% of recently infected people will be found to have active TB (CDC 2000a), so the detection of transmission is based largely on the diagnosis of LTBI.

Diagnosing Latent Tuberculosis Infection

Recently acquired LTBI is detected by conversion of a tuberculin skin test (TST) from negative to positive 2-10 weeks after exposure (CDC 2000a). In development are gamma-interferon release assays that measure cell-mediated immunity to *M. tuberculosis* protein products more specifically than the TST. The US Food and Drug Administration in 2004 approved the QuantiFERON®-TB GOLD in vitro assay by Cellestis Inc. for diagnosing LTBI (FDA 2005). While noting the need for further research, CDC has recommended that the QuantiFERON-TB GOLD be used in place of the TST (CDC 2005d). The new assay is more specific than TST because it uses antigens that are absent from bacillus Calmette-Guérin (BCG) vaccines and nontuberculous mycobacteria (such antigens can cross-react with the TST to produce false-positive results). In addition, the QuantiFERON-TB GOLD requires only a single draw of blood. Its main limitation is expense. The QuantiFERON-TB GOLD could be used as a confirmatory assay, particularly in TST-positive, BCG-vaccinated people.

Risk Factors for Transmission

TB is not a highly infectious disease, so most transmission occurs in such places where people have close and frequent contact such as households and closed community settings. Occasionally, however, infection follows brief, casual contact in airplanes, buses, hospitals, or prisons. Outbreaks of tuberculosis in closed populations where there is crowding, poor air exchange, or both, may lead to substantial transmission. Exposure to corpses who had active TB has also been identified as posing a high risk for the transmission of the disease.

For US military personnel, the risk of becoming infected with *M. tuberculosis* depends on occupation, living quarters, exposure to TB-endemic populations, chance exposure in an epidemic setting, and other factors. Cases of TB among active-duty military personnel have the potential to cause extensive TB infection (defined by a positive TST) and outbreaks of active TB among deployed troops, especially shipboard personnel.

The closed shipboard environment and extended periods at sea increase the risk of TB transmission to a level at or above that for most household contacts (Kelley 2005). Notable outbreaks of TB occurred aboard Navy ships in 1966, 1987, and 1998 (Kelley 2005). The most recent of those outbreaks occurred after a US marine with acid-fast bacilli (AFB) smear-positive cavitary pulmonary disease was deployed to a US Navy amphibious ship. More than 18% of the crew and 25% of embarked marines—696 people—converted to TST-positive (Kelley 2005).

Endemicity in Southwest and South-Central Asia

TB is a global disease. An estimated 33% of the world's population is infected with *M. tuberculosis*, although the incidence of infection has wide geographic variation (WHO 2006b; Wilson 1991).

In southwest and south-central Asia, TB is highly endemic. WHO estimated the regional incidence in 2004 to be 206 cases per 100,000 population (WHO 2006b). In that year, the estimated incidence in Iraq was 200 cases per 100,000, and in Afghanistan, 661 cases per 100,000 (WHO. 2006a). The burden of TB is particularly severe in Afghanistan, which in 2004 had the 12th highest per capita rate of TB cases in the world (Table 5.5) (WHO 2006a). The United States, in contrast, had only 3.6 cases per 100,000 in 2004 (WHO 2006a).

Thus, for US military personnel, the risk of exposure to TB is much greater in south-central and southwest Asia than domestically. Shipboard personnel and people who have extensive close contact with local populations—in prisons or hospitals, for instance—would be at higher risk than other troops for acquisition of TB during military service.

TABLE 5.5 The 12 Countries with the Highest Rate of TB, 2004

Country	Incidence of TB (All Forms), No. Cases per 100,000 Population	Rank
Djibouti	1,137	1
Swaziland	1,120	2
Kenya	888	3
Sierra Leone	847	4
Togo	718	5
Cambodia	709	6
Zambia	707	7
Timor-Leste	692	8
Somalia	673	9
Zimbabwe	673	10
South Africa	670	11
Afghanistan	661	12

SOURCE: Adapted with permission from WHO 2006a.

Risk of Progression from Latent Tuberculosis Infection to Active Tuberculosis

Persons with LTBI face a 5-10% lifetime risk of developing active TB. The risk is greatest during the first 2 years after infection (Figure 5.1). In general, the likelihood that TB infection will produce active disease varies with the intensity and duration of exposure, size of induration, and age (Figure 5.2) (Comstock et al. 1974a; Mandell et al. 2005; Vynnycky and Fine 1997). Infants, 15- to 25-year-olds, and the elderly are at greatest risk for progression from LTBI to active TB (Comstock et al. 1974b; Stead and Dutt 1991; Stead and Lofgren 1983; Stead and To 1987).

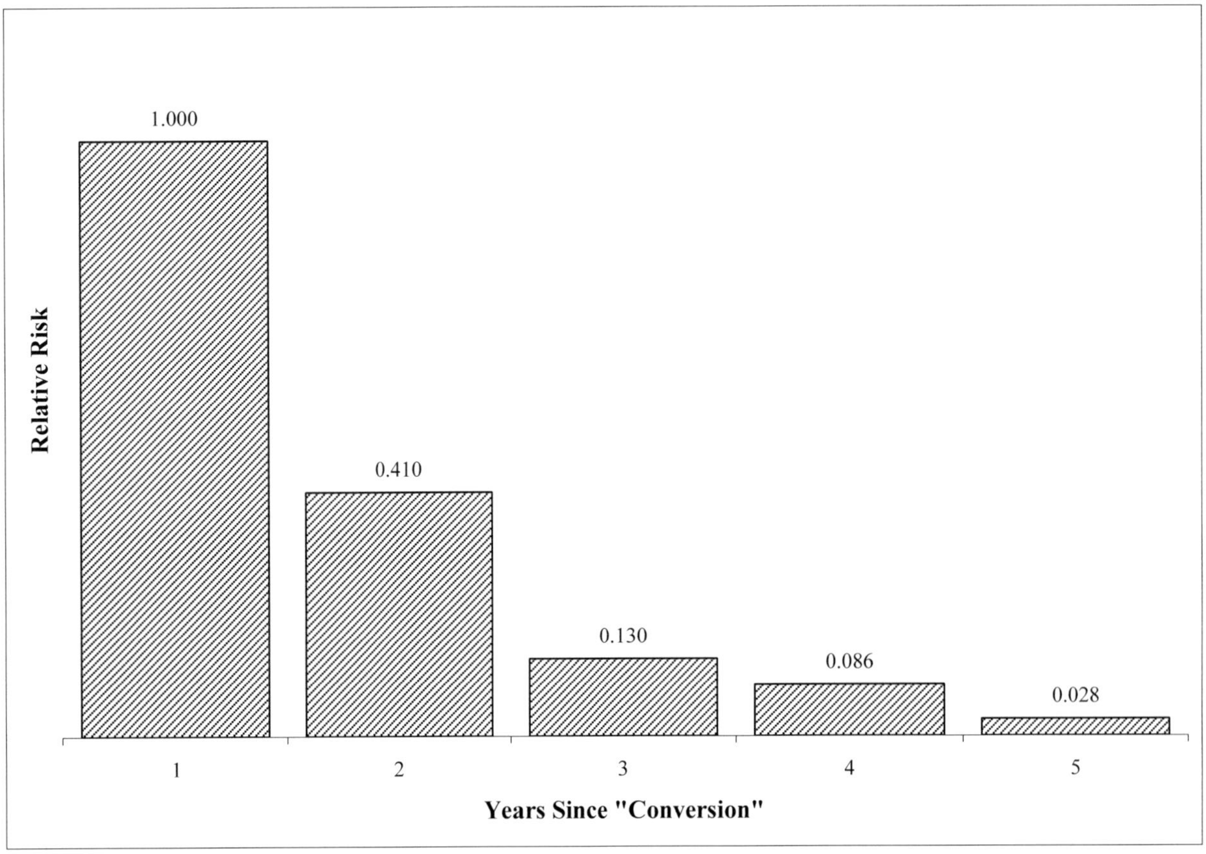

FIGURE 5.1 Relationship between rate at which people experience their first episode of active TB in each year following infection or reinfection and rate at which people experience their first episode of active TB during first year after infection or reinfection. Estimated from distribution of interval between TST conversion and onset of active TB in those who were tuberculin-negative at start of UK Medical Research Council's trial of BCG vaccine in 1950-1952 (Hart and Sutherland 1977). Relative risk for given year after TST conversion is ratio of (a) proportion of total disease incidence among initially tuberculin-negative people that occurred in that year after conversion to (b) corresponding proportion that occurred during first year after conversion.
SOURCE: Adapted with permission from Vynnycky and Fine 1997.

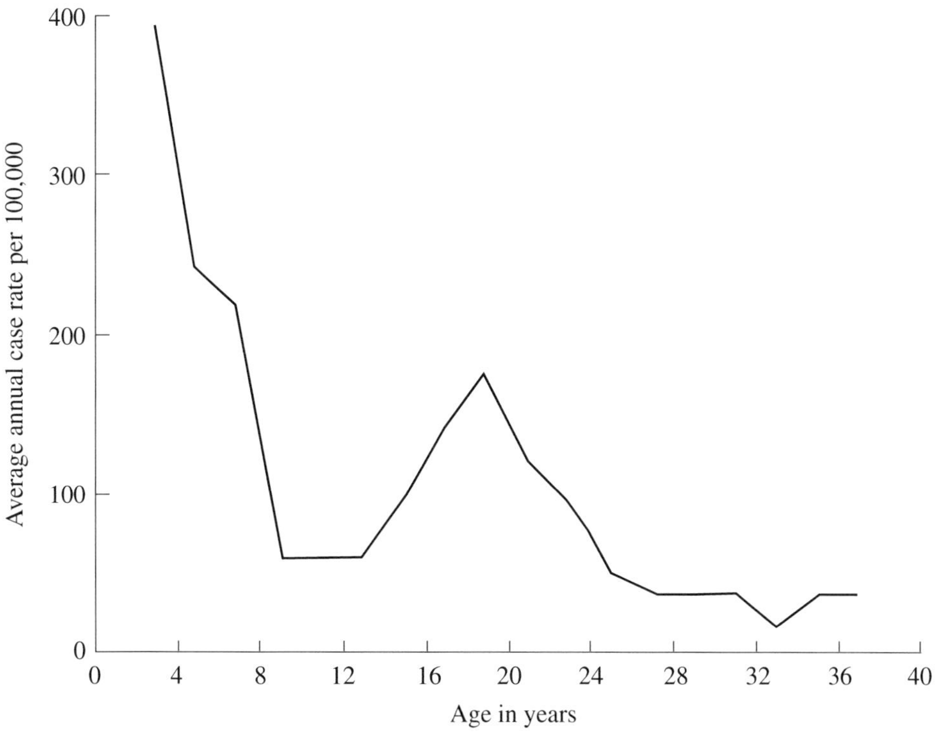

FIGURE 5.2 Incidence of tuberculosis among initial reactors to tuberculin, by age when tuberculosis was first diagnosed. From 1949 to 1951, investigators administered TSTs to nearly 200,000 Puerto Rican children ages 1-19; 82,269 children tested positive. The investigators followed this cohort through June 1969. During that 18- to 20-year period, 1,400 tuberculin-reactors progressed to active TB. Age was the most important risk factor for progression to active disease, the researchers found. This figure illustrates the age distribution of the 1,400 tuberculin-reactors who progressed to active TB. Incidence rates were highest among children less than 4 years old and second-highest among individuals around 20 years old.
SOURCE: Reprinted with permission from Comstock et al. 1974b.

Another risk factor for progression to active TB is the degree of tuberculin sensitivity, as measured by the size of induration. A 4-year study of 1.2 million recruits to the US Navy found the risk for progression from LTBI to active TB was greater for sailors whose induration at enlistment measured ≥10 mm than for those whose induration was <10 mm (Comstock et al. 1974a). The investigators found that a history of household exposure to TB further increased the risk for progression to active disease. Tuberculin reactors whose induration measured ≥5 mm at enlistment and who had a history of household exposure to TB were more likely to progress to active TB than sailors who lacked such a history.

HIV infection dramatically increases the risk of both primary TB and reactivation TB (Davies 2005). People with LTBI who become infected with HIV face a 5-10% *annual* risk of developing reactivation TB (Glynn 1998). HIV-infected people exposed to *M. tuberculosis* have an approximate 40% risk of acquiring the infection and progressing to the active disease within 3 months. Some other conditions also increase the risk of progression to active TB: disorders associated with defects in cell-mediated immunity, such as hematologic malignancies and lymphatic malignancies; diabetes mellitus; renal dialysis; weight loss; intestinal bypass; and gastrectomy. Medical conditions that increase the risk of TB are silicosis, diabetes mellitus, chronic renal failure, leukemias and lymphomas, carcinoma of the head or neck and lung, loss of at least 10% of ideal body weight, gastrectomy and jejunoileal bypass, radiation therapy, treatment with tumor-necrosis-factor inhibitors, immunosuppression associated with organ transplantation, and corticosteroid therapy. In many cases the stimulating factor is unknown.

Treatment for Latent Tuberculosis Infection to Prevent Active Tuberculosis

To mitigate the risk of LTBI's becoming active TB, such infections are treated with isoniazid for 9 months. Completing the treatment regimen reduces the risk of active TB by 70-90% (CDC 2000b), but asymptomatic people frequently fail to comply with the regimen.

Active Tuberculosis

Primary Tuberculosis vs Reactivation Tuberculosis

If a chest x-ray picture is taken during initial TB infection, it often shows features of a condition called primary TB: patchy alveolar opacities in the middle- and lower-lung fields, common with unilateral hilar adenopathy. Occasionally, patients with primary TB have fever, nonproductive cough, dyspnea, and—rarely—erythema nodosum. Compression by enlarged lymph nodes may lead to upper- or middlelung collapse. Primary TB generally resolves without treatment. In some patients, however, the immune system cannot contain the infection, and active disease develops, as discussed below. Patients who recover from primary TB (including pleural disease)—particularly those with prior pleuritis—remain at risk for recurrence of active TB.

Historically, a distinction has been made between primary TB occurring at the time of initial TB infection and the more typical adult manifestation of disease, called reactivation TB, developing later. Yet the overlapping temporal and clinical features of the two forms often blur the distinctions between them. One reason for the apparent overlap is uncertainty as to when the primary infection occurred. Therefore, to be consistent with US diagnostic standards, the committee's discussion of active TB below pertains to both primary and reactivation TB (CDC 2000a).

Diagnosing Active Tuberculosis

The standard approach to diagnosing active TB is through an AFB smear of expectorated sputum. The presence of such mycobacteria as *M. tuberculosis* in a bodily secretion or tissue specimen can be visually confirmed with the so-called acid-fast test, which exploits the unique properties of the mycobacterial cell envelope. Cells in a specimen are first stained with red carbol fuchsin, then washed with an acidic alcohol solution. The wash decolorizes almost all organisms except mycobacteria because mycobacterial cell envelopes contain mycolic acid, high-molecular-weight lipids, and waxes that prevent the wash from penetrating the cell.

About half of patients with newly diagnosed pulmonary TB have AFB-positive smears. In addition to establishing the likely diagnosis, AFB-positive smears signal highly infectious cases that must be managed through strict isolation. Smears are more likely to be negative in patients with minimal TB or noncavitary TB.

Cultures are performed on such specialized media as Lowenstein-Jensen (an egg-based media), Middlebrook 7H10 (an agar-based media), and Middlebrook 7H102 (a liquid-based media) (CDC 2000a). Using a combination of solid and liquid media will yield positive results in 85-90% of cultures that contain *M. tuberculosis*. Culture- and smear-negative cases of suspect TB are treated empirically on the basis of clinical suspicion and lack of an alternative diagnosis.

PCR-based diagnostics provide the diagnosis of TB and, to a lesser extent, extrapulmonary TB, rapidly and with greater sensitivity and specificity compared with sputum smears. Such diagnostics are expensive, however, and offer fewer advantages in cases of paucibacillary (that is, having few bacilli) TB.

Clinical Manifestations of Active Tuberculosis

Pulmonary Tuberculosis

TB presents as pulmonary disease in 80% of reported cases in the United States (CDC 2005c). Similarly, pulmonary TB accounted for 70.7% of cases among hospitalized active-duty US Army personnel from 1980 to 1996 (Table 5.6). The difference in age distribution between the civilian population and the military population probably accounts for much of the 9% difference in the proportion of pulmonary TB between the two groups.

The most common symptoms of pulmonary TB are cough that produces purulent sputum for at least 2 weeks, night sweats, weight loss, and anorexia. Hemoptysis and pleurisy also may occur. Half of patients with pulmonary TB are afebrile, and one-fifth lack pulmonary symptoms altogether.

TABLE 5.6 First Hospitalization Discharge Diagnoses for Tuberculosis Among Active-Duty US Army Personnel, by *ICD-9-CM* Code, 1980-1996

Tuberculosis Classification	ICD-9-CM Code	No.	%
Pulmonary tuberculosis	011	662	70.7
Other respiratory tuberculosis	012	82	8.8
Tuberculosis of other organs	017	62	6.6
Tuberculosis of the bones and joints	015	44	4.7
Primary tuberculosis	010	35	3.7
Tuberculosis of the genitourinary system	016	20	2.1
Tuberculosis of the meninges and central nervous system	013	11	1.2
Tuberculosis of the gastrointestinal tract	014	11	1.2
Miliary tuberculosis	018	9	1.0
Total		936	

NOTE: *ICD-9-CM = International Classification of Diseases, Ninth Revision, Clinical Modification.*
SOURCE: Adapted with permission from Camarca and Krauss 2001.

Signs of consolidation may be present on physical examination. Chest radiographs most frequently show opacities localized to apical and posterior segments of the upper lobes and the superior (dorsal) segment of the lower lobes. Early cavities may be present; these typically are thin-walled and surrounded by opacities, and 10% have air-fluid levels. TB may present atypically in some patients, particularly diabetics, immunocompromised people, and people with HIV infection. In such cases, chest radiographic findings are variable, ranging from dense lobar or segmental consolidation to atelectasis, large-mass lesions, or cavities.

Extrapulmonary Tuberculosis

About 20% of reported cases of active TB occur outside the lungs in such regions as the lymph nodes (9%), pleura (4%), bones and joints (2%), meninges (1%), genitourinary tract (1%), and peritoneal cavity (1%) (CDC 2005c). Disseminated extrapulmonary TB, known as miliary TB, consists of 1-3 mm nodules throughout the lungs and other tissues.

Tuberculosis Pleurisy

Primary TB is sometimes manifested as an infection of the pleural space, and TB pleurisy may develop later as a progression of LTBI to pleural TB with or without pulmonary TB. The typical presentation is acute onset of fever, cough, and pleuritic chest pains, although there may be a chronic course characterized by fever, general malaise, and loss of up to 10% of body weight. The pleural effusions usually are small to moderate. Concurrent parenchymal disease occurs in one-third to one-half of cases. Diagnosing TB pleurisy usually requires a pleural biopsy, which has a diagnostic yield of 85-95%. The initial TST is negative one-third of the time. Although pleural fluid is exudative, it usually tests negative with an AFB smear and, in 75% of cases, in cultures.

> **The committee concludes that there is sufficient evidence of a causal relationship between infection with *Mycobacterium tuberculosis* and occurrence of active tuberculosis months to decades after infection.**

Coinfection with Tuberculosis and Human Immunodeficiency Virus

HIV alters the clinical manifestations of TB. For example, pulmonary TB may occur in a lower lobe in a noncavitary fashion. There may be hilar or mediastinal adenopathy, pleural disease, or a normal chest x-ray picture. Extrapulmonary TB is more common among patients coinfected with HIV than among other patients, and it may occur with pulmonary disease or alone. The interactions between chemotherapeutic drugs for TB with antiretroviral drugs for HIV challenge the clinician to treat TB-HIV coinfections effectively.

Treatment for Active Tuberculosis

Treatment for drug-sensitive active TB consists of isoniazid, rifampin, pyrazinamide, and ethambutol for 2 months followed by isoniazid and rifampin for 4 months. That regimen is 95% effective, although about 5% of patients will experience relapses of active TB, most of them in the first 1-2 years after treatment completion (CDC 2003a).

Multiple-drug-resistant TB is more difficult to cure. Regimens should be tailored to known drug susceptibility of the isolates. If an isolate is resistant to isoniazid and rifampin but susceptible to other drugs, treatment regimens would consist of ethambutol, pyrazinamide, and levofloxacin for 12-18 months and an injectible aminoglycoside for the first 2-3 months.

Late Manifestations of Active Tuberculosis

Even after highly effective treatment for acute TB, affected tissues and organs may be functionally impaired or destroyed. Functional impairment may range from imperceptible to severe. The paucity of data on long-term health outcomes of acute TB and the ability of *M. tuberculosis* to infect and damage virtually any organ of the body challenged the committee to address the late manifestations of this disease comprehensively. This discussion addresses the notable late manifestations of acute TB and the committee's conclusions about the strength of the association between acute and long-term adverse health outcomes.

Late Manifestations of Pulmonary Tuberculosis

It is well accepted in the biomedical community that disability occurs after pulmonary TB. The most common adverse health outcomes are chronic disabling scarring of the lungs, long-term pulmonary dysfunction, secondary infection of residual cavities, empyema, bronchiectasis, bronchopleural fistulas, and aspergilloma. Rarely, scar carcinoma occurs. Despite the centuries-old history of TB, however, the published data on long-term manifestations are inadequate for the committee to comment on their duration, range, or severity of adverse health outcomes.

A number of studies have compared pulmonary function tests (PFTs) at diagnosis of and after treatment for active TB. For instance, a study of 25 TB patients in Canada found abnormal PFTs (reduced 1-second forced expiratory volume and forced vital capacity) in individuals with cavitary TB but not in those with noncavitary TB (Long et al. 1998). Another study, of 74 TB patients in South Africa, showed a restrictive lung function pattern in 57% of cases and an obstructive lung function pattern in 11%. After treatment for TB, 53% of patients still had abnormal PFTs (Plit et al. 1998). Although neither study commented on the potential disability associated with the findings, none of the patients had residual impairment of oxygenation at rest.

Multiple case reports have been published of patients who have developed "scar cancer", lung cancer associated with lung scars from TB or other causes (Ardies 2003). The risk of cancer after TB has not been quantified, nor has the percentage of TB patients left with pulmonary scarring. One report from Japan indicated a 2% prevalence of lymphoma of the pleural space among patients with chronic pyothorax, which is associated with tuberculosis (Iuchi et al. 1987). Because pyothorax is a rare complication of TB, the authors could not quantify the overall risk of cancer posed by TB. In summary, the available data are insufficient for the committee to determine whether an association exists between cancer and active TB. If such an association does exist, cancer is undoubtedly a very rare consequence of TB.

Late Manifestations of Extrapulmonary Tuberculosis

The long-term adverse health outcomes of extrapulmonary TB occur with varied frequency depending on the site of active disease. The more common forms of extrapulmonary TB, pleural and lymphatic disease, rarely have long-term adverse health outcomes. Two of the less common forms, TB meningitis and skeletal TB, are more likely to result in irreversible tissue damage. In general, estimates of the long-term prognoses for uncommon forms of TB are based on relatively small series of patients.

Tuberculosis Meningitis and Long-Term Neurologic Disability

It is well accepted in the biomedical community that TB meningitis is associated with long-term neurologic outcomes. The extent of disability depends on the duration and severity of acute symptoms, the age of the patient, and the neurologic deficits (Dube et al. 1992; Kennedy and Fallon 1979). Of TB meningitis patients with stupor or dense paraplegia or hemiplegia, about half either die or recover with severe residual neurologic deficits (Kennedy and Fallon 1979). Until the 1990s, most reports of outcomes for adult patients with TB meningitis focused on mortality. As the recovery rate increased, more studies about the long-term prognoses for these patients emerged. Table 5.7 summarizes the findings of seven studies about long-term neurologic deficits of TB meningitis.

TABLE 5.7 Proportion of Patients Diagnosed with TB Meningitis Who Have Long-Term Neurologic Deficits

Study	No. Patients	All Adults?	No. Survivors	Time of Followup	No. (%) Survivors with Neurologic Deficits
Prospective Analyses					
Lau et al. 2005	156[a]	no[b]	130	3 years	20 (15)
Kalita and Misra 1999	56	no	44	1 year	4 (9)
Retrospective Analyses					
Sutlas et al. 2003	61	yes	44	24 months-6 years (mean, 3 years)	19 (31)
Hosoglu et al. 1998	96[a]	yes	52	9 months[c]	21 (40)
Yechoor et al. 1996	30	yes	17	9 months	5 (29)
Verdon et al. 1996	48	yes	17	1 year	4 (24)
Bergin et al. 1989	28[a]	no	24	unspecified	7 (29)

[a] Patients not followed for the entire period are excluded from this table.
[b] Only seven patients were >15 years old during the acute phase of illness.
[c] A minimum followup period of 9 months is not directly stated in the article, but is inferred from the minimum duration of treatment reported. The committee was unable to obtain confirmation from the authors of the study.

In a recent study of the influence of HIV infection on the outcome of TB meningitis, the authors reported severe neurologic deficits in 5.9% (2/34) of HIV-positive survivors and 17% (53/310) of HIV-negative survivors (Thwaites et al. 2005). HIV status did not alter the neurologic presentation of TB meningitis but significantly reduced the survival rate.

Spinal Tuberculosis and Long-Term Neurologic Disability

It is well accepted in the biomedical community that spinal TB is associated with spinal deformity and neurologic outcomes. A review of 694 patients in Turkey, most of whom were treated both surgically and medically, reported that only 41% had improved after treatment (Turgut 2001). A series of 70 patients in India, of whom only one underwent surgery, reported that 74% had excellent to good results (Nene and Bhojraj 2005).

> **The committee concludes that there is sufficient evidence of an association between severe forms of pulmonary and extrapulmonary tuberculosis and long-term adverse health outcomes due to irreversible tissue damage.**

Relapse of Active Tuberculosis

Even with current therapy under direct observation by health-care providers, relapse can occur in about 5% of treated patients and create a potential for additional late adverse health outcomes (CDC 2003a).

Potential Relationships Between Tuberculosis and Military Service

TB is potentially connected to military service in two ways. First, people who are TST-positive before deployment have LTBI and are at risk for developing active TB during deployment; troops with active TB in the field place other troops at risk for infection and disease. Second, troops who are TST-negative before deployment may become infected with TB during deployment. Such people occasionally manifest active TB shortly after infection but more frequently have LTBI.

Promotion of Tuberculin Skin Testing

The most effective way to mitigate TB transmission and activation is to identify and treat LTBI. That is a compelling argument for testing all military personnel for TB before and after every deployment. Table 5.8 summarizes the policies of each branch of the military regarding TSTs and treatment for LTBI.

Available data suggest that prior *M. tuberculosis* infection and exposure in the theater of operations contribute about equally to the prevalence of LTBI and the risk of disease among US military personnel. The Department of Defense (DOD) estimates that 2.5% of military personnel deployed to southwest and south-central Asia during OEF and OIF acquired new *M. tuberculosis* infections during deployments (Kilpatrick 2005). In comparison, the prevalence of TST reactivity among young adults entering the Navy in 1997 and 1998 was 3.5% (Smith et al. 2002); among military police who participated in refugee and humanitarian operations in Guantanamo Bay in 1995, it was 3.7% (Kortepeter and Krauss 2001). No case of active TB has been recognized in troops deployed to the Persian Gulf during Operation Desert Shield or Operation Desert Storm (Hyams et al. 1995).

TABLE 5.8 US Military Requirements Regarding Who Must Receive TSTs and When Tests Must Be Administered

Branch of Military	Name of Policy	Requirements (Abbreviated)	Effective Date
Army	Army LTBI Surveillance and Control Program	For personnel not previously known to have a positive TST, skin tests will be administered to • Personnel on initial entry for active duty of 30 days or more. • Military personnel, civilian employees, contractors, or family members who travel to and reside in a geographic area of the world where the endemic incidence of active TB disease is high (at least 25 new cases per 100,000 persons annually). Deploying personnel should have a TST performed before travel, at the time of redeployment, and again 3-6 months after redeployment. • Prospective employees (military and civilian), students, and volunteers as a condition of employment in health-care facilities, schools, or other facilities where tuberculosis transmission is of substantial concern, as defined by CDC, state law, or local ordinance. Additional periodic screening will be based on occupational risk. • Contracting officers and their representatives will include requirements in all contracts to ensure that contractors and their employees undergo tuberculin skin testing whenever said employees are working in an environment in which DOD employees would normally be required to undergo testing. Tuberculin skin testing will be paid for by the contractor. • Inmates of detention and confinement facilities in accordance with CDC guidelines For personnel known to have a positive TST previously, per CDC guidelines based on risk, no further TSTs will be applied. Exceptions include clinically valid doubt about previously recorded result, borderline result characterized as positive at prior test time and cases in which a 10-mm increase in reaction size or other factors might warrant treatment.	May 27, 2003
Navy and Marines	Tuberculosis Control Program (Bureau of Medicine and Surgery Instruction 6224.8)	Each commander, commanding officer, or officer-in-charge is responsible for the maintenance of an effective TB-control program in his or her command. The TST with PPD administered with the Mantoux method is the most sensitive and specific test available for identifying persons infected with M. tuberculosis. Infected persons must be evaluated periodically and kept informed about the symptoms of TB disease. TB screening on entry into Naval service: all persons first entering duty in the regular Navy, Naval Reserve, Marine Corps, or the Marine Corps Reserve for more than 30 days must have the results of TSTs documented in their medical treatment records. Annual TB screening: TSTs must be administered annually to personnel in operational units and in units with a high risk of TB exposure or outbreaks, and the test results must be recorded. The level of risk for a geographic region is based on numerous sources, including reports by, WHO, and PAHO. This policy applies to • All shipboard personnel, both active-duty and civil-service. • All members of deployable Navy and Marine Corps units, except ready reservists.	February 8, 1993

Branch of Military	Name of Policy	Requirements (Abbreviated)	Effective Date
		• All health-care workers. Annual TB screening also is required when recommended by cognizant Navy Environmental Preventive Medicine Units (for example, for personnel at some high-risk overseas duty stations). Predeployment and postdeployment screening: All service members must undergo TSTs and have the results recorded within 12 months before deploying and again within 90 days of returning. On a case-by-case basis, some personnel are required to undergo TSTs just before deploying. Triennial screening: Required for all personnel who are not required to undergo annual testing. Screening before separation from Naval service: All personnel must have TSTs (or annual clinical evaluations in the case of previously known reactors) documented within the 1-year period before separation from the naval service.	

Air Force	Air Force Surveillance, Prevention, and Control of Diseases and Conditions of Public Health or Military Significance (Air Force Instruction 48-105)	The Air Force uses a targeted LTBI screening program. Except for an initial test on accession, personnel are tested only when they have high risk exposures, high risk occupations, or clinical indications for testing. (Air Force Instruction [AFI] 48-105, March 1, 2005).
		The Mantoux TST is the current standard test for identifying LTBI (AFI48-105).
		The Air Force uses WHO data to determine the prevalence of TB in each country. A country is considered to have a high prevalence if WHO has found the incidence to be at least 30 cases per 100,000 of population (personal communication). The Air Force routinely issues a TB country risk assessment for commanders of bases outside the continental United States.
		<u>A TST is administered and the results are recorded</u>
		• When a person joins the Air Force (AFI48-105).
		• For people who are at high risk for TB infection per CDC guidelines, these including
		  • People in high-risk occupations (for example, health-care workers); the interval of TB testing is based on risk assessment and classification of the facility of employment, CDC guidelines, or consultation with the Air Force Institute of Operational Health.
		  • Air Force employees with clinical indications for TB testing per local Aerospace Medicine Council recommendation (for example, child-care workers).
		• Annually for all people stationed in a high-prevalence overseas area (as indicated by the country risk assessment) who have direct and prolonged contact with high-risk populations or face a high risk of exposure; another TST is administered 3-6 months after return to the continental United States or on transfer to a location with lower TB prevalence (AFI48-105).
		• When a person is transferred from one country to another (personal communication).
		• When a person is transferred back to the United States from a country with a higher incidence of TB than the United States, according to WHO data (personal communication).
			March 1, 2005

Branch of Military	Name of Policy	Requirements (Abbreviated)	Effective Date
		• For family members and other beneficiaries of AF personnel before relocating to a high-prevalence country if they have not previously been tested (AFI48-105). After deployment, Air Force personnel must complete a questionnaire for assessing their risk of exposure to TB (personal communication). The questionnaire enables health-care personnel to determine whether people were in high-prevalence locations, high-risk settings, or both (AFMS Deployment Health Surveillance Implementation Instructions, Appendix 4—TB Risk Assessment, May 2003). People receive a TST within 3 months after deployment if, during deployment, they • Were exposed to a known or suspect case of active TB. • Had direct and prolonged contact with a refugee, displaced person, hospital population, homeless-shelter population, or prison population. • Were deployed to a high-prevalence country. Criterion for further evaluation: People with induration of at least 5 mm are evaluated by primary-care management teams for active TB.	

NOTE: AFMIC = Armed Forces Medical Intelligence Command; CDC = Centers for Disease Control and Prevention; DOD = Department of Defense; LTBI; Latent Tuberculosis Infection; PAHO = Pan-American Health Organization; PPD = Purified Protein Derivative; TST = Tuberculin Skin Test; TB = Tuberculosis; US = United States; WHO = World Health Organization.

SOURCE: Air Force Office of the Surgeon General 2003; Department of the Army 2003; Department of the Army 2005; Department of the Army 2006; Department of the Navy 1993; Department of the Navy 2001; Lamar 2006; Luke 2006; Navy Environmental Health Center 2006; Secretary of the Air Force 2005; Shibukawa-Kent 2006.

Given those data, the only way to determine whether military personnel and reservists have become infected with *M. tuberculosis* during their service is to test all personnel for TB shortly before and after deployment. Such testing would make it possible to trace cases of active TB to periods of military service if that is when infection occurred.

Anticipating Multiple Drug-Resistant *Mycobacterium tuberculosis* Infection

Some *M. tuberculosis* strains are resistant to one or more drugs commonly used to treat LTBI and active TB (WHO 2004). The military's medical corps should obtain the results of available drug-susceptibility tests for *M. tuberculosis* in regions where troops are. WHO periodically publishes a report of such data, *Resistance in the World: Anti-TB Drug Prevalence and Trends*. Those reports could help the military to estimate the likelihood that a person who acquires a TB infection harbors a drug-resistant strain.

WEST NILE VIRUS INFECTION

First isolated in 1937 from a febrile woman in the West Nile Province of Uganda, West Nile virus (WNV) belongs to the Japanese encephalitis virus antigenic complex in the family Flaviviridae (genus *Flavivirus*) and is closely related to St. Louis encephalitis virus. WNV is a 50-nm-diameter single-stranded RNA virus with a nucleocapsid core surrounded by a host-derived lipid membrane (Campbell et al. 2002).

The first human epidemics of West Nile fever were reported in Israel and occurred in 1951-1954; 2 decades later, an outbreak was reported in South Africa. By 1991, the disease had occurred throughout Africa, south Asia, and Europe. WNV has also occurred in Australia and New Zealand, but cases there were poorly documented (Wilson 1991). Later outbreaks were reported in Tunisia (1997), the Czech Republic (1997), Italy (1998), Romania (1996, 1999), the United States (1999), France (2000), and Israel (1997-2000) (Petersen and Roehrig 2001).

The US outbreak of WNV in 1999 marked the virus's debut in the Western Hemisphere (CDC 2005e). WNV spread rapidly from its epicenter in New York City; by 2004, 48 states and the District of Columbia had reported human cases (Table 5.9) (CDC 2005a; Nash et al. 2001). It has been found in Canada and Mexico as well (Gould and Fikrig 2004).

TABLE 5.9 Statistics on US Cases of West Nile Neurologic Disease,[a] 2005

Characteristic	No.
Cases of West Nile neurologic disease	1,165
Median age	57 years (range, 3 months-98 years)
Male	665 (57.1 % of WNND cases)
Deaths	85 (7.3 % of WNND cases)
Median age	75 years (range, 36-98 years)
Acute flaccid paralysis	68 (5.8%)
Median age	53 years (range, 9-84 years)
Male	39 (57.4% of paralysis cases)
Deaths	5 (7.4 % of paralysis cases)

[a] Defined as meningitis, encephalitis, or acute flaccid paralysis.
SOURCE:CDC 2005a.

West Nile virus was considered relatively benign to humans before the 1990s (Solomon and Cardosa 2000). WNV usually causes a self-limited illness, West Nile fever, which is manifested as fever with a variety of other conditions, including rash, arthralgia, myalgia, headaches, and gastrointestinal symptoms.

Since the 1990s, however, there have been reports of increased incidence and severity of WNV illness (Solomon and Cardosa 2000). New neurologic and ophthalmologic manifestations of West Nile encephalitis have been recognized each year since the virus first reached North America in 1999 (Cunha 2004). A small but significant proportion of cases of West Nile neurologic disease (WNND) have led to death, particularly among the elderly. These recent, marked changes in the epidemiology of WNV illness led the committee to include it in this chapter even though the long-term adverse health outcomes of WNV usually are manifest during the acute illness.

Alarm triggered by the sudden change in the incidence and severity of WNV illness must be tempered by the understanding that severe WNV disease remains rare. Only 0.7% of people who become infected with West Nile virus in the United States develop severe neurologic disease, and more than one-third of these recover fully within a year (Klee et al. 2004; Mostashari et al. 2001). About 20% of infected people develop traditional, self-limited West Nile fever, and about 80% are asymptomatic, whereas only 1 in 150 develops neurologic manifestations.

Transmission of West Nile Virus Infection

Although WNV is found in several species of mosquitoes, the vast majority of infections are transmitted by *Culex* spp. (Campbell et al. 2002). These highly ornithophilic vectors transmit the virus among its natural reservoir: birds. Detected in more than 275 species of birds, WNV is particularly virulent for the family *Corvidae*, which includes crows and jays. The virus amplifies itself in birds' bloodstream to a trillion or more virions per milliliter. Mammals are end-stage hosts and may develop disease but do not develop high enough viremia to contribute significantly to the virus's epidemic spread.

WNV is transmissible from human to human through blood transfusions, transplanted organs, the placenta, and breastfeeding (CDC 2002). Between June and December 2003, WNV nucleic acid amplification testing (NAT) was performed on about 6 million units of blood, which resulted in the removal of at least 818 viremic blood donations. However, even with NAT testing, there were 6 cases of transfusion-associated WNV infection due to low levels of virus not detected by the testing method (minipools from 6-16 donations were used rather than individual testing) (CDC 2004c).

Endemicity in Southwest and South-Central Asia

WNV has been reported in Afghanistan, Pakistan, Iran, and other countries in southwest and south-central Asia (Arsen'eva 1982; Hubalek and Halouzka 1999; Naficy and Saidi 1970; Sugamata et al. 1988; Wilson 1991). In Afghanistan, antibodies to WNV were found in Kunduz, Heart, Bamyan, and Helmand provinces (Arsen'eva 1982). In neighboring Pakistan, 50-65% of the population of Karachi reportedly had antibodies to WNV in 1983 and 1985; new infections were identified in 13% of the population during those years (Sugamata et al. 1988). Similarly, a serum survey conducted in northeastern Iran in the late 1960s found that 30% of surveyed subjects had antibodies to WNV (Naficy and Saidi 1970).

Acute West Nile Fever

Most persons infected with WNV are asymptomatic. A seroepidemiologic study of 677 people who lived in New York City during the 1999 outbreak found that 80% of seropositive subjects never developed symptoms (Mostashari et al. 2001). After an incubation period of 2-14 days, 20% of infected subjects developed a nonspecific febrile illness that lasted 3-6 days. Nausea, vomiting, myalgia, and headache are typical symptoms. A generalized maculopapular rash may occur in up to 20% of patients.

About 1 in 150 symptomatic patients in New York City developed WNND (Mostashari et al. 2001), which is often manifested as meningitis (WNM) or encephalitis (WNE) and sometimes as acute flaccid paralysis (AFP). Patients with WNND frequently have movement disorders with tremor, myoclonus, or Parkinsonism (Sejvar et al. 2003). Muscle weakness is also common. Investigators have reported paresis in about 50% of WNND cases and complete flaccid paralysis in 10%; the latter cases lack deep tendon reflexes and mimick GBS. Seizures and focal neurologic findings have been uncommon.

The development of WNND has been directly correlated with age. Of those over 65 years old, 1 in 50 developed WNM or WNE vs 1 in 300 of those under 65 (Mostashari et al. 2001). In fact, in those over 80 years old, the risk of symptomatic neurologic disease was 43 times higher than in those under 19.

West Nile fever without meningitis is more likely in younger patients. Among those with neurologic involvement, meningitis is more common in younger patients (mean age, 35 years), and encephalitis is more common in older patients (mean age, 70 years) (Sejvar et al. 2003).

Patients with West Nile fever who do not have neurologic manifestations might have residual fatigue, muscle weakness, and headache that can persist for months after resolution of the acute febrile illness (Watson et al. 2004). Of 98 patients with laboratory-confirmed West Nile infection but no clinical evidence of WNM, WNE, or AFP, 96% had fatigue for a median of 36 days, 61% had muscle weakness for a median of 28 days, and 71% had headache for a median of 10 days. The median time for recovery to a point that the patients considered "back to normal" was 60 days.

Diagnosis of West Nile Fever

For patients with acute symptomatic WNV infection, relative lymphocytopenia (less then 20%) is common. The cerebrospinal fluid (CSF) reveals a mild lymphocytic pleocytosis with a mean of 38 white cells/mm^3 (range, 0-525) (Nash et al. 2001). Up to one-third may have more then 50% neutrophils on initial evaluation of the CSF. Increased protein with a mean of 104 mg/dL (range, 38-899) can be found. CSF glucose is usually normal.

Imaging studies of the brain usually are normal on computed tomography without evidence of inflammation. Even magnetic resonance imaging scan reveals enhancement of the meninges or periventricular areas in only about 30% of people (Nash et al. 2001). Electromyography reveals a motor axonal polyneuropathy with sparing of the sensory fibers very similar to the findings in poliomyelitis. WNV has a propensity to involve the anterior horn cells of the spinal cord in a manner very similar to poliomyelitis.

Acute infection is diagnosed by demonstration of WNV IgM in serum, which has been found in close to 100% of patients (Tardei et al. 2000). In one study, CSF samples from 94% of patients were WNV-IgM positive (Nash et al. 2001). No cases had virus isolation from CSF, and only 57% of CSF samples and 14% of serum samples were positive with PCR. Patients with WNV may have persistent IgM antibodies for WNV. In a study by Roehrig et al. (2003), seven of 12 patients with serial samples had IgM persistently positive for WNV for 500 or more days.

Prior infection can be detected with measurement of WNV IgG. However, in a survey of 865 deployed front-line troops, 30 had both predeployment and postdeployment IgG antibodies against WNV. There was no evidence of acquisition of infection during deployment: there were no fourfold rises between predeployment and postdeployment samples, and no IgM antibodies were detected. Infection with dengue virus and prior yellow fever virus vaccine may result in detection of cross-reactive antibodies and make interpretation of serologic tests difficult. The above 30 persons' serum samples were also reactive to St. Louis encephalitis, dengue, and yellow fever viruses. Because of the high cross-reactivity with St. Louis encephalitis virus, dengue and yellow fever viruses, confirmation of a positive WNV IgG requires testing with the plaque-reduction neutralization test, which requires a biosafety level 3 facility (Gea-Banacloche et al. 2004). Prior WNV can be confidently diagnosed if the WNV neutralizing-antibody titers are 4 times higher than all the other flavivirus titers.

Treatment of West Nile Virus Infection

There is no known effective treatment for WNV infection. Ribavirin, a guanosine analogue with broad-spectrum antiviral activity, has been shown to have activity against WNV in vitro (Jordan et al. 2000). Ribavirin also has concentrations in CSF that are 70% of those in serum. Ribavirin has been used successfully to treat related viruses including LaCrosse encephalitis, Hantaan, Lassa fever, and hepatitis C viruses (Jordan et al. 2000). However, in an outbreak in Israel, patients treated with ribavirin had a higher mortality than those who were not treated (Petersen and Roehrig 2001). The poor outcomes could have been due to patient selection, with sicker patients being treated with ribavirin, inasmuch as this was a nonrandomized study. If it is effective, the predicted required dose would be high, around 4 g intravenously every day, similar to that for treatment of Lassa fever. Interferon has also been noted to have in vitro activity against WNV and has been used in individual cases (Kalil et al. 2005).

A chimeric WNV vaccine with a type 4 dengue virus backbone (an attenuated deletion mutant) with an attached WNV envelop glycoprotein has been tested in Rhesus monkeys with development of high levels of neutralizing antibodies which protected them from infection (Platonov 2001). Clinical trials in humans are in progress.

Long-Term Adverse Health Outcomes of Infection with West Nile Virus

The scientific community is just beginning to unveil the long-term adverse health outcomes of WNV infection. Two teams of investigators have conducted long-term followup studies of the self-reported health outcomes of people who suffered acute episodes of W est Nile fever, WNM, WNE, or West Nile meningoencephalitis (Gottfried et al. 2005; Klee et al. 2004). All cases were diagnosed clinically and confirmed with laboratory analysis. A rigorous study by Klee and colleagues reports the health status at 6, 12, and 18 months of 42 New York City residents whose acute illnesses were manifested in 1999 and required hospitalization in all but two cases. A less rigorous study by Gottfried and colleagues reports the health status at 12 months of 24 Tennessee residents whose acute illnesses were diagnosed and reported to the state's Department of Health in 2002; all but two of those cases had been hospitalized. About

63% of the New York City patients (22 of 35 patients who participated in a follow-up interview) and 37.5% of the Tennessee patients (nine of 24) suffered persistent cognitive, physical, or functional impairment 12 months after the onset of severe WNV infection (Box 5.2).

BOX 5.2 Persistent Signs and Symptoms of WNV Illness 1 year After Onset

New York cohort ($p \leq 0.002$ relative to baseline function):

- Muscle weakness
- Difficulty in walking
- Fatigue
- Loss of concentration
- Lightheadedness
- Memory loss
- Need for assistance with meal preparation, light housekeeping, and shopping

Tennessee cohort (five most commonly reported symptoms):

- Fatigue
- Muscle weakness
- Difficulty in walking
- Joint weakness
- Headaches

Klee and colleagues followed the New York cohort for 18 months. At that time, 30% of the patients continued to report persistent memory loss, confusion, depression, irritability, and the need for assistance with activities of daily living (mostly those requiring increased strength). Many patients continued to report difficulty in walking, muscle weakness, fatigue, and insomnia; more than 40% reported some combination of these symptoms.

The most important risk factor for long-term morbidity in both cohorts was advanced age, defined as over 50 years by Gottfried et al and at least 65 years by Klee et al. Neither the clinical manifestation of acute WN illness nor the prior presence of underlying disease was predictive of physical or cognitive recovery, Klee et al. found, even after adjusting for age. In the Gottfried et al. study, two of the five patients whose acute illness lacked neurologic involvement reported a full recovery during the 1-year followup interview; the degree of recovery of the other three patients, who moved to nursing facilities after their WNV infection, was not ascertained.

Unlike the retrospective case-series studies based on self-reported symptoms, a prospective, clinical case series of long-term morbidity associated with WNND was conducted with 39 suspect cases of acute WNV infection in Louisiana (Sejvar et al. 2003). The patients all resided in the same parish and presented from August 1 to September 2, 2002.

Hospitalized for their acute conditions, the 39 patients were examined by a neurologist and underwent neuroimaging and electrophysiologic and serologic tests. A second neurologist verified the findings in seven patients. Sixteen subjects tested positive for WNV: five had a diagnosis of WNM, eight WNE, AFP, and one classified AFP and WNE. One subject with WNE died after 2.5 months of hospitalization in a comatose state. Five patients—three with AFP and two with WNE—were discharged to long-term rehabilitation facilities. The other 10 subjects who tested positive went home on discharge.

Eight months later, a neurologist re-examined the 15 surviving patients with WNND, who also answered a standardized questionnaire about their symptoms and functional status. The most commonly reported adverse health outcomes were fatigue, tremor, and mild parkinsonism. Eleven subjects were home and functioning independently; three were home but dependent, and one was still undergoing rehabilitation. The five patients with WNM functioned at normal or nearly normal levels, according to the results of Barthel and modified Rankin scoring systems. Five patients with severe WNE also had recovered premorbid levels of functioning without residual disability; two WNE patients relied on walkers.

The three patients with AFP were faring poorly 8 months after onset. All continued to experience profound muscle weakness; they required wheelchairs and had difficulty in accomplishing such daily activities as grooming and housekeeping. Clinical findings and electrodiagnostic data on two of them suggested a poliomyelitis-like syndrome with involvement of anterior horn cells of the spinal cord. Electromyographic data suggested chronic denervation and permanent loss of motor axons in affected limbs.

Long-Term Prognosis of West Nile Virus-Positive Patients with Focal Neurologic Deficits

A number of studies have been conducted to elucidate the outcomes of patients infected with West Nile virus who develop focal neurologic deficits, especially AFP. Saad and colleagues (2005) reviewed all cases of AFP related to WNV reported in the English-language literature from January 1999 to March 2004 whose clinical characteristics were described in sufficient detail (53 subjects, including the three described above); they added three cases of their own. Forty of the 56 subjects survived the acute phase of disease had a known long-term health outcome. All 40 suffered some degree of persistent neurologic impairment or weakness at the time of long-term followup. As a case in point, the authors noted a survivor who remained quadriplegic and ventilator-dependent after 20 months of followup.

In cases of WNV-induced focal neurologic deficits, the rate and degree of recovery of muscle strength appears to vary by limb and patient; the initial severity of paralysis may not predict the final outcome (Cao et al. 2005). Cao and colleagues reached those conclusions by measuring the muscle strength and overall motor function of 11 subjects for 6-21 months after the onset of AFP. A 36-year-old woman paralyzed in one leg recovered minimal strength during the 21-month period. In contrast, a 44-year-old man with severe four-limb paralysis who was hospitalized for respiratory distress started to walk within 1 month and recovered full strength in all limbs after 9 months (with decreased endurance). Between those extremes, a third patient became paralyzed to various degrees in four limbs and was partially recovered at 21 months. A small case-control study suggested a correlation between the estimated numbers of surviving motor units in a muscle and the degree of improvement of muscle strength (Cao et al. 2005).

Pathologic Plausibility of Long-Term Neurologic Deficits in Patients with West Nile Neurologic Disease

Neurophysiologic, radiologic, and pathologic studies in humans and animals indicate that the underlying mechanism of WNV AFP is damage to the anterior horn cells of the spinal cord akin to the damage caused by poliomyelitis virus (Saad et al. 2005). That suggests that most patients with WNV AFP will not recover completely.

As Klee et al. (2004) noted, WNV infection is clinically similar to St. Louis encephalitis. Patients with the latter disease have reported disability up to 5 years after the acute illness. Persistent symptoms of St. Louis encephalitis have included fatigue, headache, nervousness, inability to concentrate, depression, and problems with gait and balance throughout the convalescent period of 6 months to 3 years.

The committee concludes that there is sufficient evidence of an association between acute West Nile virus infection and variable levels of physical, functional, or cognitive disability that may persist for months, years, or permanently.

Recommendation

It has been just 10 years since the potential long-term adverse health outcomes of WNV infection became an international public-health concern. The body of evidence on which this committee can base its conclusions is small. Future investigators will be able to conduct more robust studies on the long-term adverse health outcomes of patients who suffer acute infection by WNV, and create a broader foundation for conclusions about the acute illness and its long-term adverse health outcomes. The committee recommends that the Department of Veterans Affairs (VA) periodically review the literature on long-term adverse health outcomes of WNV infection to supplement the conclusions of this committee.

REFERENCES

Abo-Shehada MN, Odeh JS, Abu-Essud M, Abuharfeil N. 1996. Seroprevalence of brucellosis among high risk people in northern Jordan. *International Journal of Epidemiology* 25(2):450-454.

Air Force Office of the Surgeon General. 2003. AFMS Deployment Health Surveillance Implementation Instructions.

Akritidis N, Pappas G. 2001. Ascites caused by brucellosis: A report of two cases. *Scandinavian Journal of Gastroenterology* 36(1):110-112.

Al Dahouk S, Tomaso H, Nockler K, Neubauer H, Frangoulidis D. 2003. Laboratory-based diagnosis of brucellosis—a review of the literature. Part II: Serological tests for brucellosis. *Clinica y Laboratorio* 49(11-12):577-589.

al Deeb SM, Yaqub BA, Sharif HS, Phadke JG. 1989. Neurobrucellosis: Clinical characteristics, diagnosis, and outcome. *Neurology* 39(4):498-501.

al-Harthi SS. 1989. The morbidity and mortality pattern of Brucella endocarditis. *International Journal of Cardiology* 25(3):321-324.

al-Kaff AS. 1995. Ocular brucellosis. *International Ophthalmology Clinics* 35(3):139-145.

Alarcon GS, Bocanegra TS, Gotuzzo E, Hinostroza S, Carrillo C, Vasey FB, Germain BF, Espinoza LR. 1981. Reactive arthritis associated with brucellosis: HAL studies. *Journal of Rheumatology* 8(4):621-625.

Allos BM. 1997. Association between Campylobacter infection and Guillain-Barre syndrome. *Journal of Infectious Diseases* 176 (2 Suppl):S125-S128.

Allos BM. 2001. Campylobacter jejuni infections: Update on emerging issues and trends. *Clinical Infectious Diseases* 32(8):1201-1206.

Almuneef M, Memish ZA. 2003. Prevalence of Brucella antibodies after acute brucellosis. *Journal of Chemotherapy* 15(2):148-151.

Amino R, Menard R, Frischknecht F. 2005. In vivo imaging of malaria parasites—Recent advances and future directions. *Current Opinion in Microbiology* 8(4):407-414.

Araj GF, Lulu AR, Khateeb MI, Saadah MA, Shakir RA. 1988. ELISA versus routine tests in the diagnosis of patients with systemic and neurobrucellosis. *APMIS: Acta Pathologica, Microbiologica et Immunologica Scandinavica* 96(2):171-176.

Ardies CM. 2003. Inflammation as cause for scar cancers of the lung. *Integrative Cancer Therapies* 2(3):238-246.

Ariza J, Gudiol F, Valverde J, Pallares R, Fernandez-Viladrich P, Rufi G, Espadaler L, Fernandez-Nogues F. 1985. Brucellar spondylitis: A detailed analysis based on current findings. *Reviews of Infectious Diseases* 7(5):656-664.

Ariza J, Pellicer T, Pallares R, Foz A, Gudiol F. 1992. Specific antibody profile in human brucellosis. *Clinical Infectious Diseases* 14(1):131-140.

Ariza J, Pujol M, Valverde J, Nolla JM, Rufi G, Viladrich PF, Corredoira JM, Gudiol F. 1993. Brucellar sacroiliitis: Findings in 63 episodes and current relevance. *Clinical Infectious Diseases* 16(6):761-765.

Ariza J, Pigrau C, Canas C, Marron A, Martinez F, Almirante B, Corredoira JM, Casanova A, Fabregat J, Pahissa A. 2001. Current understanding and management of chronic hepatosplenic suppurative brucellosis. *Clinical Infectious Diseases* 32(7):1024-1033.

Aronson NE, Wortmann GW, Johnson SC, Jackson JE, Gasser RA Jr, Magill AJ, Endy TP, Coyne PE, Grogl M, Benson PM, Beard JS, Tally JD, Gambel JM, Kreutzer RD, Oster CN. 1998. Safety and efficacy of intravenous sodium stibogluconate in the treatment of leishmaniasis: Recent US military experience. *Clinical Infectious Diseases* 27(6):1457-1464.

Arsen'eva LP. 1982. Natural-focus zoonoses in Afghanistan: A review of the literature. *Meditsinskaia Parazitologiia i Parazitarnye Bolezni* 51(3):54-59.

Ayres JG, Flint N, Smith EG, Tunnicliffe WS, Fletcher TJ, Hammond K, Ward D, Marmion BP. 1998. Post-infection fatigue syndrome following Q fever. *QJM* 91(2):105-123.

Baird JK. 2005. Effectiveness of antimalarial drugs. *New England Journal of Medicine* 352(15):1565-1577.

Bajiya HN, Kochar DK. 1996. Incidence and outcome of neurological sequelae in survivors of cerebral malaria. *Journal of the Association of Physicians of India* 44(10):679-681.

Baldi PC, Miguel SE, Fossati CA, Wallach JC. 1996. Serological follow-up of human brucellosis by measuring IgG antibodies to lipopolysaccharide and cytoplasmic proteins of Brucella species. *Clinical Infectious Diseases* 22(3):446-455.

Balo KP, Mensah A, Mihluedo H. 1996. Chloroquine maculopathy and prevention of malaria. *Journal Francais d Ophtalmologie* 19(12):770-776.

Bashir R, Al-Kawi MZ, Harder EJ, Jinkins J. 1985. Nervous system brucellosis: Diagnosis and treatment. *Neurology* 35(11):1576-1581.

Basset D, Faraut F, Marty P, Dereure J, Rosenthal E, Mary C, Pratlong F, Lachaud L, Bastien P, Dedet JP. 2005. Visceral leishmaniasis in organ transplant recipients: 11 new cases and a review of the literature. *Microbes and Infection* 7(13):1370-1375.

Beare NA, Lewis DK, Kublin JG, Harding SP, Zijlstra EE, Molyneux ME. 2003. Retinal changes in adults with cerebral malaria. *Annals of Tropical Medicine and Parasitology* 97(3):313-315.

Begue JJ. 1964. Ocular complications observed during synthetic antimalarial treatment. *Clinique* 59:287-291.

Bennish ML. 1991. Potentially lethal complications of shigellosis. *Reviews of Infectious Diseases* 13 (4 Suppl):S319-S324.

Bergin PS, Haas LF, Miller DH. 1989. Tuberculous meningitis at Wellington Hospital 1962-88. *New Zealand Medical Journal* 102(878):554-556.

Bernit E, Pouget J, Janbon F, Dutronc H, Martinez P, Brouqui P, Raoult D. 2002. Neurological involvement in acute Q fever: A report of 29 cases and review of the literature. *Archives of Internal Medicine* 162(6):693-700.

Bernstein HN. 1967. Chloroquine ocular toxicity. *Survey of Ophthalmology* 12(5):415-447.

Berry A, Fabre R, Benoit-Vical F, Cassaing S, Magnaval JF. 2005. Contribution of PCR-based methods to diagnosis and management of imported malaria. *Medecine Tropicale* 65(2): 176-183.

Bhattacharya SK, Sur D. 2003. An evaluation of current shigellosis treatment. *Expert Opinion on Pharmacotherapy* 4(8):1315-1320.

Biswas J, Fogla R, Srinivasan P, Narayan S, Haranath K, Badrinath V. 1996. Ocular malaria. A clinical and histopathologic study. *Ophthalmology* 103(9):1471-1475.

Blaser MJ. 2000. *Campylobacter jejuni* and related species. In: Mandell GL, Bennett JE, Dolin R, Editors. *Principles and Practice of Infectious Diseases*. 5th ed. New York: Churchill Livingstone. Pp. 2276-2285.

Blaser MJ. 2005. Infections due to *Campylobacter* and related species. In: Kasper DL, Braunwald E, Fauci A, Hauser SL, Longo DL, Jameson JL, Editors. *Harrison's Principles of Internal Medicine*. 16th ed. New York: McGraw-Hill. Pp. 907-909.

Blaser MJ, Perez GP, Smith PF, Patton C, Tenover FC, Lastovica AJ, Wang WI. 1986. Extraintestinal Campylobacter jejuni and Campylobacter coli infections: Host factors and strain characteristics. *Journal of Infectious Diseases* 153(3):552-559.

Bloom PD, MacPhail AP, Klugman K, Louw M, Raubenheimer C, Fischer C. 1994. Haemolytic-uraemic syndrome in adults with resistant Shigella dysenteriae type I. *Lancet* 344(8916):206.

Bodur H, Erbay A, Akinci E, Colpan A, Cevik MA, Balaban N. 2003. Neurobrucellosis in an endemic area of brucellosis. *Scandinavian Journal of Infectious Diseases* 35(2):94-97.

Bouza E, Garcia de la Torre M, Parras F, Guerrero A, Rodriguez-Creixems M, Gobernado J. 1987. Brucellar meningitis. *Reviews of Infectious Diseases* 9(4):810-822.

Bravo MJ, Colmenero Jde D, Alonso A, Caballero A. 2003. HLA-B*39 allele confers susceptibility to osteoarticular complications in human brucellosis. *Journal of Rheumatology* 30(5):1051-1053.

Breman JG. 2001. The ears of the hippopotamus: Manifestations, determinants, and estimates of the malaria burden. *American Journal of Tropical Medicine and Hygiene* 64(1-2 Suppl):1-11.

Bremell T, Bjelle A, Svedhem A. 1991. Rheumatic symptoms following an outbreak of campylobacter enteritis: A five year follow up. *Annals of the Rheumatic Diseases* 50(12):934-938.

Brouqui P, Dupont HT, Drancourt M, Berland Y, Etienne J, Leport C, Goldstein F, Massip P, Micoud M, Bertrand A, et al. 1993. Chronic Q fever. Ninety-two cases from France, including 27 cases without endocarditis. *Archives of Internal Medicine* 153(5):642-648.

Butcher GA. 2005. T-cell depletion and immunity to malaria in HIV-infections. *Parasitology* 130(Pt 2):141-150.

Buxton JA, Fyfe M, Berger S, Cox MB, Northcott KA. 2002. Reactive arthritis and other sequelae following sporadic Salmonella typhimurium infection in British Columbia, Canada: A case control study. *Journal of Rheumatology* 29(10):2154-2158.

Calin A, Fries JF. 1976. An "experimental" epidemic of Reiter's syndrome revisited. Follow-up evidence on genetic and environmental factors. *Annals of Internal Medicine* 84(5):564-566.

Camarca MM, Krauss MR. 2001. Active tuberculosis among US Army personnel, 1980 to 1996. *Military Medicine: International Journal of AMSUS* 166(5):452-456.

Campbell GL, Marfin AA, Lanciotti RS, Gubler DJ. 2002. West Nile virus. *The Lancet Infectious Diseases* 2(9):519-529.

Cao NJ, Ranganathan C, Kupsky WJ, Li J. 2005. Recovery and prognosticators of paralysis in West Nile virus infection. *Journal of the Neurological Sciences* 236(1-2):73-80.

CDC (Centers for Disease Control and Prevention). 1986. Annual summary 1984. Reported morbidity and mortality in the United States. *Morbidity and Mortality Weekly Report* 33(54):1-135.

CDC. 1992. 1993 revised classification system for HIV infection and expanded surveillance case definition for AIDS among adolescents and adults. *Morbidity and Mortality Weekly Report* 41(RR-17):1-19.

CDC. 2000a. Diagnostic Standards and Classification of Tuberculosis in Adults and Children. This official statement of the American Thoracic Society and the Centers for Disease Control and Prevention was adopted by the ATS Board of Directors, July 1999. This statement was endorsed by the Council of the Infectious Disease Society of America, September 1999. *American Journal of Respiratory and Critical Care Medicine* 161(4 Pt 1):1376-1395.

CDC. 2000b. Targeted tuberculin testing and treatment of latent tuberculosis infection. American Thoracic Society. *Morbidity and Mortality Weekly Report: Recommendations and Reports* 49(RR-6):1-51.

CDC. 2002. Update: Investigations of West Nile virus infections in recipients of organ transplantation and blood transfusion. *Morbidity and Mortality Weekly Report* 51(37):833-836.

CDC. 2003a. Treatment of tuberculosis. *Morbidity and Mortality Weekly Report: Recommendations and Reports* 52(RR-11):1-77.

CDC. 2003b. Cutaneous leishmaniasis in US military personnel—Southwest/Central Asia, 2002-2003. *Morbidity and Mortality Weekly Report* 52(42):1009-1012.

CDC. 2004a. Two cases of visceral leishmaniasis in US military personnel—Afghanistan, 2002-2004. *Morbidity and Mortality Weekly Report* 53 (12):265-268.

CDC. 2004b. Update: Cutaneous leishmaniasis in US military personnel—Southwest/Central Asia, 2002-2004. *Morbidity and Mortality Weekly Report* 53(12):264-265.

CDC. 2004c. Update: West Nile virus screening of blood donations and transfusion-associated transmission—United States, 2003. *Morbidity and Mortality Weekly Report* 53(13):281-284.

CDC. 2005a. *Statistics, Surveillance, and Control, 2005 West Nile Virus Activity in the United States*. [Online]. Available: http://www.cdc.gov/ncidod/dvbid/westnile/surv&controlCaseCount05_detailed.htm [accessed April 26, 2006].

CDC. 2005b. *Typhoid Fever: Fequently Asked Questions*. [Online]. Available: http://www.cdc.gov/ncidod/dbmd/diseaseinfo/files/typhoid_fever_FAQ.pdf [accessed April 26, 2006].

CDC. 2005c. Reported Tuberculosis in the United States, 2004. US Department of Health and Human Services.

CDC. 2005d. Guidelines for the investigation of contacts of persons with infectious tuberculosis. Recommendations from the National Tuberculosis Controllers Association and CDC. *Morbidity and Mortality Weekly Report: Recommendations and Reports* 54(RR-15):1-47.

CDC. 2005e. West Nile Virus Activity—United States, January 1—December 1, 2005. *Morbidity and Mortality Weekly Report* 54(49):1253-1256.

Center for Infectious Disease Research and Policy, University of Minnesota. 2006. *Salmonellosis*. [Online]. Available: http://www.cidrap.umn/edu/cidrap/content/fs/food-disease/causes/salmoview.html [accessed April 26, 2006].

Cetinkaya B, Kalender H, Ertas HB, Muz A, Arslan N, Ongor H, Gurcay M. 2000. Seroprevalence of coxiellosis in cattle, sheep and people in the east of Turkey. *Veterinary Record* 146(5):131-136.

Chakravarty A, Ghosh B, Bhattacharyya R, Sengupta S, Mukherjee S. 2004. Acute inflammatory demyelinating polyneuropathy following plasmodium vivax malaria. *Neurology India* 52(1):130-131.

Chen M, Delpech V, O'Sullivan B, Donovan B. 2002. Shigella sonnei: Another cause of sexually acquired reactive arthritis. *International Journal of STD and AIDS* 13(2):135-136.

Choi CM, Lerner EA. 2002. Leishmaniasis: Recognition and management with a focus on the immunocompromised patient. *American Journal of Clinical Dermatology* 3(2):91-105.

Choi HJ, Lee SY, Yang H, Bang JK. 2004. Retinal haemorrhage in vivax malaria. *Transactions of the Royal Society of Tropical Medicine and Hygiene* 98(6):387-389.

Chomel BB, DeBess EE, Mangiamele DM, Reilly KF, Farver TB, Sun RK, Barrett LR. 1994. Changing trends in the epidemiology of human brucellosis in California from 1973 to 1992: A shift toward foodborne transmission. *Journal of Infectious Diseases* 170(5):1216-1223.

Colmenero JD, Reguera JM, Martos F, Sanchez-De-Mora D, Delgado M, Causse M, Martin-Farfan A, Juarez C. 1996. Complications associated with Brucella melitensis infection: A study of 530 cases. *Medicine* 75(4):195-211.

Colmenero JD, Queipo-Ortuno MI, Maria Reguera J, Angel Suarez-Munoz M, Martin-Carballino S, Morata P. 2002. Chronic hepatosplenic abscesses in Brucellosis. Clinico-therapeutic features and molecular diagnostic approach. *Diagnostic Microbiology and Infectious Disease* 42(3):159-167.

Comstock GW, Edwards LB, Livesay VT. 1974a. Tuberculosis morbidity in the US Navy: Its distribution and decline. *American Review of Respiratory Disease* 110(5):572-580.

Comstock GW, Livesay VT, Woolpert SF. 1974b. The prognosis of a positive tuberculin reaction in childhood and adolescence. *American Journal of Epidemiology* 99(2):131-138.

Cope SE, Schultz GW, Richards AL, Savage HM, Smith GC, Mitchell CJ, Fryauff DJ, Conlon JM, Corneil JA, Hyams KC. 1996. Assessment of arthropod vectors of infectious diseases in areas of US troop deployment in the Persian Gulf. *American Journal of Tropical Medicine and Hygiene* 54(1):49-53.

Crosby E, Llosa L, Miro Quesada M, Carrillo C, Gotuzzo E. 1984. Hematologic changes in brucellosis. *Journal of Infectious Diseases* 150(3):419-424.

Cunha BA. 2004. Differential diagnosis of West Nile encephalitis. *Current Opinion in Infectious Diseases* 17(5):413-420.

Cunningham AC. 2002. Parasitic adaptive mechanisms in infection by leishmania. *Experimental and Molecular Pathology* 72(2):132-141.

Dalrymple-Champneys W. 1950. Undulant fever, a neglected problem. *Lancet* 1:429-777.

Davies NE, Haverty JR, Boatwright M. 1969. Reiter's disease associated with shigellosis. *Southern Medical Journal* 62(8):1011-1014.

Davies PD. 2005. Risk Factors for Tuberculosis. *Monaldi Archives of Chest Disease* 63(1):37-45.

Department of the Army. 2003. Army Latent Tuberculosis Infection (LTBI) Surveillance and Control Program. Office of the Surgeon General.

Department of the Army. 2005. *Army Regulation 40-5 Medical Services: Preventive Medicine*. [Online]. Available: http://www.usapa.army.mil/pdffiles/r40_5.pdf [accessed May 8, 2006].

Department of the Army. 2006. *Personnel Policy Guidance (PPG) of Operations Iraqi Freedom (OIF), Enduring Freedom (OEF) and Noble Eagle (ONE)*. [Online]. Available: http://www.armyg1.army.mil/MilitaryPersonnel/ppg.asp [accessed May 8, 2006].

Department of the Navy. 1993. *Bumed Instruction 6224.8 Change Transmittal: Tuberculosis Control Program*. [Online]. Available: http://www.nehc.med.navy.mil/nepmu2/pmttoolbox/IMMUNIZATIONS1_files/Instructions%20&%20Notices/BUMEDINST%206224.8%20CH-1.pdf [accessed May 8, 2006].

Department of the Navy. 2001. *BUMED, Tuberculosis Control Program - Clarification*. [Online]. Available: http://www.nehc.med.navy.mil/nepmu2/pmttoolbox/IMMUNIZATIONS1_files/Immunization%20Messages/TB%20clar%204-01%20241350Z.txt [accessed May 8, 2006].

Derrick E. 1937. Q Fever, a new fever entity: Clinical features, diagnosis and laboratory investigation. *Medical Journal of Australia* 2:281-299.

Desjeux P. 2004. Leishmaniasis: Current situation and new perspectives. *Comparative Immunology, Microbiology and Infectious Diseases* 27(5):305-318.

Dey AB, Trikha I, Banerjee M, Jain R, Nagarkar KM . 2001. Acute disseminated encephalomyelitis—another cause of post malaria cerebellar ataxia. *Journal of the Association of Physicians of India* 49:756-758.

Digre KB. 2003. Not so benign intracranial hypertension. *British Medical Journal (Clinical Research Ed.)* 326(7390):613-614.

Digre KB, Corbett JJ. 2001. Idiopathic intracranial hypertension (pseudotumor cerebri): A reappraisal. *The Neurologist* 7:2-68.

Dingle KE, Van Den Braak N, Colles FM, Price LJ, Woodward DL, Rodgers FG, Endtz HP, Van Belkum A, Maiden MC. 2001. Sequence typing confirms that Campylobacter jejuni strains associated with Guillain-Barre and Miller-Fisher syndromes are of diverse genetic lineage, serotype, and flagella type. *Journal of Clinical Microbiology* 39(9):3346-3349.

Doganay M, Aygen B, Inan M, Ozbakir O. 1993. Brucella peritonitis in a cirrhotic patient with ascites. *European Journal of Medicine* 2(7):441-442.

Doyle TJ, Bryan RT. 2000. Infectious disease morbidity in the US region bordering Mexico, 1990-1998. *Journal of Infectious Diseases* 182(5):1503-1510.

Drancourt M, Raoult D, Xeridat B, Milandre L, Nesri M, Dano P. 1991. Q fever meningoencephalitis in five patients. *European Journal of Epidemiology* 7(2):134-138.

Dube MP, Holtom PD, Larsen RA. 1992. Tuberculous meningitis in patients with and without human immunodeficiency virus infection. *American Journal of Medicine* 93(5):520-524.

Dworkin MS, Shoemaker PC, Goldoft MJ, Kobayashi JM. 2001. Reactive arthritis and Reiter's syndrome following an outbreak of gastroenteritis caused by Salmonella enteritidis. *Clinical Infectious Diseases* 33(7):1010-1014.

Easterbrook M. 1999. Detection and prevention of maculopathy associated with antimalarial agents. *International Ophthalmology Clinics* 39(2):49-57.

Eastmond CJ, Rennie JA, Reid TM. 1983. An outbreak of Campylobacter enteritis—A rheumatological followup survey. *Journal of Rheumatology* 10(1):107-108.

Eiam-Ong S. 2003. Malarial nephropathy. *Seminars in Nephrology* 23(1):21-33.

El Hassan AM, Ali MS, Zijlstra E, Eltoum IA, Ghalib HW, Ahmed HM. 1992. Post-kala-azar dermal leishmaniasis in the Sudan: Peripheral neural involvement. *International Journal of Dermatology* 31(6):400-403.

Eliades MJ, Shah S, Nguyen-Dinh P, Newman RD, Barber AM, Nguyen-Dinh P, Roberts JM, Mali S, Parise ME, Barber AM, Steketee R. 2005. Malaria surveillance—United States, 2003. *Morbidity and Mortality Weekly Report: Surveillance Summaries* 54(2):25-40.

Enders U, Karch H, Toyka KV, Michels M, Zielasek J, Pette M, Heesemann J, Hartung HP. 1993. The spectrum of immune responses to Campylobacter jejuni and glycoconjugates in Guillain-Barre syndrome and in other neuroimmunological disorders. *Annals of Neurology* 34(2):136-144.

Falchook GS, Malone CM, Upton S, Shandera WX. 2003. Postmalaria neurological syndrome after treatment of Plasmodium falciparum malaria in the United States. *Clinical Infectious Diseases* 37(2):e22-e24.

Fasanaro AM, Scoleri G, Pizza V, Gaeta GB, Fasanaro A. 1991. Guillain-Barre syndrome as presenting manifestation of visceral leishmaniasis. *Lancet* 338(8775):1142.

FDA (Food and Drug Administration). 2005. *PMA Final Decisions Rendered for December 2004*. [Online]. Available: http://fda.gov/cdrh/pma/pmadec04.html [accessed May 8, 2006].

Fenollar F, Fournier PE, Carrieri MP, Habib G, Messana T, Raoult D. 2001. Risks factors and prevention of Q fever endocarditis. *Clinical Infectious Diseases* 33(3):312-316.

Fenollar F, Thuny F, Xeridat B, Lepidi H, Raoult D. 2006. Endocarditis after acute Q fever in patients with previously undiagnosed valvulopathies. *Clinical Infectious Diseases* 42(6): 818-821.

Ferrante MA, Dolan MJ. 1993. Q fever meningoencephalitis in a soldier returning from the Persian Gulf War. *Clinical Infectious Diseases* 16(4):489-496.

Finch M, Rodey G, Lawrence D, Blake P. 1986. Epidemic Reiter's syndrome following an outbreak of shigellosis. *European Journal of Epidemiology* 2(1):26-30.

Fosgate GT, Carpenter TE, Chomel BB, Case JT, DeBess EE, Reilly KF. 2002. Time-space clustering of human brucellosis, California, 1973-1992. *Emerging Infectious Diseases* 8(7):672-678.

Fournier PE, Casalta JP, Piquet P, Tournigand P, Branchereau A, Raoult D. 1998. Coxiella burnetii infection of aneurysms or vascular grafts: Report of seven cases and review. *Clinical Infectious Diseases* 26(1):116-121.

Fox KF, Fox A, Nagpal M, Steinberg P, Heroux K. 1998. Identification of Brucella by ribosomal-spacer-region PCR and differentiation of Brucella canis from other Brucella spp. pathogenic for humans by carbohydrate profiles. *Journal of Clinical Microbiology* 36(11):3217-3222.

Fryauff DJ, Modi GB, Mansour NS, Kreutzer RD, Soliman S, Youssef FG. 1993. Epidemiology of cutaneous leishmaniasis at a focus monitored by the multinational force and observers in the northeastern Sinai Desert of Egypt. *American Journal of Tropical Medicine and Hygiene* 49(5):598-607.

Gami AS, Antonios VS, Thompson RL, Chaliki HP, Ammash NM. 2004. Q fever endocarditis in the United States. *Mayo Clinic Proceedings* 79(2):253-257.

Gardner K, Cox T, Digre KB. 1995. Idiopathic intracranial hypertension associated with tetracycline use in fraternal twins: Case reports and review. *Neurology* 45(1):6-10.

Gea-Banacloche J, Johnson RT, Bagic A, Butman JA, Murray PR, Agrawal AG. 2004. West Nile virus: Pathogenesis and therapeutic options. *Annals of Internal Medicine* 140(7):545-553.

Geyik MF, Gur A, Nas K, Cevik R, Sarac J, Dikici B, Ayaz C. 2002. Musculoskeletal involvement of brucellosis in different age groups: A study of 195 cases. *Swiss Medical Weekly* 132(7-8):98-105.

Giles CL, Henderson JW. 1965. The ocular toxicity of chloroquine therapy. *American Journal of the Medical Sciences* 249:230-235.

Glynn, JR. Resurgence of tuberculosis and the impact of HIV infection. *British Medical Bulletin* 54(3): 579-593.

Gokul BN, Paul A, Hussein I. 2000. Neurobrucellosis. *Saudi Medical Journal* 21(6):577-580.

Good AE. 1979. Shigellae and Reiter's syndrome. *Annals of the Rheumatic Diseases* 38 (1 Suppl):S119-S122.

Goossens H, Marcelis L, Dekeyser P, Butzler JP. 1983. Brucella melitensis: Person-to-person transmission? *Lancet* 1(8327):773.

Gordon JD, MacKeen AD, Marrie TJ, Fraser DB. 1984. The radiographic features of epidemic and sporadic Q fever pneumonia. *Journal of the Canadian Association of Radiologists* 35(3):293-296.

Gottesman G, Vanunu D, Maayan MC, Lang R, Uziel Y, Sagi H, Wolach B. 1996. Childhood brucellosis in Israel. *Pediatric Infectious Disease Journal* 15(7):610-615.

Gottfried K, Quinn R, Jones T. 2005. Clinical description and follow-up investigation of human West Nile virus cases. *Southern Medical Journal* 98(6):603-606.

Gotuzzo E, Alarcon GS, Bocanegra TS, Carrillo C, Guerra JC, Rolando I, Espinoza LR. 1982. Articular involvement in human brucellosis: A retrospective analysis of 304 cases. *Seminars in Arthritis and Rheumatism* 12(2):245-255.

Gotuzzo E, Carrillo C, Guerra J, Llosa L. 1986. An evaluation of diagnostic methods for brucellosis—the value of bone marrow culture. *Journal of Infectious Diseases* 153(1): 122-125.

Gotuzzo E, Seas C, Guerra JG, Carrillo C, Bocanegra TS, Calvo A, Castaneda O, Alarcon GS. 1987. Brucellar arthritis: A study of 39 Peruvian families. *Annals of the Rheumatic Diseases* 46(7):506-509.

Gould LH, Fikrig E. 2004. West Nile virus: A growing concern? *Journal of Clinical Investigation* 113(8):1102-1107.

Gruenewald R, Ropper AH, Lior H, Chan J, Lee R, Molinaro VS. 1991. Serologic evidence of Campylobacter jejuni/coli enteritis in patients with Guillain-Barre syndrome. *Archives of Neurology* 48(10):1080-1082.

Guerrant RL, Walker DH, Weller PF. 1999. *Tropical Infectious Diseases: Principles, Pathogens, and Practice.* 1st ed. Philadelphia, PA: Churchill Livingstone.

Gungor K, Bekir NA, Namiduru M. 2002. Ocular complications associated with brucellosis in an endemic area. *European Journal of Ophthalmology* 12(3):232-237.

Gur A, Geyik MF, Dikici B, Nas K, Cevik R, Sarac J, Hosoglu S. 2003. Complications of brucellosis in different age groups: A study of 283 cases in southeastern Anatolia of Turkey. *Yonsei Medical Journal* 44(1):33-44.

Halpern Z, Dan M, Giladi M, Schwartz I, Sela O, Levo Y. 1989. Shigellosis in adults: Epidemiologic, clinical, and laboratory features. *Medicine* 68(4):210-217.

Hannu T, Leirisalo-Repo M. 1988. Clinical picture of reactive salmonella arthritis. *Journal of Rheumatology* 15(11):1668-1671.

Hannu T, Mattila L, Rautelin H, Pelkonen P, Lahdenne P, Siitonen A, Leirisalo-Repo M. 2002. Campylobacter-triggered reactive arthritis: A population-based study. *Rheumatology* 41(3):312-318.

Hannu T, Kauppi M, Tuomala M, Laaksonen I, Klemets P, Kuusi M. 2004a. Reactive arthritis following an outbreak of Campylobacter jejuni infection. *Journal of Rheumatology* 31(3):528-30.

Hannu T, Sihto-Kauppi K, Kotaniemi K, Kauppi M. 2004b. Acute anterior uveitis in association with an outbreak of Campylobacter jejuni infection. *Scandinavian Journal of Rheumatology* 33(1):55-57.

Hannu T, Mattila L, Siitonen A, Leirisalo-Repo M. 2005. Reactive arthritis attributable to Shigella infection: A clinical and epidemiological nationwide study. *Annals of the Rheumatic Diseases* 64(4):594-598.

Hariharan H, Naseema K, Kumaran C, Shanmugam J, Nair MD, Radhakrishnan K. 1996. Detection of Campylobacter jejuni/C.coli infection in patients with Guillain-Barre syndrome by serology and culture. *New Microbiologica* 19(3):267-271.

Harrington PT, Gutierrez JJ, Ramirez-Ronda CH, Quinones-Soto R, Bermudez RH, Chaffey J. 1982. Granulomatous hepatitis. *Reviews of Infectious Diseases* 4(3):638-655.

Hart PD, Sutherland I. 1977. BCG and vole bacillus vaccines in the prevention of tuberculosis in adolescence and early adult life. *British Medical Journal* 2(6082):293-295.

Hasanjani Roushan MR, Mohrez M, Smailnejad Gangi SM, Soleimani Amiri MJ, Hajiahmadi M. 2004. Epidemiological features and clinical manifestations in 469 adult patients with brucellosis in Babol, Northern Iran. *Epidemiology and Infection* 132(6):1109-1114.

Hatchette TF, Hayes M, Merry H, Schlech WF, Marrie TJ. 2003. The effect of C. burnetii infection on the quality of life of patients following an outbreak of Q fever. *Epidemiology and Infection* 130(3):491-495.

Hawker JI, Ayres JG, Blair I, Evans MR, Smith DL, Smith EG, Burge PS, Carpenter MJ, Caul EO, Coupland B, Desselberger U, Farrell ID, Saunders PJ, Wood MJ. 1998. A large outbreak of Q fever in the West Midlands: Windborne spread into a metropolitan area? *Communicable Disease and Public Health* 1(3):180-187.

Helbig KJ, Heatley SL, Harris RJ, Mullighan CG, Bardy PG, Marmion BP. 2003. Variation in immune response genes and chronic Q fever. Concepts: Preliminary test with post-Q fever fatigue syndrome. *Genes and Immunity* 4(1):82-85.

Helbig K, Harris R, Ayres J, Dunckley H, Lloyd A , Robson J, Marmion BP. 2005. Immune response genes in the post-Q-fever fatigue syndrome, Q fever endocarditis and uncomplicated acute primary Q fever. *QJM* 98(8):565-574.

Hertig M, Sabin AB. 1964. Sandfly fever (pappataci, Phlebotomus, three-day fever). In: Hoff EC, Editor. *Preventive Medicine in World War II: Communicable Diseases*. Volume 7. Office of the Surgeon General, US Department of the Army. Pp. 109-174.

Hewitt S, Reyburn H, Ashford R, Rowland M. 1998. Anthroponotic cutaneous leishmaniasis in Kabul, Afghanistan: Vertical distribution of cases in apartment blocks. *Transactions of the Royal Society of Tropical Medicine and Hygiene* 92(3):273-274.

Heymann DL. 2004. *Control of Communicable Diseases Manual*. Washington, DC: American Public Health Association.

Hidayat AA, Nalbandian RM, Sammons DW, Fleischman JA, Johnson TE. 1993. The diagnostic histopathologic features of ocular malaria. *Ophthalmology* 100(8):1183-1186.

Hosoglu S, Ayaz C, Geyik MF, Kokoglu OF, Ceviz A. 1998. Tuberculous meningitis in adults: An eleven-year review. *International Journal of Tuberculosis and Lung Disease* 2(7):553-557.

Howard RS, Sarkies NJ, Sanders MD. 1987. Anterior uveitis associated with Campylobacter jejuni infection. *Journal of Infection* 14(2):186-187.

Hubalek Z, Halouzka J. 1999. West Nile fever—A reemerging mosquito-borne viral disease in Europe. *Emerging Infectious Diseases* 5(5):643-650.

Hyams KC, Hanson K, Wignall FS, Escamilla J, Oldfield EC, 3rd. 1995. The impact of infectious diseases on the health of US troops deployed to the Persian Gulf during operations Desert Shield and Desert Storm. *Clinical Infectious Diseases* 20(6):1497-1504.

Ibero I, Vela P, Pascual E. 1997. Arthritis of shoulder and spinal cord compression due to Brucella disc infection. *British Journal of Rheumatology* 36(3):377-381.

Ibrahim AI, Awad R, Shetty SD, Saad M, Bilal NE. 1988. Genito-urinary complications of brucellosis. *British Journal of Urology* 61(4):294-298.

Idro R, Jenkins NE, Newton CR. 2005. Pathogenesis, clinical features, and neurological outcome of cerebral malaria. *Lancet Neurology* 4(12):827-840.

Ilnyckyj A, Balachandra B, Elliott L, Choudhri S, Duerksen DR. 2003. Post-traveler's diarrhea irritable bowel syndrome: A prospective study. *American Journal of Gastroenterology* 98(3):596-599.

Imboden JB, Canter A, Cluff LE, Trever RW. 1959. Brucellosis. III. Psychologic aspects of delayed convalescence. *AMA Archives of Internal Medicine* 103(3):406-414.

IOM (Institute of Medicine). 2000. *Ending Neglect: The Elimination of Tuberculosis in the United States*. Washington, DC: National Academy Press.

Islam MZ, Itoh M, Shamsuzzaman SM, Mirza R, Matin F, Ahmed I, Shamsuzzaman Choudhury AK, Hossain MA, Qiu XG, Begam N, Furuya M, Leafasia JL, Hashiguchi Y, Kimura E. 2002. Diagnosis of visceral leishmaniasis by enzyme-linked immunosorbent assay using urine samples. *Clinical and Diagnostic Laboratory Immunology* 9(4):789-794.

Iuchi K, Ichimiya A, Akashi A, Mizuta T, Lee YE, Tada H, Mori T, Sawamura K, Lee YS, Furuse K, et al. 1987. Non-Hodgkin's lymphoma of the pleural cavity developing from long-standing pyothorax. *Cancer* 60(8):1771-1775.

Jordan I, Briese T, Fischer N, Lau JY, Lipkin WI. 2000. Ribavirin inhibits West Nile virus replication and cytopathic effect in neural cells. *Journal of Infectious Diseases* 182(4):1214-1217.

Kalil AC, Devetten MP, Singh S, Lesiak B, Poage DP, Bargenquast K, Fayad P, Freifeld AG. 2005. Use of interferon-alpha in patients with West Nile encephalitis: Report of 2 cases. *Clinical Infectious Diseases* 40(5):764-766.

Kalita J, Misra UK. 1999. Outcome of tuberculous meningitis at 6 and 12 months: A multiple regression analysis. *International Journal of Tuberculosis and Lung Disease* 3(3):261-265.

Kanjalkar M, Karnad DR, Narayana RV, Shah PU. 1999. Guillain-Barre syndrome following malaria. *Journal of Infection* 38(1):48-50.

Karmali MA, Fleming PC. 1979. Campylobacter enteritis in children. *Journal of Pediatrics* 94(4):527-533.

Kaslow RA RRCA. 1979. Search for Reiter's syndrome after an outbreak of Shigella sonnei dysentery. *Journal of Rheumatology* 6:562-566.

Kelley PW. 2005. *Military Preventive Medicine: Mobilization and Deployment.* Volume 2. Washington, DC: Walter Reed Army Medical Center.

Kennedy DH, Fallon RJ. 1979. Tuberculous meningitis. *Journal of the American Medical Association* 241(3):264-268.

Khan MY, Mah MW, Memish ZA. 2001. Brucellosis in pregnant women. *Clinical Infectious Diseases* 32(8):1172-1177.

Khandpur S, Ramam M, Sharma VK, Salotra P, Singh MK, Malhotra A. 2004. Nerve involvement in Indian post kala-azar dermal leishmaniasis. *Acta Dermato-Venereologica* 84:245-246.

Khateeb MI, Araj GF, Majeed SA, Lulu AR. 1990. Brucella arthritis: A study of 96 cases in Kuwait. *Annals of the Rheumatic Diseases* 49(12):994-998.

Kibukamusoke JW. 1986. The hazard of malarial nephropathy. *Parasitology Today* 2(4): 119-121.

Kilpatrick ME. 2005. *Presentation to IOM Committee on Gulf War and Health: Infectious Diseases*. Washington, DC.

Kim AY, Goldberg MB, Rubin RH. 2004. *Salmonella* infections. In: Gorbach SL, Bartlett JG, Blacklow NR, Editors. *Infectious Diseases*. 3rd ed. Philadelphia, PA: Lippincott Williams and Wilkins. Pp. 618-633.

Klee AL, Maidin B, Edwin B, Poshni I, Mostashari F, Fine A, Layton M, Nash D. 2004. Long-term prognosis for clinical West Nile virus infection. *Emerging Infectious Diseases* 10(8):1405-1411.

Kochar DK, Agarwal N, Jain N, Sharma BV, Rastogi A, Meena CB. 2000a. Clinical profile of neurobrucellosis—a report on 12 cases from Bikaner (north-west India). *Journal of the Association of Physicians of India* 48(4):376-380.

Kochar DK, Shubhakaran, Kumawat BL, Vyas SP. 2000b. Prognostic significance of eye changes in cerebral malaria. *Journal of the Association of Physicians of India* 48(5):473-477.

Kolaczinski J, Graham K, Fahim A, Brooker S, Rowland M. 2005. Malaria control in Afghanistan: Progress and challenges. *Lancet* 365(9469):1506-1512.

Kortepeter MG, Krauss MR. 2001. Tuberculosis infection after humanitarian assistance, Guantanamo Bay, 1995. *Military Medicine* 166(2):116-120.

Koster F, Levin J, Walker L, Tung KS, Gilman RH, Rahaman MM, Majid MA, Islam S, Williams RC Jr. 1978. Hemolytic uremic syndrome after shigellosis. Relation to endotoxemia and circulating immune complexes. *New England Journal of Medicine* 298(17):927-933.

Kurcer MA, Simsek Z, Kurcer Z. 2006. The decreasing efficacy of chloroquine in the treatment of Plasmodium vivax malaria, in Sanliurfa, south-eastern Turkey. *Annals of Tropical Medicine and Parasitology* 100(2):109-113.

Kuroki S, Saida T, Nukina M, Haruta T, Yoshioka M, Kobayashi Y, Nakanishi H. 1993. Campylobacter jejuni strains from patients with Guillain-Barre syndrome belong mostly to Penner serogroup 19 and contain beta-N-acetylglucosamine residues. *Annals of Neurology* 33(3):243-247.

Kuwabara S, Ogawara K, Misawa S, Koga M, Mori M, Hiraga A, Kanesaka T, Hattori T, Yuki N. 2004. Does Campylobacter jejuni infection elicit "demyelinating" Guillain-Barre syndrome? *Neurology* 63(3):529-533.

Lamar J. 2006. Navy Environmental Health Center. Personal communication.

Lau KK, Yu IT, Chan AC, Wong LK, Tam CM, Sheng B, Li HL. 2005. A registry of tuberculous meningitis in Hong Kong. *International Journal of Tuberculosis and Lung Disease* 9(12):1391-1397.

Lauhio A, Lahdevirta J, Janes R, Kontiainen S, Repo H. 1988. Reactive arthritis associated with Shigella sonnei infection. *Arthritis and Rheumatism* 31(9):1190-1193.

Lee AT, Hall RG, Pile KD. 2005. Reactive joint symptoms following an outbreak of Salmonella typhimurium phage type 135a. *Journal of Rheumatology* 32(3):524-527.

Leirisalo-Repo M, Helenius P, Hannu T, Lehtinen A, Kreula J, Taavitsainen M, Koskimies S. 1997. Long-term prognosis of reactive salmonella arthritis. *Annals of the Rheumatic Diseases* 56(9):516-520.

Lever AM, Dolby JM, Webster AD, Price AB. 1984. Chronic campylobacter colitis and uveitis in patient with hypogammaglobulinaemia. *British Medical Journal (Clinical Research Ed.)* 288(6416):531.

Lewallen S. 1998. The fundus in severe malaria. *Archives of Ophthalmology* 116(4):542-543.

Lewis RB. 1982. The absence of reactive arthritis after Shigella sonnei infection. *Arthritis and Rheumatism* 25(10):1267.

Liu GF, Wu ZL, Wu HS, Wang QY, Zhao-Ri GT, Wang CY, Liang ZX, Cui SL, Zheng JD. 2003. A case-control study on children with Guillain-Barre syndrome in North China. *Biomedical and Environmental Sciences* 16(2):105-111.

Lochhead J, Elston JS. 2003. Doxycycline induced intracranial hypertension. *British Medical Journal (Clinical Research Ed.)* 326(7390):641-642.

Locht H, Kihlstrom E, Lindstrom FD. 1993. Reactive arthritis after Salmonella among medical doctors—Study of an outbreak. *Journal of Rheumatology* 20(5):845-848.

Locht H, Molbak K, Krogfelt KA. 2002. High frequency of reactive joint symptoms after an outbreak of Salmonella enteritidis. *Journal of Rheumatology* 29(4):767-771.

Long R, Maycher B, Dhar A, Manfreda J, Hershfield E, Anthonisen N. 1998. Pulmonary tuberculosis treated with directly observed therapy: Serial changes in lung structure and function. *Chest* 113(4):933-943.

Lozier JR, Friedlaender MH. 1989. Complications of antimalarial therapy. *International Ophthalmology Clinics* 29(3):172-178.

Lubani MM, Dudin KI, Araj GF, Manandhar DS, Rashid FY. 1989a. Neurobrucellosis in children. *Pediatric Infectious Disease Journal* 8(2):79-82.

Lubani MM, Dudin KI, Sharda DC, Ndhar DS, Araj GF, Hafez HA, al-Saleh QA, Helin I, Salhi MM. 1989b. A multicenter therapeutic study of 1100 children with brucellosis. *Pediatric Infectious Disease Journal* 8(2):75-78.

Luke T. 2006. Department of the Navy Bureau of Medicine and Surgery. Personal communication.

Lulu AR, Araj GF, Khateeb MI, Mustafa MY, Yusuf AR, Fenech FF. 1988. Human brucellosis in Kuwait: A prospective study of 400 cases. *Quarterly Journal of Medicine* 66(249):39-54.

Lyall M. 1973. Ocular brucellosis. *Transactions of the Ophthalmological Societies of the United Kingdom* 93(0):689-697.

Madariaga MG, Pulvirenti J, Sekosan M, Paddock CD, Zaki SR. 2004. Q fever endocarditis in HIV-infected patient. *Emerging Infectious Diseases* 10(3):501-504.

Magill AJ, Grogl M, Gasser RA Jr, Sun W, Oster CN. 1993. Visceral infection caused by Leishmania tropica in veterans of Operation Desert Storm. *New England Journal of Medicine* 328(19):1383-1387.

Magill AJ, Grogl M, Johnson SC, Gasser RA Jr. 1994. Visceral infection due to Leishmania tropica in a veteran of Operation Desert Storm who presented 2 years after leaving Saudi Arabia. *Clinical Infectious Diseases* 19(4):805-806.

Makhseed M, Harouny A, Araj G, Moussa MA, Sharma P. 1998. Obstetric and gynecologic implication of brucellosis in Kuwait. *Journal of Perinatology* 18(3):196-199.

Maki-Ikola O, Granfors K. 1992. Salmonella-triggered reactive arthritis. *Scandinavian Journal of Rheumatology* 21(6):265-270.

Maki-Ikola O, Leirisalo-Repo M, Kantele A, Toivanen P, Granfors K. 1991. Salmonella-specific antibodies in reactive arthritis. *Journal of Infectious Diseases* 164(6):1141-1148.

Maki-Ikola O, Yli-Kerttula U, Saario R, Toivanen P, Granfors K. 1992. Salmonella specific antibodies in serum and synovial fluid in patients with reactive arthritis. *British Journal of Rheumatology* 31(1):25-29.

Malviya G, Sinha MK, Bhattacharya SK. 2005. Post-malarial neuropsychiatric syndrome. *Journal of the Association of Physicians of India* 53:227.

Mandell GL, Bennett JE, Dolin R. 2005. *Principles and Practice of Infectious Diseases*. 6th ed. Philadelphia, PA: Elsevier Churchill Livingstone

Marmion BP, Shannon M, Maddocks I, Storm P, Penttila I. 1996. Protracted debility and fatigue after acute Q fever. *Lancet* 347(9006):977-978.

Marmion BP, Storm PA, Ayres JG, Semendric L, Mathews L, Winslow W, Turra M, Harris RJ. 2005. Long-term persistence of Coxiella burnetii after acute primary Q fever. *QJM* 98(1): 7-20.

Marrie TJ. 1990. *Q Fever: The Disease.* Volume 1. Boca Raton, FL: CRC Press.

Marrie TJ. 2000. *Coxiella burnetti* (Q Fever). In: Mandell GL, Bennett JE, Dolin R, Editors. *Principles and Practice of Infectious Diseases*. 5th ed. New York: Churchill Livingstone. Pp. 2043-2049.

Martin WJ, Nichols DR, Beahrs OH. 1961. Chronic localized brucellosis. *Archives of Internal Medicine* 107:43.

Mattila L, Leirisalo-Repo M, Koskimies S, Granfors K, Siitonen A. 1994. Reactive arthritis following an outbreak of Salmonella infection in Finland. *British Journal of Rheumatology* 33(12):1136-1141.

Mattila L, Leirisalo-Repo M, Pelkonen P, Koskimies S, Granfors K, Siitonen A. 1998. Reactive arthritis following an outbreak of Salmonella Bovismorbificans infection. *Journal of Infection* 36(3):289-295.

Maurin M, Raoult D. 1999. Q fever. *Clinical Microbiology Reviews* 12(4):518-553.

McCarthy N, Giesecke J. 2001. Incidence of Guillain-Barre syndrome following infection with Campylobacter jejuni. *American Journal of Epidemiology* 153(6):610-614.

McLean DR, Russell N, Khan MY. 1992. Neurobrucellosis: Clinical and therapeutic features. *Clinical Infectious Diseases* 15(4):582-590.

McQuiston JH, Childs JE. 2002. Q fever in humans and animals in the United States. *Vector Borne Zoonotic Disease* 2(3):179-191.

MedlinePlus Medical Encyclopedia. 2006. *MedlinePlus Medical Encyclopedia: Uveitis*. [Online]. Available: http://www.nlm.nih.gov/medlineplus/print/ency/article/001005.htm [accessed May 1, 2006].

Meier CR, Wilcock K, Jick SS. 2004. The risk of severe depression, psychosis or panic attacks with prophylactic antimalarials. *Drug Safety* 27(3):203-213.

Memish ZA, Venkatesh S. 2001. Brucellar epididymo-orchitis in Saudi Arabia: A retrospective study of 26 cases and review of the literature. *BJU International* 88(1):72-76.

Metha SR, Joshi V, Lazar AI. 1996. Unusual acute and chronic complications of malaria. *Journal of the Association of Physicians of India* 44(7):451-453.

Milazzo A, Hall R, Storm PA, Harris RJ, Winslow W, Marmion BP. 2001. Sexually transmitted Q fever. *Clinical Infectious Diseases* 33(3):399-402.

Mishu B, Ilyas AA, Koski CL, Vriesendorp F, Cook SD, Mithen FA, Blaser MJ. 1993. Serologic evidence of previous Campylobacter jejuni infection in patients with the Guillain-Barre syndrome. *Annals of Internal Medicine* 118(12):947-953.

Montes M, Cilla G, Marimon JM, Diaz de Tuesta JL, Perez-Trallero E. 1995. Coxiella burnetii infection in subjects with HIV infection and HIV infection in patients with Q fever. *Scandinavian Journal of Infectious Diseases* 27(4):344-346.

Morata P, Queipo-Ortuno MI, Reguera JM, Miralles F, Lopez-Gonzalez JJ, Colmenero JD. 2001. Diagnostic yield of a PCR assay in focal complications of brucellosis. *Journal of Clinical Microbiology* 39(10):3743-3746.

Mostashari F, Bunning ML, Kitsutani PT, Singer DA, Nash D, Cooper MJ, Katz N, Liljebjelke KA, Biggerstaff BJ, Fine AD, Layton MC, Mullin SM, Johnson AJ, Martin DA, Hayes EB, Campbell GL. 2001. Epidemic West Nile encephalitis, New York, 1999: Results of a household-based seroepidemiological survey. *Lancet* 358(9278):261-264.

Mousa AR, Koshy TS, Araj GF, Marafie AA, Muhtaseb SA, Al-Mudallal DS, Busharetulla MS. 1986. Brucella meningitis: Presentation, diagnosis and treatment—a prospective study of ten cases. *Quarterly Journal of Medicine* 60(233):873-885.

Mousa AR, Muhtaseb SA, Almudallal DS, Khodeir SM, Marafie AA. 1987. Osteoarticular complications of brucellosis: A study of 169 cases. *Reviews of Infectious Diseases* 9(3):531-543.

Murray HW. 2000. Treatment of visceral leishmaniasis (kala-azar): A decade of progress and future approaches. *International Journal of Infectious Diseases* 4(3):158-177.

Murray HW. 2004. Treatment of visceral leishmaniasis in 2004. *American Journal of Tropical Medicine and Hygiene* 71(6):787-794.

Murray HW, Berman JD, Davies CR, Saravia NG. 2005. Advances in leishmaniasis. *Lancet* 366(9496):1561-1577.

Nachamkin I. 2002. Chronic effects of Campylobacter infection. *Microbes and Infection* 4(4):399-403.

Nachamkin I, Allos BM, Ho T. 1998. Campylobacter species and Guillain-Barre syndrome. *Clinical Microbiology Reviews* 11(3):555-567.

Nachamkin I, Engberg J, Gutacker M, Meinersman RJ, Li CY, Arzate P, Teeple E, Fussing V, Ho TW, Asbury AK, Griffin JW, McKhann GM, Piffaretti JC. 2001. Molecular population genetic analysis of Campylobacter jejuni HS: 19 associated with Guillain-Barre syndrome and gastroenteritis. *Journal of Infectious Diseases* 184(2):221-226.

Naficy K, Saidi S. 1970. Serological survey on viral antibodies in Iran. *Tropical and Geographical Medicine* 22(2):183-188.

Namiduru M, Karaoglan I, Gursoy S, Bayazit N, Sirikci A. 2004. Brucellosis of the spine: Evaluation of the clinical, laboratory, and radiological findings of 14 patients. *Rheumatology International* 24(3):125-129.

Nash D, Mostashari F, Fine A, Miller J, O'Leary D, Murray K, Huang A, Rosenberg A, Greenberg A, Sherman M, Wong S, Layton M. 2001. The outbreak of West Nile virus infection in the New York City area in 1999. *New England Journal of Medicine* 344(24):1807-1814.

Nathoo KJ, Sanders JA, Siziya S, Mucheche C. 1995. Haemolytic uraemic syndrome following Shigella dysenteriae type 1 outbreak in Zimbabwe: A clinical experience. *Central African Journal of Medicine* 41(9):267-274.

Navarro-Martinez A, Solera J, Corredoira J, Beato JL, Martinez-Alfaro E, Atienzar M, Ariza J. 2001. Epididymoorchitis due to Brucella mellitensis: A retrospective study of 59 patients. *Clinical Infectious Diseases* 33(12):2017-2022.

Navy Environmental Health Center. 2006. *Preventive Medicine - Tuberculosis*. [Online]. Available: http://www-nehc.med.navy.mil/prevmed/PM/PM_Tuberculosis.htm [accessed May 8, 2006].

Neithercut WD, Hudson MA, Smith CC. 1984. Can erythema nodosum and reactive arthritis be a sequel to Shigella flexneri gastroenteritis? *Scottish Medical Journal* 29(3):197-199.

Nene A, Bhojraj S. 2005. Results of nonsurgical treatment of thoracic spinal tuberculosis in adults. *The Spine Journal* 5(1):79-84.

Newman RD, Parise ME, Barber AM, Steketee RW. 2004. Malaria-related deaths among US travelers, 1963-2001. *Annals of Internal Medicine* 141(7):547-555.

Niemeyer G, Fruh B. 1989. Examination strategies in the diagnosis of drug-induced retinal damage. *Klinische Monatsblatter Fur Augenheilkunde* 194(5):355-358.

NIH (National Institutes of Health). 2002. *Questions and Answers About Reactive Arthritis*. National Institute of Arthritis and Musckuloskeletal Diseases (NIAMS), Public Health Service, US Department of Health and Human Services.

Nikkari S, Rantakokko K, Ekman P, Mottonen T, Leirisalo-Repo M, Virtala M, Lehtonen L, Jalava J, Kotilainen P, Granfors K, Toivanen P. 1999. Salmonella-triggered reactive arthritis: Use of polymerase chain reaction, immunocytochemical staining, and gas chromatography-mass spectrometry in the detection of bacterial components from synovial fluid. *Arthritis and Rheumatism* 42(1):84-89.

Noer HR. 1966. An "experimental" epidemic of Reiter's syndrome. *Journal of the American Medical Association* 198(7):693-698.

Norton WL. 1984. Brucellosis and rheumatic syndromes in Saudi Arabia. *Annals of the Rheumatic Diseases* 43(6):810-815.

Nourse C, Allworth A, Jones A, Horvath R, McCormack J, Bartlett J, Hayes D, Robson JM. 2004. Three cases of Q fever osteomyelitis in children and a review of the literature. *Clinical Infectious Diseases* 39(7):e61-e66.

Oh MD, Shin H, Shin D, Kim U, Lee S, Kim N, Choi MH, Chai JY, Choe K. 2001. Clinical features of vivax malaria. *American Journal of Tropical Medicine and Hygiene* 65(2):143-146.

Ohl CA, Hyams KC, Malone JD, Oldfield EC 3rd. 1993. Leishmaniasis among Desert Storm veterans: A diagnostic and therapeutic dilemma. *Military Medicine* 158(11):726-729.

Okhuysen PC, Jiang ZD, Carlin L, Forbes C, DuPont HL. 2004. Post-diarrhea chronic intestinal symptoms and irritable bowel syndrome in North American travelers to Mexico. *American Journal of Gastroenterology* 99(9):1774-1778.

Oldfield EC 3rd, Wallace MR, Hyams KC, Yousif AA, Lewis DE, Bourgeois AL. 1991. Endemic infectious diseases of the Middle East. *Reviews of Infectious Diseases* 13(3 Suppl):S199-S217.

Oliveri R, Matera G, Foca A, Zappia M, Aguglia U, Quattrone A. 1996. Polyradiculoneuropathy with cerebrospinal fluid albuminocytological dissociation due to neurobrucellosis. *Clinical Infectious Diseases* 23(4):833-834.

Olsen SJ, Bleasdale SC, Magnano AR, Landrigan C, Holland BH, Tauxe RV, Mintz ED, Luby S. 2003. Outbreaks of typhoid fever in the United States, 1960-99. *Epidemiology and Infection* 130(1):13-21.

Oren I, Kraoz Z, Hadani Y, Kassis I, Zaltzman-Bershadsky N, Finkelstein R. 2005. An outbreak of Q fever in an urban area in Israel. *European Journal of Clinical Microbiology and Infectious Diseases* 24(5):338-341.

Papatsoris AG, Mpadra FA, Karamouzis MV, Frangides CY. 2002. Endemic brucellar epididymo-orchitis: A 10-year experience. *International Journal of Infectious Diseases* 6(4):309-313.

Pappas G, Bosilkovski M, Akritidis N, Mastora M, Krteva L, Tsianos E. 2003. Brucellosis and the respiratory system. *Clinical Infectious Diseases* 37(7):e95-e99.

Pappas G, Kitsanou M, Christou L, Tsianos E. 2004. Immune thrombocytopenia attributed to brucellosis and other mechanisms of Brucella-induced thrombocytopenia. *American Journal of Hematology* 75(3):139-141.

Pappas G, Akritidis N, Bosilkovski M, Tsianos E. 2005. Brucellosis. *New England Journal of Medicine* 352(22):2325-2336.

Parker NR, Barralet JH, Bell AM. 2006. Q fever. *Lancet* 367(9511):679-688.

Parsonnet J, Griffin PM. 1993. Hemolytic uremic syndrome: Clinical picture and bacterial connection. *Current Clinical Topics in Infectious Diseases* 13:172-187.

Parsonnet J, Greene KD, Gerber AR, Tauxe RV, Vallejo Aguilar OJ, Blake PA. 1989. Shigella dysenteriae type 1 infections in US travellers to Mexico, 1988. *Lancet* 2(8662):543-545.

Pascual J, Combarros O, Polo JM, Berciano J. 1988. Localized CNS brucellosis: Report of 7 cases. *Acta Neurologica Scandinavica* 78(4):282-289.

Pegues DA, Ohl ME, Miler SI. 2005. *Salmonella* species, including *Salmonella typhi*. In: Mandell GL, Bennett JE, Dolin R, Editors. *Principles and Practice of Infectious Diseases*. 6th ed. Philadelphia, PA: Elsevier. Pp. 2636-2654.

Petersen LR, Roehrig JT. 2001. West Nile virus: A reemerging global pathogen. *Emerging Infectious Diseases* 7(4):611-614.

Platonov AE. 2001. West Nile encephalitis in Russia 1999-2001: Were we ready? Are we ready? *Annals of the New York Academy of Sciences* 951:102-116.

Plit ML, Anderson R, Van Rensburg CE, Page-Shipp L, Blott JA, Fresen JL, Feldman C. 1998. Influence of antimicrobial chemotherapy on spirometric parameters and pro-inflammatory indices in severe pulmonary tuberculosis. *European Respiratory Journal* 12(2):351-356.

Portnoy JZ, Callen JP. 1983. Ophthalmologic aspects of chloroquine and hydroxychloroquine therapy. *International Journal of Dermatology* 22(5):273-278.

Queipo-Ortuno MI, Morata P, Ocon P, Manchado P, Colmenero JD. 1997. Rapid diagnosis of human brucellosis by peripheral-blood PCR assay. *Journal of Clinical Microbiology* 35 (11):2927-2930.

Rabinowitz R, Schneck M, Levy J, Lifshitz T. 2005. Bilateral multifocal choroiditis with serous retinal detachment in a patient with Brucella infection: Case report and review of the literature. *Archives of Ophthalmology* 123(1):116-118.

Rahaman MM, JamiulAlam AK, Islam MR, Greenough WB 3rd. 1975. Shiga bacillus dysentery associated with marked leukocytosis and erythrocyte fragmentation. *Johns Hopkins Medical Journal* 136(2):65-70.

Raoult D. 2003. Use of macrolides for Q fever. *Antimicrobial Agents and Chemotherapy* 47(1):446.

Raoult D, Piquet P, Gallais H, de Micco C, Drancourt M, Casanova P. 1986. Coxiella burnetii infection of a vascular prosthesis. *New England Journal of Medicine* 315(21):1358-1359.

Raoult D, Levy PY, Dupont HT, Chicheportiche C, Tamalet C, Gastaut JA, Salducci J. 1993. Q fever and HIV infection. *AIDS* 7(1):81-86.

Raoult D, Houpikian P, Tissot-Dupont H, Riss JM, Arditi-Djiane J, Brouqui P. 1999. Treatment of Q fever endocarditis: Comparison of 2 regimens containing doxycycline and ofloxacin or hydroxychloroquine. *Archives of Internal Medicine* 159(2):167-173.

Raoult D, Tissot-Dupont H, Foucault C, Gouvernet J, Fournier PE, Bernit E, Stein A, Nesri M, Harle JR, Weiller PJ. 2000. Q fever 1985-1998. Clinical and epidemiologic features of 1,383 infections. *Medicine* 79(2):109-123.

Raoult D, Fenollar F, Stein A. 2002. Q fever during pregnancy: Diagnosis, treatment, and follow-up. *Archives of Internal Medicine* 162(6):701-704.

Raoult D, Marrie T, Mege J. 2005. Natural history and pathophysiology of Q fever. *The Lancet Infectious Diseases* 5(4):219-226.

RBM (Roll Back Malaria). 2005a. *Roll Back Malaria - Epidemiology*. [Online]. Available: http://www.emro.who.int/rbm/Epidemiology-current.htm [accessed May 4, 2006].

RBM. 2005b. *Roll Back Malaria - Regional Office for the Eastern Mediterranean: Epidemiological Situation*. [Online]. Available: http://www.emro.who.int/rbm/epidemiology-2004.htm [accessed July 17, 2006].

RBM. 2005c. *Roll Back Malaria - World Malaria Report: Afghanistan Country Profile*. [Online]. Available: http://www.rbm.who.int/wmr2005/profiles/afghanistan.pdf [accessed May 4, 2006].

RBM. 2005d. *Roll Back Malaria - World Malaria Report: Iran Country Profile*. [Online]. Available at: http://www.rbm.who.int/wmr2005/profiles/iran.pdf [accessed May 5, 2006].

RBM. 2005e. *Roll Back Malaria - World Malaria Report: Iraq Country Profile*. [Online]. Available: http://www.rbm.who.int/wmr2005/profiles/iraq.pdf [accessed May 4, 2006].

RBM. 2005f. *Roll Back Malaria - World Malaria Report: Pakistan Country Profile*. [Online]. Available: http://www.rbm.who.int/wmr2005/profiles/pakistan.pdf [accessed May 4, 2006].

RBM. 2005g. *Roll Back Malaria - World Malaria Report: Saudi Arabia Country Profile*. [Online]. Available: http://www.rbm.who.int/wmr2005/profiles/saudiarabia.pdf [accessed May 4, 2006].

RBM. 2005h. *Roll Back Malaria - World Malaria Report 2005 - Malaria Control, By Region*. [Online]. Available: http://rbm.who.int/wmr2005/html/2-2.htm [accessed June 27, 2006].

Rees JH, Soudain SE, Gregson NA, Hughes RA. 1995. Campylobacter jejuni infection and Guillain-Barre syndrome. *New England Journal of Medicine* 333(21):1374-1379.

Rees JR, Pannier MA, McNees A, Shallow S, Angulo FJ, Vugia DJ. 2004. Persistent diarrhea, arthritis, and other complications of enteric infections: A pilot survey based on California FoodNet surveillance, 1998-1999. *Clinical Infectious Diseases* 38(3 Suppl):S311-S17.

Renia L, Potter SM, Mauduit M, Rosa DS, Kayibanda M, Deschemin JC, Snounou G, Gruner AC. 2006. Pathogenic T cells in cerebral malaria. *International Journal for Parasitology* 36(5):547-554.

Rhodes KM, Tattersfield AE. 1982. Guillain-Barre syndrome associated with Campylobacter infection. *British Medical Journal (Clinical Research Ed.)* 285(6336):173-174.

Riestra-Castaneda R, Gonzalez-Garrido A, Gonzalez-Cornejo S. 1996. Brucellosis and polyneuroradiculomyeloencephalitis. A case report. *Archives of Medical Research* 27(3):331-333.

Roehrig JT, Nash D, Maldin B, Labowitz A, Martin DA, Lanciotti RS, Campbell GL. 2003. Persistence of virus-reactive serum immunoglobulin m antibody in confirmed west nile virus encephalitis cases. *Emerging Infectious Diseases* 9(3):376-379.

Roiz MP, Peralta FG, Valle R, Arjona R. 1998. Microbiological diagnosis of brucellosis. *Journal of Clinical Microbiology* 36(6):1819.

Rolando I, Carbone A, Gotuzzo E, Carillo CP. 1985a. Circulating immune complexes in the pathogenesis of human brucellar uveitis. *Chibret International Journal of Ophthalmology* 3:30-38.

Rolando I, Carbone A, Haro D, Gotuzzo E, Carrillo C. 1985b. Retinal detachment in chronic brucellosis. *American Journal of Ophthalmology* 99(6):733-734.

Rolando I, Tobaru L, Hinostruza S. 1987. Clinical manifestations of 25 Brucella uveitis. *Ophthalmic Practice* 5:12-17.

Rongnoparat C, Panpanit R. 1987. Hemolytic uremic syndrome associated with shigellosis: Report of two cases. *Southeast Asian Journal of Tropical Medicine and Public Health* 18(2):226-228.

Ropper AH. 1988. Campylobacter diarrhea and Guillain-Barre syndrome. *Archives of Neurology* 45(6):655-656.

Ruben B, Band JD, Wong P, Colville J. 1991. Person-to-person transmission of Brucella melitensis. *Lancet* 337(8732):14-15.

Rubin M. 1968. Prolonged pharmacotherapy and the eye. A symposium. The antimalarials and the tranquilizers. *Diseases of the Nervous System* 29(3):S67-S76.

Ruiz RS, Saatci OA. 1991. Chloroquine and hydroxychloroquine retinopathy: How to follow affected patients. *Annals of Ophthalmology* 23(8):290-291.

Russo R, Laguna F, Lopez-Velez R, Medrano FJ, Rosenthal E, Cacopardo B, Nigro L. 2003. Visceral leishmaniasis in those infected with HIV: Clinical aspects and other opportunistic infections. *Annals of Tropical Medicine and Parasitology* 97(1 Suppl):99-105.

Rynes RI, Bernstein HN. 1993. Ophthalmologic safety profile of antimalarial drugs. *Lupus* 2 (1 Suppl):S17-S19.

Saad M, Youssef S, Kirschke D, Shubair M, Haddadin D, Myers J, Moorman J. 2005. Acute flaccid paralysis: The spectrum of a newly recognized complication of West Nile virus infection. *Journal of Infection* 51(2):120-127.

Saah AJ. 2000. Introduction to rickettsioses and ehrlichioses. In: Mandell GL, Bennett JE, Dolin R, Editors. *Principles and Practice of Infectious Diseases*. 5th ed. New York: Churchill Livingstone. Pp. 2033-2035.

Sacks N, Van Rensburg AJ. 1976. Clinical aspects of chronic brucellosis. *South African Medical Journal* 50(19):725-728.

Sanchez-Sousa A, Torres C, Campello MG, Garcia C, Parras F, Cercenado E, Baquero F. 1990. Serological diagnosis of neurobrucellosis. *Journal of Clinical Pathology* 43(1):79-81.

Schlagenhauf P, Tschopp A, Johnson R, Nothdurft HD, Beck B, Schwartz E, Herold M, Krebs B, Veit O, Allwinn R, Steffen R. 2003. Tolerability of malaria chemoprophylaxis in non-immune travellers to sub-Saharan Africa: Multicentre, randomised, double blind, four arm study. *British Medical Journal (Clinical Research Ed.)* 327(7423):1078.

Scrimgeour EM, Al-Ismaily SI, Rolain JM, Al-Dhahry SH, El-Khatim HS, Raoult D. 2003. Q Fever in human and livestock populations in Oman. *Annals of the New York Academy of Sciences* 990:221-225.

Secretary of the Air Force. 2005. *Air Force Instruction 48-105: Surveillance, Prevention, and Control of Diseases and Conditions of Public Health or Military Significance.*

Sejvar JJ, Haddad MB, Tierney BC, Campbell GL, Marfin AA, Van Gerpen JA, Fleischauer A, Leis AA, Stokic DS, Petersen LR. 2003. Neurologic manifestations and outcome of West Nile virus infection. *Journal of the American Medical Association* 290(4):511-515.

Senanayake N, de Silva HJ. 1994. Delayed cerebellar ataxia complicating falciparum malaria: A clinical study of 74 patients. *Journal of Neurology* 241(7):456-459.

Shamo FJ. 2001. Malaria in Iraq. *Meditsinskaia Parazitologiia i Parazitarnye Bolezni* (1):46-47.

Shanks GD, Edstein MD. 2005. Modern malaria chemoprophylaxis. *Drugs* 65(15):2091-2110.

Shears P. 1996. Shigella infections. *Annals of Tropical Medicine and Parasitology* 90(2):105-114.

Shibukawa-Kent R. 2006. Air Force Institute for Operational Health. Personal communication.

Shubhakaran, Sharma CM. 2003. Acute inflammatory demyelinating polyneuropathy with P. falciparum malaria. *Journal of the Association of Physicians of India* 51:223-224.

Shute PG, Lupascu G, Branzei P, Maryon M, Constantinescu P, Bruce-Chwatt LJ, Draper CC, Killick-Kendrick R, Garnham PC. 1977. A strain of Plasmodium vivax characterized by prolonged incubation: The effect of numbers of sporozoites on the length of the prepatent period. *Transactions of the Royal Society of Tropical Medicine and Hygiene* 70(5-6):474-481.

Siegman-Igra Y, Kaufman O, Keysary A, Rzotkiewicz S, Shalit I. 1997. Q fever endocarditis in Israel and a worldwide review. *Scandinavian Journal of Infectious Diseases* 29(1):41-49.

Sieper J, Braun J, Wu P, Hauer R, Laitko S. 1993. The possible role of Shigella in sporadic enteric reactive arthritis. *British Journal of Rheumatology* 32(7):582-585.

Simon DG, Kaslow RA, Rosenbaum J, Kaye RL, Calin A. 1981. Reiter's syndrome following epidemic shigellosis. *Journal of Rheumatology* 8(6):969-973.

Sinha R, Aggarwal A, Prasad K, Misra R. 2003. Sporadic enteric reactive arthritis and undifferentiated spondyloarthropathy: Evidence for involvement of Salmonella typhimurium. *Journal of Rheumatology* 30(1):105-113.

Sinha S, Prasad KN, Pradhan S, Jain D, Jha S. 2004. Detection of preceding Campylobacter jejuni infection by polymerase chain reaction in patients with Guillain-Barre syndrome. *Transactions of the Royal Society of Tropical Medicine and Hygiene* 98(6):342-346.

Skirrow MB, Blaser MJ. 2002. Campylobacter jejuni. In: Blaser MJ, Smith PD, Raudin JI, Greenberg HB, Guerrant RL, Editors. *Infections of the Gastrointestinal Tract*. 2nd ed. Philadelphia, PA: Lippincott. Pp. 719-739.

Smith B, Ryan MA, Gray GC, Polonsky JM, Trump DH. 2002. Tuberculosis infection among young adults enlisting in the United States Navy. *International Journal of Epidemiology* 31(5):934-939.

Smith DL, Ayres JG, Blair I, Burge PS, Carpenter MJ, Caul EO, Coupland B, Desselberger U, Evans M, Farrell ID, et al. 1993. A large Q fever outbreak in the West Midlands: Clinical aspects. *Respiratory Medicine* 87(7):509-516.

Solera J, Rodriguez-Zapata M, Geijo P, Largo J, Paulino J, Saez L, Martinez-Alfaro E, Sanchez L, Sepulveda MA, Ruiz-Ribo MD. 1995. Doxycycline-rifampin versus doxycycline-streptomycin in treatment of human brucellosis due to Brucella melitensis. The GECMEI Group. Grupo de Estudio de Castilla-la Mancha de Enfermedades Infecciosas. *Antimicrobial Agents and Chemotherapy* 39(9):2061-2067.

Solera J, Lozano E, Martinez-Alfaro E, Espinosa A, Castillejos ML, Abad L. 1999. Brucellar spondylitis: Review of 35 cases and literature survey. *Clinical Infectious Diseases* 29(6):1440-1449.

Solomon T, Cardosa MJ. 2000. Emerging arboviral encephalitis. Newsworthy in the West but much more common in the East. *British Medical Journal (Clinical Research Ed.)* 321(7275):1484-1485.

Speed B, Kaldor J, Cavanagh P. 1984. Guillain-Barre syndrome associated with Campylobacter jejuni enteritis. *Journal of Infection* 8(1):85-86.

Spink WW. 1951. What is chronic brucellosis? *Annals of Internal Medicine* 35(2):358-374.

Spink WW. 1954. Family studies on brucellosis. *American Journal of the Medical Sciences* 227(2):128-133.

Stead WW, Dutt AK. 1991. Tuberculosis in elderly persons. *Annual Review of Medicine* 42: 267-276.

Stead WW, Lofgren JP. 1983. Does the risk of tuberculosis increase in old age? *Journal of Infectious Diseases* 147(5):951-955.

Stead WW, To T. 1987. The significance of the tuberculin skin test in elderly persons. *Annals of Internal Medicine* 107(6):837-842.

Stein A, Raoult D. 1995. Q fever endocarditis. *European Heart Journal* 16(B Suppl):19-23.

Sugamata M, Ahmed A, Miura T, Takasu T, Kono R, Ogata T, Kimura-Kuroda J, Yasui K. 1988. Seroepidemiological study of infection with West Nile virus in Karachi, Pakistan, in 1983 and 1985. *Journal of Medical Virology* 26(3):243-247.

Sugiyama T, Okazaki T, Yabe Y, Suda H, Saito T. 1967. Basic and clinical study on chloroquine therapy of rheumatic diseases. Eye disorders due to chloroquine. *Saishin Igaku. Recent Medicine* 22(10):2331-2335.

Sundar S, Agrawal S, Pai K, Chance M, Hommel M. 2005. Detection of leishmanial antigen in the urine of patients with visceral leishmaniasis by a latex agglutination test. *American Journal of Tropical Medicine and Hygiene* 73(2):269-271.

Sutlas PN, Unal A, Forta H, Senol S, Kirbas D. 2003. Tuberculous meningitis in adults: Review of 61 cases. *Infection* 31(6):387-391.

Svedhem A, Kaijser B. 1980. Campylobacter fetus subspecies jejuni: A common cause of diarrhea in Sweden. *Journal of Infectious Diseases* 142(3):353-359.

Tabbara KF. 1990. Brucellosis and nonsyphilitic treponemal uveitis. *International Ophthalmology Clinics* 30(4):294-296.

Tam CC, Rodrigues LC, O'Brien SJ. 2003. Guillain-Barre syndrome associated with Campylobacter jejuni infection in England, 2000-2001. *Clinical Infectious Diseases* 37(2):307-310.

Tardei G, Ruta S, Chitu V, Rossi C, Tsai TF, Cernescu C. 2000. Evaluation of immunoglobulin M (IgM) and IgG enzyme immunoassays in serologic diagnosis of West Nile Virus infection. *Journal of Clinical Microbiology* 38(6):2232-2239.

Tasova Y, Saltoglu N, Sahin G, Aksu HS. 1999. Osteoarthricular involvement of brucellosis in Turkey. *Clinical Rheumatology* 18(3):214-219.

Tauxe RV, Blake PA. 1992. Epidemic cholera in Latin America. *Journal of the American Medical Association* 267(10):1388-1390.

Taylor JP, Perdue JN. 1989. The changing epidemiology of human brucellosis in Texas, 1977-1986. *American Journal of Epidemiology* 130(1):160-165.

Taylor WR, White NJ. 2004. Antimalarial drug toxicity: A review. *Drug Safety* 27(1):25-61.

Taylor DN, Echeverria P, Pitarangsi C, Seriwatana J, Bodhidatta L, Blaser MJ. 1988. Influence of strain characteristics and immunity on the epidemiology of Campylobacter infections in Thailand. *Journal of Clinical Microbiology* 26(5):863-868.

Taylor DN, Bodhidatta L, Echeverria P. 1991. Epidemiologic aspects of shigellosis and other causes of dysentery in Thailand. *Reviews of Infectious Diseases* 13(4):S226-S230.

Teixeira MJ, Teixeira CR, Andrade BB, Barral-Netto M, Barral A. 2006. Chemokines in host-parasite interactions in leishmaniasis. *Trends in Parasitology* 22(1):32-40.

Thomas MF, Hedayati H. 1986. Reactive arthropathy (Reiter's syndrome) after salmonellosis: Report of two cases and review of the literature. *Journal of the American Osteopathic Association* 86(8):504-507.

Thomas R, Kameswaran M, Murugan V, Okafor BC. 1993. Sensorineural hearing loss in neurobrucellosis. *Journal of Laryngology and Otology* 107(11):1034-1036.

Thomson GT, Chiu B, De Rubeis D, Falk J, Inman RD. 1992. Immunoepidemiology of post-Salmonella reactive arthritis in a cohort of women. *Clinical Immunology and Immunopathology* 64(3):227-232.

Thomson GT, Alfa M, Orr K, Thomson BR, Olson N. 1994. Secretory immune response and clinical sequelae of Salmonella infection in a point source cohort. *Journal of Rheumatology* 21(1):132-137.

Thomson GT, DeRubeis DA, Hodge MA, Rajanayagam C, Inman RD. 1995. Post-Salmonella reactive arthritis: Late clinical sequelae in a point source cohort. *American Journal of Medicine* 98(1):13-21.

Thwaites GE, Duc Bang N, Huy Dung N, Thi Quy H, Thi Tuong Oanh D, Thi Cam Thoa N, Quang Hien N, Tri Thuc N, Ngoc Hai N, Thi Ngoc Lan N, Ngoc Lan N, Hong Duc N, Ngoc Tuan V, Huu Hiep C, Thi Hong Chau T, Phuong Mai P, Thi Dung N, Stepniewska K, Simmons CP, White NJ, Tinh Hien T, Farrar JJ. 2005. The influence of HIV infection on clinical presentation, response to treatment, and outcome in adults with Tuberculous meningitis. *Journal of Infectious Diseases* 192(12):2134-2141.

Tissot-Dupont H, Raoult D, Brouqui P, Janbon F, Peyramond D, Weiller PJ, Chicheportiche C, Nezri M, Poirier R. 1992. Epidemiologic features and clinical presentation of acute Q fever in hospitalized patients: 323 French cases. *American Journal of Medicine* 93(4):427-434.

Tissot-Dupont H, Amadei MA, Nezri M, Raoult D. 2004. Wind in November, Q fever in December. *Emerging Infectious Diseases* 10(7):1264-1269.

Toler SM. 2004. Oxidative stress plays an important role in the pathogenesis of drug-induced retinopathy. *Experimental Biology and Medicine (Maywood, NJ)* 229(7):607-615.

Travis LB, Travis WD, Li CY, Pierre RV. 1986. Q fever. A clinicopathologic study of five cases. *Archives of Pathology and Laboratory Medicine* 110(11):1017-1020.

Tripathi BM, Dube S, Biseria S. 1995. Ophthalmic involvement in severe malaria. *Journal of the Association of Physicians of India* 43(6):441-442.

Trujillo IZ, Zavala AN, Caceres JG, Miranda CQ. 1994. Brucellosis. *Infectious Disease Clinics of North America* 8(1):225-241.

Turck WP, Howitt G, Turnberg LA, Fox H, Longson M, Matthews MB, Das Gupta R. 1976. Chronic Q fever. *Quarterly Journal of Medicine* 45(178):193-217.

Turgut M. 2001. Spinal tuberculosis (Pott's disease): Its clinical presentation, surgical management, and outcome. A survey study on 694 patients. *Neurosurgical Review* 24(1): 8-13.

Tzekov R. 2005. Ocular toxicity due to chloroquine and hydroxychloroquine: Electrophysiological and visual function correlates. *Documenta Ophthalmologica* 110(1):111-120.

Vallejo JG, Stevens AM, Dutton RV, Kaplan SL. 1996. Hepatosplenic abscesses due to Brucella melitensis: Report of a case involving a child and review of the literature. *Clinical Infectious Diseases* 22(3):485-489.

van Woerden HC, Mason BW, Nehaul LK, Smith R, Salmon RL, Healy B, Valappil M, Westmoreland D, de Martin S, Evans MR, Lloyd G, Hamilton-Kirkwood M, Williams NS. 2004. Q fever outbreak in industrial setting. *Emerging Infectious Diseases* 10(7):1282-9.

Varney NR, Roberts RJ, Springer JA, Connell SK, Wood PS. 1997. Neuropsychiatric sequelae of cerebral malaria in Vietnam veterans. *Journal of Nervous and Mental Disease* 185(11):695-703.

Verdon R, Chevret S, Laissy JP, Wolff M. 1996. Tuberculous meningitis in adults: Review of 48 cases. *Clinical Infectious Diseases* 22(6):982-988.

Vynnycky E, Fine PE. 1997. The natural history of tuberculosis: The implications of age-dependent risks of disease and the role of reinfection. *Epidemiology and Infection* 119(2):183-201.

Walker J, Sharma OP, Rao NA. 1992. Brucellosis and uveitis. *American Journal of Ophthalmology* 114(3):374-375.

Wallace MR, Hale BR, Utz GC, Olson PE, Earhart KC, Thornton SA, Hyams KC. 2002. Endemic infectious diseases of Afghanistan. *Clinical Infectious Diseases* 34(Suppl 5):S171-S207.

Watson JT, Pertel PE, Jones RC, Siston AM, Paul WS, Austin CC, Gerber SI. 2004. Clinical characteristics and functional outcomes of West Nile Fever. *Annals of Internal Medicine* 141(5):360-365.

Wei LC, Chen SN, Ho CL, Kuo YH, Ho JD. 2001. Progression of hydroxychloroquine retinopathy after discontinuation of therapy: Case report. *Chang Gung Medical Journal* 24(5):329-334.

Weil Y, Mattan Y, Liebergall M, Rahav G. 2003. Brucella prosthetic joint infection: A report of 3 cases and a review of the literature. *Clinical Infectious Diseases* 36(7):e81-e86.

Weina PJ, Neafie RC, Wortmann G, Polhemus M, Aronson NE. 2004. Old world leishmaniasis: An emerging infection among deployed US military and civilian workers. *Clinical Infectious Diseases* 39(11):1674-1680.

WHO (World Health Organization). 1986. Joint FAO/WHO expert committee on brucellosis. *World Health Organization Technical Report Series* 740:1-132.

WHO. 2002. Strategic Direction for Research: Leishmaniasis. Geneva: World Health Organization.

WHO. 2003. *Africa Malaria Report 2003*. [Online]. Available: http://www.rbm.who.int/amd2003/amr2003/amr_toc.htm [accessed May 2, 2005].

WHO. 2004. Anti-Tuberculosis Drug Resistance in the World Report No. 3. Geneva: World Health Organization.

WHO. 2006a. WHO Report 2006: Global Tuberculosis Control Surveillance, Planning, Financing. Geneva: World Health Organization.

WHO. 2006b. *Tuberculosis Fact Sheet No 104*. [Online]. Available: http://www.who.int/mediacentre/factsheets/fs104/en/print.html [accessed May 1, 2006].

Wildman MJ, Smith EG, Groves J, Beattie JM, Caul EO, Ayres JG. 2002. Chronic fatigue following infection by Coxiella burnetii (Q fever): Ten-year follow-up of the 1989 UK outbreak cohort. *QJM* 95(8):527-538.

Willard RJ, Jeffcoat AM, Benson PM, Walsh DS. 2005. Cutaneous leishmaniasis in soldiers from Fort Campbell, Kentucky returning from Operation Iraqi Freedom highlights diagnostic and therapeutic options. *Journal of the American Academy of Dermatology* 52(6):977-987.

Williams RK, Crossley K. 1982. Acute and chronic hepatic involvement of brucellosis. *Gastroenterology* 83(2):455-458.

Wilson ME. 1991. *A World Guide to Infections: Diseases, Distribution, Diagnosis*. New York: Oxford University Press.

Wilson PE, Alker AP, Meshnick SR. 2005. Real-time PCR methods for monitoring antimalarial drug resistance. *Trends in Parasitology* 21(6):278-283.

Wortmann G. 2004. Pulmonary manifestations of other agents: Brucella, Q fever, tularemia and smallpox. *Respiratory Care Clinics of North America* 10(1):99-109.

Yebra M, Marazuela M, Albarran F, Moreno A. 1988. Chronic Q fever hepatitis. *Reviews of Infectious Diseases* 10(6):1229-1230.

Yechoor VK, Shandera WX, Rodriguez P, Cate TR. 1996. Tuberculous meningitis among adults with and without HIV infection. Experience in an urban public hospital. *Archives of Internal Medicine* 156(15):1710-1716.

Young EJ. 1983. Human brucellosis. *Reviews of Infectious Diseases* 5(5):821-842.

Young EJ. 1991. Serologic diagnosis of human brucellosis: Analysis of 214 cases by agglutination tests and review of the literature. *Reviews of Infectious Diseases* 13(3):359-372.

Young EJ, Tarry A, Genta RM, Ayden N, Gotuzzo E. 2000. Thrombocytopenic purpura associated with brucellosis: Report of 2 cases and literature review. *Clinical Infectious Diseases* 31(4):904-909.

Yu D, Kuipers JG. 2003. Role of bacteria and HLA-B27 in the pathogenesis of reactive arthritis. *Rheumatic Diseases Clinics of North America* 29(1):21-36, v-vi.

Zaks N, Sukenik S, Alkan M, Flusser D, Neumann L, Buskila D. 1995. Musculoskeletal manifestations of brucellosis: A study of 90 cases in Israel. *Seminars in Arthritis and Rheumatism* 25(2):97-102.

Zijlstra EE, Musa AM, Khalil EA, el-Hassan IM, el-Hassan AM. 2003. Post-kala-azar dermal leishmaniasis. *The Lancet Infectious Dieases* 3(2):87-98.

Zinneman HH, Glenchur H, Hall WH. 1961. Chronic renal brucellosis. *New England Journal of Medicine* 265:872-875.

6

DISEASES AND AGENTS OF SPECIAL CONCERN TO VETERANS OF THE GULF WAR, OPERATION IRAQI FREEDOM, AND OPERATION ENDURING FREEDOM

Several diseases and agents have been reported in the published literature or in the popular press to have infectious components and to have caused illnesses in veterans of the Gulf War, Operation Iraqi Freedom (OIF), and Operation Enduring Freedom (OEF). This chapter provides information on each of those diseases and agents—Al Eskan disease, idiopathic acute eosinophilic pneumonia, wound and nosocomial infections (for example, infections caused by *Acinetobacter baumannii*), mycoplasmas, and biologic-warfare agents.

AL ESKAN DISEASE

In the early 1980s, King Khalid of Saudi Arabia attempted to settle Bedouins in a group of villages, including one in Riyadh called Al Eskan (Korenyi-Both et al. 1992). However, the villages were never used until the US military came to the region for Operation Desert Shield (ODSh) and Operation Desert Storm (ODSt). The 316th Station Hospital personnel lived in Al Eskan village from January 12 until March 12, 1991. Korenyi-Both and colleagues observed among the troops a vague systemic illness (causing primarily respiratory symptoms) that they termed Al-Eskan disease or Desert Storm pneumonitis (Korenyi-Both et al. 1997; Korenyi-Both et al. 1992; Korenyi-Both et al. 2000). Their investigations ascribe the illness to an immune response to sand-particle exposure (Korenyi-Both et al. 1997; Korenyi-Both et al. 2000). However, the hypotheses and conclusions of those researchers have not been uniformly accepted and have generated considerable debate (Clooman et al. 2000; Kilpatrick 2000).

During ODSh and ODSt, about 697,000 US troops were deployed. It is not possible to determine the exact number of troops affected by Al Eskan disease. However, data on respiratory illnesses in troops are available; those data are summarized in detail in Chapter 4. Respiratory symptoms were more common in those with a history of lung disease, smoking, and longer deployment and they were more common in those with less outdoor exposure and most prominent in personnel who slept in air-conditioned facilities.

Among the 282 316th Station Hospital personnel who lived in the Al Eskan village, the prevalence of respiratory illness was 43% (Korenyi-Both et al. 1992). During the period September-March of 1992, the marines reported respiratory illness in 2.3% of troops, and the Air Force reported 2.6%. A brigade of a separate mechanized infantry (1,800 soldiers) conducted training in the same region of Saudi Arabia over five summer seasons and reported respiratory illness in 0.2% of the soldiers. Al Eskan disease or a similar illness has not been reported in troops deployed to OIF or OEF.

Description of Acute Illness

Al Eskan disease was first reported in 1992 (Korenyi-Both et al. 1992). The disease is characterized by sudden or insidious onset of chills, fever, sore throat, hoarseness, nausea and vomiting, and generalized malaise and then respiratory tract complaints, including increasingly severe dry cough or expectoration of tan sputum. Some patients experience symptoms of gastroenteritis. Physical findings are minimal, and x-ray pictures on occasion reveal "atypical pneumonitis". The disease appears to be self-limited, and less than 1% of patients with the complaints had a relapse. Systematic description and precise case definition of Al Eskan disease are unavailable.

Long-Term Adverse Health Outcomes

No data link Al Eskan disease to any specific chronic illness. In their initial report, Korenyi-Both et al. (1992) indicated that most patients had recovered within 6 weeks and that the relapse rate was less than 1%. They argued later that exposure to sand particles can serve as a source of pneumoconiosis and can stimulate a severe and perhaps chronic allergic immune response (Korenyi-Both et al. 1997; Korenyi-Both et al. 2000). They refer to such a chronic immune response as the "second phase of Al Eskan disease", which they imply might explain some of the health problems noted in Gulf War veterans (Korenyi-Both et al. 1997).

Pathogenesis

Military personnel deployed to the Persian Gulf are inevitably exposed to sand. Working at the Armed Forces Institute of Pathology, Irey (1994) reported birefringent sand particles in the lungs of some of 86 casualties from the Kuwait theater of operations. However, the author found no long-term lung inflammation.

Korenyi-Both et al. demonstrated that although many sand grains were agglomerated, 18% of the sample included dispersed particles in the range of 0.1-0.25 μm; such particles would be expected to bypass lung defenses (Korenyi-Both et al. 1992). The sand material was extremely rich in calcium and silicon. Sand from Iraq had a calcium-to-silicon ratio of 4.2:1, and sand from Kuwait had a ratio of 3.75:1 (Korenyi-Both et al. 1997). Both the size of the sand grains and their composition differ considerably from those of sand samples harvested from other sites (for example, sand taken from Hawaii). Cultures of the sand showed some filamentous fungi, yeast, and staphylococcal species. No mycobacteria or chlamydia specimens were recovered. Contamination of sand with weapons of chemical warfare has been proposed but not studied (Korenyi-Both et al. 2000).

Korenyi-Both et al. have argued that Al Eskan disease is most likely a form of acute silicosis aggravated by the pulmonary immune response and perhaps other genetic and environmental factors (Korenyi-Both et al. 1997; Korenyi-Both et al. 1992; Korenyi-Both et al. 2000). However, there are no clinical data to support that hypothesis and no reports of chronic lung disease consistent with silicosis in veterans.

Treatment

Korenyi-Both et al. (1992) indicate that cephalosporin antibiotics and expectorants were useful and that no response to the quinolone antibiotic ciprofloxacin was observed. Supporting data were not presented.

Summary

There is no evidence that the syndrome or disease observed in troops in Al Eskan village was caused by a communicable microbial pathogen. Indeed, Koryeni-Both et al. have argued that the disease is caused by exposure to the unique sand dust of the central and eastern Arabian Peninsula and in particular to the silica in the sand. They note that given the sand-mediated damage to helicopters in the fields and silicosis in Somali camels, sand-mediated disease in humans would be expected. More than 13 years have passed since the initial description of Al Eskan disease appeared in the literature, but little progress has been made in linking chronic respiratory diseases in military personnel to exposure to Persian Gulf sand.

IDIOPATHIC ACUTE EOSINOPHILIC PNEUMONIA

Idiopathic acute eosinophilic pneumonia (IAEP) is a syndrome characterized by a febrile illness, diffuse pulmonary infiltrates, and pulmonary eosinophila (Allen et al. 1989; Badesch et al. 1989; Philit et al. 2002). Patients with IAEP have no history of asthma, allergy, or chronic lung disease and no discernable infection. Relapse is uncommon after recovery.

Severe pneumonia was reported in 19 military personnel deployed in OIF, 10 of whom had IAEP (Shorr et al. 2004). Prospective surveillance from March 2003 to March 2004 led to detection of eight additional cases of IAEP (Shorr et al. 2004). Twelve patients required mechanical ventilation, and two died. Given that 183,000 personnel were deployed in Iraq during the study period, the incidence rate of IAEP was calculated as 9.1/100,000 person-years. Of the 18 patients, 15 were in the Army, two in the Navy, and one in the Marines; 16 were men. The peak incidence of IAEP was in the summer months.

Description of Acute Illness

Patients with IAEP present with fever, diffuse pulmonary infiltrates, cough, shortness of breath, and, not infrequently, respiratory failure. The case definition of IAEP requires recovery of pulmonary eosinophils in high concentration in bronchial lavage (Allen et al. 1989; Badesch et al. 1989; Philit et al. 2002). In six lavage specimens recovered from military recruits, eosinophils made up 24-75% of the cells recovered (Shorr et al. 2004). Peripheral blood eosinophilia may or may not be present and may increase during the course of illness (Shorr et al. 2004). Lung biopsies reveal acute and organizing alveolar damage with eosinophils filling alveolar and interstitial air spaces (Tazelaar et al. 1997).

Long-Term Adverse Health Outcomes

Most IAEP patients who survive the acute illness make a complete recovery. Twelve of 16 military IAEP survivors were evaluated 1-4 months after diagnosis; none required corticosteroid therapy (Shorr et al. 2004). Three patients reported mild residual dyspnea and one had wheezing. Pulmonary-function tests showed that forced vital capacity was 97% of predicted, and forced expiratory volume 94% of predicted. However, mean carbon monoxide diffusing capacity was 82% of predicted.

Pathogenesis

In many cases, IAEP has been associated with cigarette smoking and exposure to dust (Badesch et al. 1989; Pope-Harman et al. 1996; Rom et al. 2002). Shorr et al. (2004) found that the most common exposures in the IAEP-diagnosed military patients were cigarette-smoking (100%), exposure to dust or sand (94%), convoy operations (70%), and exposure to the local population (71%). However, cases were different from controls only in their tobacco exposure. All the patients were smokers and 14% were new smokers, whereas only 67% of controls were smokers and only two of seventy-two controls were new to smoking (OR 1.22, $p < 0.001$). Other investigators have related cigarette-smoking to IAEP (Badesch et al. 1989; Shintani et al. 2000; Watanabe et al. 2002).

Treatment

Corticosteroids are the mainstay of therapy for IAEP and most patients respond quickly to it (Allen et al. 1989; Badesch et al. 1989; Philit et al. 2002). Some patients with IAEP require mechanical ventilation.

Summary

Eighteen soldiers deployed to OIF developed IAEP. By definition, no causative pathogens were detected or implied by the immune response of soldiers with IAEP (Allen et al. 1989; Shorr et al. 2004). *Toxocara canis* and other helminthic pathogens known to produce eosinophilic pneumonia were specifically excluded (Roig et al. 1992; Shorr et al. 2004). Survey results failed to identify a common source of environmental, drug, or toxin exposure (Shorr et al. 2004). Rapid detection of this condition is essential for a positive outcome. IAEP would not be expected to have long-term adverse health outcomes.

WOUND AND NOSOCOMIAL INFECTIONS (INCLUDING INFECTIONS WITH *ACINETOBACTER* SPP.)

Soldiers can experience a wide variety of exposures to pathogens from explosives or combat (wound infections) or in health-care settings (nosocomial infections). Trends in casualty rates in modern US military warfare indicate rising wounded-to-killed ratios in the most recent wars (Department of Defense, 2005). Military personnel who might have been killed in an earlier era may now live to be hospitalized because of the use of body armor, better helmets, and more rapid emergency care. These soldiers with serious wounds can carry organisms of environmental origin (for example, from soil or water) into the hospital setting. Organisms of environmental origin that are prevalent in wound infections can colonize fomites and be transmitted to others via hospital personnel.

Nosocomial infections in military hospitals may have different microbial profiles from those in civilian hospitals in that they represent soil or water organisms prevalent in wounds suffered in explosions or combat. Nosocomial organisms that are familiar in civilian settings can also be seen in soldiers, given the conditions prevalent in intensive-care units (ICUs) and hospital wards when universal precautions are not adhered to.

Concerns Regarding *Acinetobacter baumannii*

One condition that is more prevalent in OEF and OIF troops than in civilian settings is infection with *Acinetobacter calcoaceticus-baumannii* complex, a well-recognized cause of wound infection in general and among military troops in particular (CDC 2004; Davis et al. 2005). The complex is also a cause of nosocomially-acquired infection when wounded, infected soldiers are intermingled with other patients in the ICU, emergency room, or hospital ward. *Acinetobacter* spp. infection has been discovered in wounds from OEF and OIF and in European and American hospitals because of nosocomial transmission (CDC 2004; Davis et al. 2005; Joly-Guillou 2005). It is likely that wound infections become a nidus for nosocomial transmission to others, particularly in an ICU setting, because of suboptimal handwashing by hospital personnel (Joly-Guillou 2005). *A. baumannii* is the species isolated most often.

Acinetobacter spp. infection was described decades ago as a cause of postsurgical urinary tract infections, but in the early 21st century is seen more often as an extremity wound infection, a respiratory tract infection, or bacteremia (CDC 2004; Davis et al. 2005; Joly-Guillou 2005). The human body louse has been reported to be a likely vector (La Scola and Raoult 2004). Multiple-drug-resistant *A. baumannii* has been reported in troops deployed in OIF and OEF (CDC 2004; Davis et al. 2005; Zapor and Moran 2005), in Israelis hospitalized in Tel-Aviv (Abbo et al. 2005), in patients in a Brazilian tertiary referral hospital (Reis et al. 2003), and in South Korean hospital patients (Lee et al. 2003). Environmental sources are ubiquitous, including soil and river water worldwide, including in the United States (Ash et al. 2002). Examples of extremity infections include osteomyelitis, postburn lesions, open fractures, and deep wounds. The origin of *Acinetobacter* spp. infection can therefore be the original soil contamination due to the injury, a hospital, or, very rarely, a community source unrelated to a known wound. A patient's history and epidemiologic circumstances can indicate which source is most likely to be responsible.

Although most *Acinetobacter* spp. infections are not life-threatening, multiple-drug-resistant strains are now prevalent among US military troops returning from OEF and OIF (CDC 2004; Davis et al. 2005). Extended use of combination antibiotics to which the organisms are sensitive was successful in curing all patients in a case series of 23 infected US soldiers reported in 2005 (Davis et al. 2005). Among the 38 isolates obtained from these 23 men, susceptibility varied from 3% to 29% for amoxicillin-clavulanate, cefepime, cefotetan, ceftazidime, ceftriaxone, ciprofloxacin, gentamicin, tobramycin, and trimethoprim and sulfamethoxazole. About half the 38 isolates were sensitive to amikacin and to ampicillin and sulbactam. Imipenem was effective against 89% of the multiple-drug-resistant strains. Colistin was effective against 100%, but only three isolates were tested (Davis et al. 2005). To minimize the risk of nosocomial *A. baumannii* spread, Iraqi-based US military facilities now isolate new wound patients until results of colonization swabs are known (Davis et al. 2005). Earlier generation antibiotics that are not in widespread current use (including colistin and polymyxin B) have been administered to multiple-drug-resistant *A. baumannii* patients. However, *A. baumannii* resistant to polymyxin B was reported in Brazil in 2003 (Reis et al. 2003).

The Brooke Army Medical Center experience in San Antonio suggested a median of 6 days and a maximum of 12 days between an OIF- or OEF-acquired war injury and the presentation of *Acinetobacter* spp. in a defined wound or bone infection (bone, draining purulence, or wound) (Davis et al. 2005). Of blood, urine, wound, or sputum specimens obtained from March 2003 to May 2004, 145 of 24,114 (0.6%) were positive for *Acinetobacter* spp. Among those sampled were 237 active-duty patients with injuries, 151 of whom had been deployed to OEF or OIF. Blood, wound, sputum, urine, and skin cultures were obtained on 84 of those deployed soldiers, and 48 of them (32%) were *Acinetobacter* spp.-positive. Thirty of the 237 patients were judged to have either wound injuries or related osteomyelitis; the wound or bone infections represented 63% of the culture positives, 36% of all OEF- or OIF-deployed men who were cultured and hospitalized, and 20% of all those with injuries who had been deployed to OEF or OIF. Those results demonstrate that *Acinetobacter* spp. is a common cause of wound infection or related osteomyelitis in men hospitalized for their war-related injuries from OEF and OIF. That no soldier had more than 12 days between injury and infection is informative, although a larger series would be needed to assess more accurately what a maximal incubation period might be.

Another contemporaneous case series of 102 patients with *A. baumannii* bacteremia was published; the cases presented in 2002-2004 at the Landstuhl Regional Medical Center (which accounted for about 78% of the patients), Walter Reed Army Medical Center (WRAMC), Brooke Army Medical Center (BAMC), National Naval Medical Center, and the US Navy hospital ship Comfort (Joly-Guillou 2005). The typical patient was a male soldier who experienced a traumatic injury in Iraq. In this multihospital series and the BAMC series, *A. baumannii* bacteremia was common in OEF and OIF returnees who were hospitalized for injuries, but it was rare before the start of OEF and OIF (CDC 2004; Davis et al. 2005; Zapor and Moran 2005). No late manifestations (months after injury) were reported in either case series (CDC 2004; Davis et al. 2005).

Death from *A. baumannii* is unusual. The only four deaths at WRAMC from 2003 to 2004 attributable to *A. baumannii* were in immunosuppressed patients whose ages were 35 years (renal transplantation and nosocomial pneumonia), 72 years (prolonged hospitalization with congestive heart failure), 78 years (diabetes and prior malignancy), and 84 years (in nursing home, mental status changes, and nosocomial pneumonia) (Zapor and Moran 2005). Fifty-three multiple-drug-resistant *A. baumannii* cases were seen at WRAMC in the 2003-2004 period, 34 in civilians and 19 in active-duty personnel. Zapor and Moran assert that successful reduction of risk to noncombatants and combatants alike who share hospital wards with infected combatants will require more rigorous universal precautions with thorough education of staff, patients, and family members.

Emerging infectious diseases, by definition, may arise from unanticipated sources. A previously unrecognized *Acinetobacter*-like organism from dog and cat bites was reported in 2002 (Kaiser et al. 2002). It is possible that organisms will emerge from southwest and south-central Asia that are not recognized as threats to soldiers or civilians. Hospital-based microbiologic and epidemiologic surveillance should be conducted on newly recognized organisms, as was done with the reports of drug-resistant *A. baumannii* in US military hospitals (CDC 2004; Davis et al. 2005).

Other Wound Infections

Nearly any war-theater injury, whether combat-derived or otherwise, may result in infection. The risk of infection is inherent in military service, training, readiness activities, transport, or combat (Zapor and Moran 2005). Men and women deployed to OEF and OIF face the risk of being injured by explosive devices of many types, including improvised explosives, mortars, and grenades. Torso injuries are less common than in prior conflicts because of widespread use of body armor, but it does not protect the extremities or head. Infections of skin and orthopedic wounds of the extremities are the most common reported causes of inpatient consultations for OEF and OIF returnees at WRAMC (Zapor and Moran 2005).

A BAMC wound-bacteriology survey was conducted in 2004 at a Combat Support Hospital in Baghdad, Iraq (Zapor and Moran 2005). It covered 49 soldiers who had 61 wounds, primarily blast injuries of the extremities. Eighteen of the soldiers (with 20 wounds) underwent wound lavage, had antibiotics administered at the time of the injury, or both. Of the 40 bacteria obtained from 30 wounds, most were obtained from soldiers before they received antibiotics. Gram-positive commensal skin bacteria, such as *Staphylococcus* spp. and *Micrococcus* spp. were found in 93% of isolates. Less common were gram-negative bacterial genera, such as *Pseudomonas, Chryseobacterium,* and *Escherichia*. Two isolates demonstrated broad antibiotic resistance; both were methicillin-resistant *Staphylococcus aureus*. To reconcile the differences in the bacteriologic profiles noted in this unpublished survey with those at stateside military hospitals (the latter see more *Acinetobacter* spp. and extended-spectrum β-lactamase-producing lactose-fermenters), Zapor and Moran recommended larger field hospital surveys from multiple locations, using best-practice sampling and microbiologic methods (Davis et al. 2005; Zapor and Moran 2005).

Wound infections occur shortly after the wounds themselves, with exceptions, such as infections associated with chronic osteomyelitis that are rare with modern medical care. Therefore, making an epidemiologic link to service in the war theater is rarely difficult. Current military medical practices include surgical debridement of wounds, probing of deep tissues, and cultures of wounds, bone, deep tissues, skin, and other fluids to find and treat infection. Such aggressive management prevents chronic osteomyelitis in the vast majority of wounded soldiers. If a stateside civilian, military, or Department of Veterans Affairs (VA) medical facility encounters chronic osteomyelitis, it is the one clear example of an infection that may result from underdetection and undertreatment or from hospital acquisition. That condition can theoretically manifest far from the war and later, although it will be rare, as judged from the near absence of modern case reports. Each case must be evaluated as to the epidemiologic, clinical, and microbiologic characteristics of the infectious disease to judge whether it is linked to the war or is community-acquired.

Other Nosocomial Infections

Many potential nosocomial organisms may go unrecognized if an outbreak is not apparent and not investigated. Observant clinical providers may reveal outbreaks that might otherwise be missed. For example, a nebulizer from a local manufacturer in Saudi Arabia caused an outbreak of *Burkholderia cepacia* in US National Guard troops deployed in the Middle East (Balkhy et al. 2005). US manufacturing adhering to Food and Drug Administration requirements would have been expected to virtually eliminate contaminated respiratory products for US troops, but the overseas pharmaceutical plant that made the inhalant medication was not under such scrutiny. Another example is a keratoconjunctivitis outbreak caused by adenovirus type 8 in troops in a hospital setting, but that may have been mistaken for a community-acquired organism if seen out of the context of the outbreak (Colon 1991). Given the relatively short time between exposure and symptoms, most nosocomial conditions would be associated temporally with active military duty in southwest and south-central Asia and would not present any confusion for stateside medical staff if the troops have not been disbursed; if they have been, the nosocomial origin of the condition might be masked by the "isolated" cases seen by many practitioners.

Other causes of nosocomial infections in OEF- and OIF-deployed troops and civilian military employees include those familiar in civilian settings, such as infections caused by methicillin-resistant *Staphylococcus aureus* (LaMar et al. 2003) and anaerobes (Brook and Frazier 1993). The origin of those infections (southwest and south-central Asia) is evident from the temporal association with deployment, as was the case in the 1991 Gulf War with Irish troops (Humphreys et al. 1988) and in the present conflicts among US troops (CDC 2004; Davis et al. 2005; Zapor and Moran 2005).

Returning soldiers may serve as a nidus of organisms that can infect others in the same hospital or rehabilitation unit. A number of prevention research projects have evaluated colonization rates, including those among family members of returning soldiers (Fishbain et al. 2003; Kenner et al. 2003). Unrecognized sources of contamination of the hands of hospital workers are also being investigated, for example, computer keyboards in an ICU (Bures et al. 2000). Nosocomial risks that have been recognized in US military facilities also may be of importance in the field setting, depending on the specific circumstances of the field hospital or clinic (Blatt et al. 1993; Conger et al. 2004; Cumberland and Jones 1987; John 1977; Lamarque et al. 1992).

Given the rarity of chronic infections related to wounds, the committee believes that unrecognized wound or nosocomial infections will pose a diagnostic dilemma for returning veterans only in the most unusual circumstances, such as a late-presenting osteomyelitis. A penetrating injury of an extremity (from stepping on a pressure-detonated mine) resulted in chronic osteomyelitis and later squamous-cell carcinoma in a Vietnam veteran in 1987 (Coy 1994). Cultures taken 20 years after the injury (and after 18 years of draining of a sinus tract) grew *Bacteroides fragilis, Proteus vulgaris, P. aeruginosa*, and *Enterococcus faecalis*; the patient had been treated with cleocin, erythromycin, and tobramycin (no culture sensitivity results were presented) (Coy 1994). No details were given as to why those complications were manifest and so unsuccessfully managed.

Regional Experiences in Non-Americans

A number of reports of *A. baumannii* and other wound infections have come from countries neighboring Iraq or Afghanistan. The reports may provide lessons that inform the care of US troops, especially in the evolution of antibiotic resistance in environmentally acquired *A. baumannii*.

In 2002, *A. baumannii* infection occurred in 21 patients in a trauma ICU in Qatar; the outbreak was attributed to poor infection-control management and environmental contamination (El Shafie et al. 2004). The organism was sensitive only to amikacin among 17 antibiotics tested, including the carbapenems (El Shafie et al. 2004). In a series of 36 patients infected with 38 strains of *A. baumannii* in January 2000-August 2001 in a Turkish teaching hospital, only the carbapenems and colistin were fully efficacious against all strains in the laboratory (Ayan et al. 2003). A devastating earthquake in the Marmara region of Turkey in 1999 resulted in the hospitalization of 630 trauma victims at one hospital, of whom 240 were hospitalized for more than 48 hours. Of the 240, 41 patients (17%) had 43 nosocomial infection episodes that resulted in analysis of 143 culture specimens. In the 48 specimens with positive results (34% of specimens), *A. baumannii* was most common (31%), followed by *S. aureus* (19%), *P. aeruginosa* (15%), *E. coli* (13%), *Klebsiella pneumoniae* (13%), other *Pseudomonas* spp. (6%), and *Stenotrophomonas (*now called *Xanthomonas) maltophilia* (4%) (Oncul et al. 2002). Mortality was high, and antibiotic resistance was common, including methicillin resistance in all nine *S. aureus* strains and resistance to all tested antibiotics, such as carbapenems, in two *A. baumannii* strains and one *P. aeruginosa* strain (Oncul et al. 2002).

In a 1999 outbreak, 12 of 170 (7%) ICU patients in a Turkish hospital acquired *A. baumannii* infection; of 25 strains isolated, all were carbapenem-resistant, and the ICU had to be closed and disinfected because of environmental contamination and continuing transmission (Aygun et al. 2002). Wound infections in a Saudi Arabian hospital were assessed in the hot summer months of an unspecified year, possibly 1994 or 1995; of 2331 wounds, 193 (8%) were infected with 283 bacterial strains, and the most prevalent organisms were *S. aureus* (35% of strains), *E. coli* (31%), *P. aeruginosa* (25%), and *Klebsiella* spp. (10%) (Abussaud 1996). Neonatal ICUs have also experienced multiple-drug-resistant *Acinetobacter* spp. infections in the Middle East; one series of seven Saudi neonates (of whom three died) demonstrated sensitivity only to imipenem and resistance to 12 other antibiotics tested (probably in 2002 or 2003) (Manzar 2004).

One hundred and fifty-seven patients (96% men) at a military hospital in Turkey in 1994-1999 were admitted because of maxillofacial fractures (Ortakoglu et al. 2004). The precipitating events were from traffic accidents (44%), combat (27%), falls (17%), work accidents (10%), and sports (3%). Infectious complications occurred in local wounds and with osteomyelitis due to delayed primary treatment or delayed evacuation. Organisms of concern were not detailed, nor were the treatment experiences of the infected patients.

In two ICUs in Saudi Arabia and Kuwait where gram-negative bacterial isolates were studied in 1994-1995, *A. baumannii* isolates made up 42 of 207 isolates from 172 patients; they were much more common in Kuwaiti isolates (33%) than in Saudi isolates (8%) (Rotimi et al. 1998). Detailed susceptibility testing suggested that all 42 *A. baumannii* isolates were sensitive to imipenem (both sites) and that all 33 isolates in Kuwait were sensitive to ciprofloxacin and 89% (eight of nine isolates) in Saudi Arabia (Rotimi et al. 1998).

War in Lebanon in 1984 was associated with *A. baumannii* infection in 36 patients with isolates obtained from sputum, wounds, blood, urine, ulcer swab, or vaginal swab (Matar et al. 1992); the organisms were largely sensitive to minocycline, imipenem, and ciprofloxacin at that time.

Osteomyelitis was common in 210 patients with maxillofacial injuries seen at the Mostafa-Khomeini Hospital in Tehran, Iran, during the 1981-1986 Iran-Iraq war (Akhlaghi and Aframian-Farnad 1997). Missile or blast hits accounted for 94% of cases, and motor-vehicle accidents 6%. Twenty-four persons (11%) had infectious complications: eight with mandibular and one with maxillary osteomyelitis, one with cervical abscess, six with foreign-body infections (four in silicone implants), and eight with other infections. The authors attributed the high incidence of osteomyelitis to the inability to evacuate and promptly treat patients with wounds, something that will occur only rarely in US military troops (such as in capture after injury with later release). No organisms or treatment approaches were presented in the Iranian series, although the surgical antibiotics used were limited to cephalotin, gentamycin, ampicillin, and penicillin.

Afghan guerrilla combatants and civilians seen in a Pakistani hospital in 1985-1987 also had very high wound- and bone-infection rates, which were attributed to the long time between injury and medical attention (Bhatnagar et al. 1992). In 1274 patient records reviewed, about 50% of the patients had musculoskeletal injuries. Comminuted fractures and foreign bodies were each seen in 6% of patients. Wound infections were seen in 14% of the men, and chronic osteomyelitis in 11%, most often in the femur or tibia. No microbiologic data or infection-treatment outcomes were reported.

Those experiences from non-Americans in Afghanistan, Iraq, and neighboring nations suggest that the experience of US military with *A. baumannii* and combat-related wound infections in southwest and south-central Asia is not unique.

Summary

Both wound infections and nosocomial infections are hazards for US personnel deployed to OEF and OIF. Given modern medical and surgical treatment and the ability to evacuate injured military personnel rapidly, most infections will be seen within days or weeks of wounds. Longer-term adverse health outcomes are possible but unlikely.

MYCOPLASMAS

Mycoplasmas are ubiquitous microorganisms found as commensal colonizers and as pathogens in plants, insects, and animals. They are the smallest known free-living organisms (150-250 nm) (Baum 2005; Murray et al. 2005). They are pleomorphic and filamentous and have a deformable membrane, which allows them to pass through filters that retain bacteria. They are fastidious and difficult to culture on cell-free media; at the same time, because of their common presence as nonpathogenic colonizers, they are common contaminants of cell cultures. The propensity for contamination of cell cultures can lead to false conclusions about the association of mycoplasmas with a variety of clinical syndromes (Baum 2005). Furthermore, the major antigenic determinants of mycoplasmas are glycolipids and proteins in the cell membrane, which are serologically cross-reactive with bacteria and human tissues (Murray et al. 2005). Mycoplasmas lack a cell wall, so they are resistant to antibiotics that inhibit cell-wall synthesis, such as penicillins, cephalosporins, and glycopeptides, for example, vancomycin. However, they have been shown to be sensitive to a variety of antibiotics that act at sites other than the cell wall, such as doxycycline, clindamycin, and quinolones (Hayes et al. 1993).

Taxonomically, mycoplasmas are assigned to their own class, Mollicutes. Mycoplasmas that can infect humans are members of the family Mycoplasmataceae. Sixteen species of mycoplasma have been found to colonize humans, and five of them have been associated with disease. *Mycoplasma pneumoniae* is a common cause of tracheobronchitis and pneumonia and can cause outbreaks in crowded settings such as would be found in military deployments (McDonough et al. 1996). *M. pneumoniae* has also been associated with numerous extrapulmonary manifestations, including a variety of rashes, cardiac abnormalities, aseptic meningitis and meningoencephalitis, and arthralgias. *M. hominis* has been associated with a variety of genitourinary infections (primarily pelvic inflammatory disease). *M. fermentans* (incognitus strain) and *M. penetrans* have been associated with a severe multisystem disease in both healthy people and people with AIDS (Lo et al. 1989). Culture of *M. fermentans* on cell-free media (which decrease the risk of contamination) has been extremely difficult, and this has led to controversy over whether the organisms are true pathogens or merely contaminants. *M. fermentans* has been found in the blood of 11% of HIV-seropositive patients but not in seronegative patients (Hawkins et al. 1992). Although Montagnier, codiscoverer of HIV, at one time postulated that *M. fermentans* and other mycoplasmas were cofactors for progression to

AIDS, no increase in prevalence of *M. fermentans* was seen with later-stage AIDS (Cotton 1990; Hawkins et al. 1992). The authors speculated that mycoplasmas may survive as colonizers of mucosal surfaces for many years and that acquisition may be related to high-risk sexual behaviors associated with acquisition of HIV infection.

Mycoplasmas and "Gulf War Illness"

There have been no reports of cases of *M. hominis* infection in troops deployed to southwest and south-central Asia. There are no published reports of cases of *M. pneumoniae* infection; however, search results from a Department of Defense Gulf War hospitalization database identified 5 cases of this infection (see Chapter 4). Nicolson and Rosenberg-Nicolson have suggested that many of the symptoms of "Gulf War Illness" (GWI) could be explained by "aggressive pathogenic mycoplasma infections, such as *Mycoplasma fermentans* or *Mycoplasma penetrans*, and they should be treatable with multiple courses of antibiotics, such as doxycycline (100-200 mg/day) or macrolides" (Nicolson and Rosenberg-Nicolson 1995). Nicolson et al. (2003) hypothesized that the source of the infections may have been contamination of the multiple vaccines received by troops before and during deployment. They noted a study by Steele (2000) that found chronic symptoms consistent with GWI in 34.2% of Gulf War veterans who reported receiving vaccines during the war, 11.5% of Gulf War-era veterans (people in the military in 1990-1991 who did not serve in the Gulf War) who reported receiving vaccines, and 3.7% of Gulf War-era veterans who did not receive vaccines. Steele suggested that vaccines used during the war may have contributed to GWI.

Nicolson et al. (2003) noted anecdotally that 55 of 73 Gulf War veterans with whom they spoke "indicated that they had good responses to doxycycline and eventually returned to normal duty." Nicolson et al. referred to an article by Lo et al. (1991), who discovered *M. fermentans* (incognitus strain), as evidence of the ability of the organism to cause chronic infections. Nicolson et al. further suggested that the presence of similar symptoms in family members supported the possibility of a transmissible agent. Nicolson and Nicolson (1996) reported a sampling of veterans with GWI and 21 healthy controls with a gene-tracking technique. The technique was designed by the authors to detect hybridization signals of *M. fermentans* DNA in nuclear fractions from the blood cells of subjects. Of 30 subjects, 14 had evidence of infection of leukocytes with this test method (65% were infected with *M. fermentans* only); 11 of the 14 responded to multiple cycles of antibiotics to which mycoplasmas are sensitive. Four of the successfully treated veterans were retested; results were negative for *M. fermentans* gene sequences. Further studies by Nicolson et al. (2002) using polymerase chain reaction (PCR) to detect mycoplasma found a 9-fold increase in mycoplasma infections and an 18-fold increase in *M. fermentans* compared with healthy control subjects. Other investigators have found similar rates of positivity in patients with chronic fatigue syndrome who had no exposure to multiple vaccinations or deployment to the Gulf War (Teixeira et al. 2006). Using their gene-tracking technique, Nicolson and Nicolson (1996) claim to have detected "highly unusual DNA sequences" that "included a portion of a retrovirus genome (the HIV-1 env gene), but not all of the genes that make up the virus." They speculated further that "the presence of the viral envelope gene in the mycoplasma could be due to genetic manipulation, or much less likely natural causes," and they went on to say that "the mycoplasmas that we have found in Gulf War veterans are not naturally occurring organisms, or to be more specific, they could have been genetically manipulated to be more invasive and pathogenic (potent biological weapons)."

Independent attempts to confirm the results of Nicolson and colleagues have been unsuccessful. Gray et al. (1999) studied serum from symptomatic and asymptomatic Gulf War veterans who had given prewar and postwar blood samples. They used immunoblot banding for *M. fermentans* at the University of Alabama Diagnostic Mycoplasma Laboratory, and none of the banding profiles was associated with reported symptoms in veterans. The study revealed that 10.9% of Gulf War veterans and 9.3% of nondeployed veterans who served in the military during the same period as the Gulf War veterans had prewar antibodies to *M. fermentans*. Of those without pre-existing antibodies, 19.2% of Gulf War veterans and 13.7% of nondeployed veterans developed serologic evidence of new *M. fermentans* infections.

A matched case-control study was conducted to determine the prevalence of *M. fermentans* antibodies in military personnel before and after Gulf War deployment and seroconversion rates in veterans with and without complaints of GWI (Lo et al. 2000). The study found a predeployment prevalence of *M. fermentans*-specific antibodies of 4.8% in veterans with GWI and 5.2% in controls; no difference in rates of seroconversion (1.1% in GWI cases and 1.2% in controls) during deployment was found. Lo et al. noted that their serologic test has been shown to be highly sensitive and specific and that most patients, including immunocompromised patients with AIDS, produce detectable species-specific antibodies to *M. fermentans*. That specificity suggests that the results are not an artifact of intracellular infections that do not yield antibody responses. Lo et al. also noted that "it is difficult to assess the validity and specificity of the NGT [nuclear gene tracking] testing [of Nicolson and colleagues, as discussed above], as there is no precedent for identifying any viral, mycoplasmal, or bacterial infection in clinical specimens using this uncommon technique."

A report prepared for the US Senate Committee on Veterans Affairs Special Investigation Unit on Persian Gulf War Illness stated in part that "*M. fermentans* has been at times suspected of causing various diseases in humans and, therefore, the center of some controversy" but that "this organism is considered to be a member of the normal human flora" (Dybvig, 1998). Dybvig noted that the NGT method used by Nicolson and colleagues was "an inappropriate diagnostic method for detection of *M. fermentans*" and that neither the specificity nor the sensitivity of the test had been established. He noted further that "*M. fermentans* DNA resides within the mycoplasmal cell and would not be present in the material assayed by this procedure, namely, host nucleoprotein." Dybvig also wrote that genetic engineering of *M. fermentans* was not technically feasible at the time of his report and certainly did not occur before the Gulf War.

Because of the conflicting data related to *M. fermentans* infections and their possible association with GWI and the suggestion of possible benefits of treatment with doxycycline, the VA conducted a randomized placebo-controlled trial to determine whether doxycycline given at 200 mg/day for 12 months could improve functional status of persons with GWI (Donta et al. 2004). In the trial, 491 deployed Gulf War veterans with GWI and detectable mycoplasma DNA in the blood were randomized to receive either doxycycline or a placebo for 12 months. Of the participants, 324 (66%) had an *M. fermentans* infection, 197 (40.1%) had an *M. genitalium* infection, and 53 (10.8%) had an *M. pneumoniae* infection, either singly or in combination as detected with PCR testing. Although a higher fraction of doxycycline participants than controls showed improvement at 3 months (21.5% vs 9.9%), there was no statistically significant difference at 9, 12, and 18 months. Overall, there was no statistically significant difference between the doxycycline-treated and placebo groups on the primary outcome measures. There was a trend toward fewer unscheduled clinic visits and hospitalizations among doxycycline-treated veterans than placebo subjects, but this was not related to the presence of mycoplasma infections. Rates of mycoplasma positivity decreased significantly during the 18-month study but did not differ between treatment and placebo groups. Specifically, 55% of the doxycycline-treated participants and 58.2% of the placebo subjects had negative results on tests for any mycoplasma species at 6 months of treatment, and 90% and 86.6%, respectively, had negative results at 18 months. Participants in the doxycycline group had a higher incidence of nausea and photosensitivity. The accompanying editorial by Wesseley (2004) noted that "we are fortunate that it was large enough and conducted diligently enough to give an unequivocal answer for both its primary and secondary end points. Doxycycline treatment has no effect on the health of symptomatic Gulf War veterans."

Summary

Several studies by Nicolson and colleagues report a link between *M. fermentans* and health problems in Gulf War veterans (Nicolson et al. 2002; Nicolson et al. 2003; Nicolson and Rosenberg-Nicolson 1995; Nicolson and Nicolson 1996). However, other investigators were not able to duplicate their work and there are concerns about the NGT technique used by Nicolson et al. (Dybvig, 1998; Gray et al. 1999; Lo et al. 2000). In addition, a well-conducted randomized placebo-controlled trial in which doxycycline was administered to veterans with GWI and mycoplasma infection did not improve the health status of the treated veterans (Donta et al. 2004). After reviewing the evidence on mycoplasmas, the committee believes that mycoplasma infection is not related to the symptoms reported by Gulf War veterans. Mycoplasmas are known to cause other types of acute and long-term adverse health outcomes, as noted in Table 3.1.

BIOLOGIC-WARFARE AGENTS

Biologic warfare (BW) is defined as the use of microorganisms or toxic products derived from microorganisms to inflict mass casualties in military and civilian populations (Horn 2003). Living microorganisms can multiply in a living target host and cause adverse health effects but require an incubation period of 24 hours to 6 weeks between infection and the appearance of symptoms (Rosenbloom et al. 2002). Toxins cannot reproduce themselves but are more lethal and act relatively quickly.

At the time of the Gulf War, Iraq had an active BW program. Iraq's BW program probably began sometime in the middle 1970s with studies on *Clostridium botulinum*, bacillus spores, and influenza virus (Leitenberg 2001; Roffey et al. 2002). In the middle 1980s, the program began "in earnest", and as many as 30 agents might have been investigated for potential use as biologic weapons (Roffey et al. 2002; Zilinskas 1997).

Iraq conducted intensive study of five bacterial strains (four strains of *Bacillus anthracis* and one of *Clostridium perfringens*), one fungal strain (wheat cover smut), five viruses (Congo-Crimean hemorrhagic virus, yellow fever virus, enterovirus 17, human rotavirus, and camelpox virus), and four toxins (aflatoxin, botulinum toxin, ricin, and tricothecenes) (Zilinskas 1997). *Bacillus anthracis*, aflatoxin, botulinum toxin, and possibly ricin were weaponized (Roffey et al. 2002; Zilinskas 1997). Iraq is reported to have manufactured almost 10,000 L of botulinum toxin during the 1980s and 1990s (Han and Zunt 2003).

Iraq developed bombs, missile warheads, aerosol generators, and helicopter and jet spray systems for dispersal of BW agents (Leitenberg 2001). Iraqi sources reported that aflatoxin, botulinum toxin, and *Bacillus anthracis* were loaded in missiles and air-delivery bombs in preparation for the Gulf War (Roffey et al. 2002). The comprehensive report of the special adviser to the director of central intelligence on Iraq's weapons of mass destruction states that "at a meeting of the Iraqi leadership immediately prior to the Gulf War in 1991, Saddam Husayn personally authorized the use of BW weapons against Israel, Saudi Arabia, and US forces" (CIA 2004). No evidence was found that Iraq deployed any weapons containing BW agents (Roffey et al. 2002; Zilinskas 1997).

After the Gulf War, Iraq was supposed to destroy all biologic agents developed for BW purposes. However, the United Nations Special Commission was not able to confirm that the destruction was complete (Zilinskas 1997). The Central Intelligence Agency reports that Iraq probably abandoned its BW program in 1995, although some BW-related seed stocks were discovered by US forces during OIF (CIA 2004).

Of the four BW agents that Iraq reportedly weaponized—aflatoxin, botulinum toxin, *Bacillus anthracis*, and ricin—only anthrax is a living microorganism and capable of multiplying in infected people. Although it is infectious, *Bacillus anthracis* has little potential for person-to-person transmission (Cieslak and Eitzen 2000). Aflatoxin, botulinum toxin, and ricin are toxins derived from microorganisms and cannot replicate.

SUMMARY

Al Eskan disease, mycoplasma infection, and exposure to BW agents have long been of concern to veterans of the Gulf War and have been proposed as possible causes of the veterans' health problems. IAEP and *A. baumannii* infections have been diagnosed in a number of military personnel serving in OIF and OEF. Having reviewed the data, the committee does not believe that Al Eskan disease and IAEP are caused by infectious organisms. Al Eskan disease might be caused by exposure to silica in the sand; the long-term adverse health outcomes of this disease are unknown. The committee does not expect that people who survive IAEP will experience long-term health outcomes related to that illness. Long-term adverse health outcomes from *A. baumannii* infections are unlikely to occur, given modern medical and surgical treatments. The evidence does not support mycoplasma infections as a cause of the symptoms reported by Gulf War veterans. No evidence has been found that Iraq deployed anthrax-containing weapons.

REFERENCES

Abbo A, Navon-Venezia S, Hammer-Muntz O, Krichali T, Siegman-Igra Y, Carmeli Y. 2005. Multidrug-resistant Acinetobacter baumannii. *Emerging Infectious Diseases* 11(1):22-29.

Abussaud MJ. 1996. Incidence of wound infection in three different departments and the antibiotic sensitivity pattern of the isolates in a Saudi Arabian hospital. *Acta Microbiologica et Immunologica Hungarica* 43(4):301-305.

Akhlaghi F, Aframian-Farnad F. 1997. Management of maxillofacial injuries in the Iran-Iraq War. *Journal of Oral and Maxillofacial Surgery* 55(9):927-930.

Allen JN, Pacht ER, Gadek JE, Davis WB. 1989. Acute eosinophilic pneumonia as a reversible cause of noninfectious respiratory failure. *New England Journal of Medicine* 321(9):569-574.

Ash RJ, Mauck B, Morgan M. 2002. Antibiotic resistance of gram-negative bacteria in rivers, United States. *Emerging Infectious Diseases* 8(7):713-716.

Ayan M, Durmaz R, Aktas E, Durmaz B. 2003. Bacteriological, clinical and epidemiological characteristics of hospital-acquired Acinetobacter baumannii infection in a teaching hospital. *Journal of Hospital Infection* 54(1):39-45.

Aygun G, Demirkiran O, Utku T, Mete B, Urkmez S, Yilmaz M, Yasar H, Dikmen Y, Ozturk R. 2002. Environmental contamination during a carbapenem-resistant Acinetobacter baumannii outbreak in an intensive care unit. *Journal of Hospital Infection* 52(4):259-262.

Badesch DB, King TE Jr, Schwarz MI. 1989. Acute eosinophilic pneumonia: A hypersensitivity phenomenon? *American Review of Respiratory Disease* 139(1):249-252.

Balkhy HH, Cunningham G, Francis C, Almuneef MA, Stevens G, Akkad N, Elgammal A, Alassiri A, Furukawa E, Chew FK, Sobh M, Daniel D, Poff G, Memish ZA. 2005. A National Guard outbreak of Burkholderia cepacia infection and colonization secondary to intrinsic contamination of albuterol nebulization solution. *American Journal of Infection Control* 33(3):182-188.

Baum S. 2005. Introduction to mycoplasma diseases. Mycoplasma diseases. In: Mandell G, Bennett J, Dolin R, Editors. *Principles and Practice of Infectious Diseases*. 6th ed. Philadelphia, PA: Churchill Livingstone. Pp. 2269-2271.

Bhatnagar MK, Curtis MJ, Smith GS. 1992. Musculoskeletal injuries in the Afghan war. *Injury* 23(8):545-548.

Blatt SP, Parkinson MD, Pace E, Hoffman P, Dolan D, Lauderdale P, Zajac RA, Melcher GP. 1993. Nosocomial Legionnaires' disease: Aspiration as a primary mode of disease acquisition. *American Journal of Medicine* 95(1):16-22.

Brook I, Frazier EH. 1993. Anaerobic osteomyelitis and arthritis in a military hospital: A 10-year experience. *American Journal of Medicine* 94(1):21-28.

Bures S, Fishbain JT, Uyehara CF, Parker JM, Berg BW. 2000. Computer keyboards and faucet handles as reservoirs of nosocomial pathogens in the intensive care unit. *American Journal of Infection Control* 28(6):465-471.

CDC (Centers for Disease Control and Prevention). 2004. Acinetobacter baumannii infections among patients at military medical facilities treating injured U.S. service members, 2002-2004. *Morbidity and Mortality Weekly Report* 53(45):1063-1066.

CIA (Central Intelligence Agency). 2004. *Comprehensive Report of the Special Advisor to the DCI on Iraq's WMD*. [Online]. Available: http://www.odci.gov/cia/reports/iraq_wmd_2004/chap6.html [accessed September 1, 2005].

Cieslak TJ, Eitzen EM Jr. 2000. Bioterrorism: Agents of concern. *Journal of Public Health Management and Practice* 6(4):19-29.

Clooman CC, Tenglin R, Butler F, Leitch RA. 2000. Six degrees of Kevin Bacon—Al Eskan disease and "dirty dust" *Military Medicine* 165(9):iv-v.

Colon LE. 1991. Keratoconjunctivitis due to adenovirus type 8: Report on a large outbreak. *Annals of Ophthalmology* 23(2):63-65.

Conger NG, O'Connell RJ, Laurel VL, Olivier KN, Graviss EA, Williams-Bouyer N, Zhang Y, Brown-Elliott BA, Wallace RJ Jr. 2004. Mycobacterium simae outbreak associated with a hospital water supply. *Infection Control and Hospital Epidemiology* 25(12):1050-1055.

Cotton P. 1990. Cofactor question divides codiscoverers of HIV. *Journal of the American Medical Association* 264(24):3111-3112.

Coy J. 1994. Combat injury with chronic osteomyelitis complicated by squamous cell carcinoma. *Military Medicine* 159(10):665-667.

Cumberland NS, Jones KP. 1987. Hospital acquired native valve endocarditis caused by Acinetobacter calcoaceticus and treated with imipenem/cilastin. *Journal of the Royal Army Medical Corps* 133(3):156-158.

Davis KA, Moran KA, McAllister CK, Gray PJ. 2005. Multidrug-resistant Acinetobacter extremity infections in soldiers. *Emerging Infectious Diseases* 11(8):1218-1224.

DOD (Department of Defense). 2005. *Principal Wars in Which the United States Participated U.S. Military Personnel Serving and Casualties A/.* [Online]. Available: http://www.dior.whs.mil/mmid/casualty/WCPRINCIPAL.pdf [accessed 2006].

Donta ST, Engel CC Jr, Collins JF, Baseman JB, Dever LL, Taylor T, Boardman KD, Kazis LE, Martin SE, Horney RA, Wiseman AL, Kernodle DS, Smith RP, Baltch AL, Handanos C, Catto B, Montalvo L, Everson M, Blackburn W, Thakore M, Brown ST, Lutwick L, Norwood D, Bernstein J, Bacheller C, Ribner B, Church LW , Wilson KH, Guduru P, Cooper R, Lentino J, Hamill RJ, Gorin AB, Gordan V, Wagner D, Robinson C, DeJace P, Greenfield R, Beck L, Bittner M, Schumacher HR, Silverblatt F, Schmitt J, Wong E, Ryan MA, Figueroa J , Nice C, Feussner JR. 2004. Benefits and harms of doxycycline treatment for Gulf War veterans' illnesses: A randomized, double-blind, placebo-controlled trial. *Annals of Internal Medicine* 141(2):85-94.

Dybvig K. 1998. Mycoplasma and illness. *Report of the Special Investigation Unit on Gulf War Illnesses*. Washington, DC: United States Senate Committee on Veterans' Affairs. Pp. 216-225.

El Shafie SS, Alishaq M, Leni Garcia M. 2004. Investigation of an outbreak of multidrug-resistant Acinetobacter baumannii in trauma intensive care unit. *Journal of Hospital Infection* 56(2):101-105.

Fishbain JT, Lee JC, Nguyen HD, Mikita JA, Mikita CP, Uyehara CF, Hospenthal DR. 2003. Nosocomial transmission of methicillin-resistant Staphylococcus aureus: A blinded study to establish baseline acquisition rates. *Infection Control and Hospital Epidemiology* 24(6):415-421.

Gray GC, Kaiser KS, Hawksworth AW, Watson HL. 1999. No serologic evidence of an association found between Gulf War service and Mycoplasma fermentans infection. *American Journal of Tropical Medicine and Hygiene* 60(5):752-757.

Han MH, Zunt JR. 2003. Bioterrorism and the nervous system. *Current Neurology and Neuroscience Reports* 3(6):476-482.

Hawkins RE, Rickman LS, Vermund SH, Carl M. 1992. Association of mycoplasma and human immunodeficiency virus infection: Detection of amplified Mycoplasma fermentans DNA in blood. *Journal of Infectious Diseases* 165(3):581-585.

Hayes MM, Foo HH, Kotani H, Wear DJ, Lo SC. 1993. In vitro antibiotic susceptibility testing of different strains of Mycoplasma fermentans isolated from a variety of sources. *Antimicrobial Agents and Chemotherapy* 37(11):2500-2503.

Horn JK. 2003. Bacterial agents used for bioterrorism. *Surgical Infections* 4(3):281-287.

Humphreys H, Bourke S, Dooley C, McKenna D, Power B, Keane CT, Sweeney EC, O'Morain C. 1988. Effect of treatment on Campylobacter pylori in peptic disease: A randomised prospective trial. *Gut* 29(3):279-283.

Irey NS. 1994. *Kuwait Casualties: Morphologic and Toxicologic Findings: The Persian Gulf Experience and Health.* NIH Technology Assessment Statement April 27-29.

John JF Jr. 1977. Nosocomial infection rates at a General Army Hospital. *American Journal of Surgery* 134(3):381-384.

Joly-Guillou ML. 2005. Clinical impact and pathogenicity of Acinetobacter. *Clinical Microbiology and Infection* 11(11):868-873.

Kaiser RM, Garman RL, Bruce MG, Weyant RS, Ashford DA. 2002. Clinical significance and epidemiology of NO-1, an unusual bacterium associated with dog and cat bites. *Emerging Infectious Diseases* 8(2):171-174.

Kenner J, O'Connor T, Piantanida N, Fishbain J, Eberly B, Viscount H, Uyehara C, Hospenthal D. 2003. Rates of carriage of methicillin-resistant and methicillin-susceptible Staphylococcus aureus in an outpatient population. *Infection Control and Hospital Epidemiology* 24(6):439-444.

Kilpatrick ME. 2000. Al Eskan disease and "dirty dust". *Military Medicine* 165(11):iii.

Korenyi-Both AL, Korenyi-Both AL, Molnar AC, Fidelus-Gort R. 1992. Al Eskan disease: Desert Storm pneumonitis. *Military Medicine* 157(9):452-462.

Korenyi-Both AL, Korenyi-Both AL, Juncer DJ. 1997. Al Eskan disease: Persian Gulf syndrome. *Military Medicine* 162(1):1-13.

Korenyi-Both AL, Sved L, Korenyi-Both GE, Juncer DJ, Korenyi-Both AL, Szekely A. 2000. The role of the sand in chemical warfare agent exposure among Persian Gulf War veterans: Al Eskan disease and "dirty dust". *Military Medicine* 165(5):321-336.

La Scola B, Raoult D. 2004. Acinetobacter baumannii in human body louse. *Emerging Infectious Diseases* 10(9):1671-1673.

LaMar JE, Carr RB, Zinderman C, McDonald K. 2003. Sentinel cases of community-acquired methicillin-resistant Staphylococcus aureus onboard a naval ship. *Military Medicine* 168(2):135-138.

Lamarque D, Garin D, Flechaire AO, Martignago C, Chapalain JC, Bartoli M. 1992. Incidence of nosocomial infections in a military hospital. *Presse Medicale* 21(24):1110-1113.

Lee K, Lee WG, Uh Y, Ha GY, Cho J, Chong Y. 2003. VIM- and IMP-type metallo-beta-lactamase-producing Pseudomonas spp. and Acinetobacter spp. in Korean hospitals. *Emerging Infectious Diseases* 9(7):868-871.

Leitenberg M. 2001. Biological weapons in the twentieth century: A review and analysis. *Critical Reviews in Microbiology* 27(4):267-320.

Lo SC, Dawson MS, Newton PB 3rd, Sonoda MA, Shih JW, Engler WF, Wang RY, Wear DJ. 1989. Association of the virus-like infectious agent originally reported in patients with AIDS with acute fatal disease in previously healthy non-AIDS patients. *American Journal of Tropical Medicine and Hygiene* 41(3):364-376.

Lo SC, Buchholz CL, Wear DJ, Hohm RC, Marty AM. 1991. Histopathology and doxycycline treatment in a previously healthy non-AIDS patient systemically infected by Mycoplasma fermentans (incognitus strain). *Modern Pathology* 4(6):750-754.

Lo SC, Levin L, Ribas J, Chung R, Wang RY, Wear D, Shih JW. 2000. Lack of serological evidence for Mycoplasma fermentans infection in army Gulf War veterans: A large scale case-control study. *Epidemiology and Infection* 125(3):609-616.

Manzar S. 2004. Outbreak of multidrug resistant Acinetobacter in the neonatal intensive care unit. *Saudi Medical Journal* 25(7):961-963.

Matar GM, Gay E, Cooksey RC, Elliott JA, Heneine WM, Uwaydah MM, Matossian RM, Tenover FC. 1992. Identification of an epidemic strain of Acinetobacter baumannii using electrophoretic typing methods. *European Journal of Epidemiology* 8(1):9-14.

McDonough C, Benjamin C, Gray GC. 1996. *Select Bibliography of Mycoplasma Pneumoniae Citations with Military Relevance*. Bethesda, MD: Naval Medical Research and Development Command.

Murray PR, Rosenthal KS, Pfaller MA. 2005. *Mycoplasma and Ureaplasma*. Medical Microbiology. 5th Edition. New York: Mosby Publishing.

Nicolson GL, Nicolson NL. 1996. Diagnosis and treatment of mycoplasmal infections in Persian Gulf War illness-CFIDS patients. *International Journal of Occupational Medicine, Immunology and Toxicology* 5:69-75.

Nicolson GL, Rosenberg-Nicolson NL. 1995. Doxycycline treatment and Desert Storm. *Journal of the American Medical Association* 273(8):618-619.

Nicolson GL, Nasralla MY, Haier J, Pomfret J. 2002. High frequency of systemic mycoplasmal infections in Gulf War veterans and civilians with Amyotrophic Lateral Sclerosis (ALS). *Journal of Clinical Neuroscience* 9(5):525-529.

Nicolson GL, Nasralla MY, Nicolson NL, Haier J. 2003. High prevalence of mycoplasma infections in symptomatic (Chronic Fatigue Syndrome) family members of mycoplasma-positive Gulf War illness patients. *Journal of the Chronic Fatigue Syndrome* 11(2):21-36.

Oncul O, Keskin O, Acar HV, Kucukardali Y, Evrenkaya R, Atasoyu EM, Top C, Nalbant S, Ozkan S, Emekdas G, Cavuslu S, Us MH, Pahsa A, Gokben M. 2002. Hospital-acquired infections following the 1999 Marmara earthquake. *Journal of Hospital Infection* 51(1): 47-51.

Ortakoglu K, Gunaydin Y, Aydintug YS, Bayar GR. 2004. An analysis of maxillofacial fractures: A 5-year survey of 157 patients. *Military Medicine* 169(9):723-727.

Philit F, Etienne-Mastroianni B, Parrot A, Guerin C, Robert D, Cordier JF. 2002. Idiopathic acute eosinophilic pneumonia: A study of 22 patients. *American Journal of Respiratory and Critical Care Medicine* 166(9):1235-1239.

Pope-Harman AL, Davis WB, Allen ED, Christoforidis AJ, Allen JN. 1996. Acute eosinophilic pneumonia. A summary of 15 cases and review of the literature. *Medicine* 75(6):334-342.

Reis AO, Luz DA, Tognim MC, Sader HS, Gales AC. 2003. Polymyxin-resistant Acinetobacter spp. isolates: What is next? *Emerging Infectious Diseases* 9(8):1025-1027.

Richards AL, Hyams KC, Watts DM, Rozmajzl PJ, Woody JN, Merrell BR. 1993. Respiratory disease among military personnel in Saudi Arabia during Operation Desert Shield. *American Journal of Public Health* 83(9):1326-1329.

Roffey R, Tegnell A, Elgh F. 2002. Biological warfare in a historical perspective. *Clinical Microbiology and Infection* 8(8):450-454.

Roig J, Romeu J, Riera C, Texido A, Domingo C, Morera J. 1992. Acute eosinophilic pneumonia due to toxocariasis with bronchoalveolar lavage findings. *Chest* 102(1):294-296.

Rom WN, Weiden M, Garcia R, Yie TA, Vathesatogkit P, Tse DB, McGuinness G, Roggli V, Prezant D. 2002. Acute eosinophilic pneumonia in a New York City firefighter exposed to World Trade Center dust. *American Journal of Respiratory and Critical Care Medicine* 166 (6):797-800.

Rosenbloom M, Leikin JB, Vogel SN, Chaudry ZA. 2002. Biological and chemical agents: A brief synopsis. *American Journal of Therapeutics* 9(1):5-14.

Rotimi VO, al-Sweih NA, Feteih J. 1998. The prevalence and antibiotic susceptibility pattern of gram-negative bacterial isolates in two ICUs in Saudi Arabia and Kuwait. *Diagnostic Microbiology and Infectious Disease* 30(1):53-59.

Shintani H, Fujimura M, Ishiura Y, Noto M. 2000. A case of cigarette smoking-induced acute eosinophilic pneumonia showing tolerance. *Chest* 117(1):277-279.

Shorr AF, Scoville SL, Cersovsky SB, Shanks GD, Ockenhouse CF, Smoak BL, Carr WW, Petruccelli BP. 2004. Acute eosinophilic pneumonia among US Military personnel deployed in or near Iraq. *Journal of the American Medical Association* 292(24):2997-3005.

Steele L. 2000. Prevalence and patterns of Gulf War illness in Kansas veterans: Association of symptoms with characteristics of person, place, and time of military service. *American Journal of Epidemiology* 152(10):992-1002.

Tazelaar HD, Linz LJ, Colby TV, Myers JL, Limper AH. 1997. Acute eosinophilic pneumonia: Histopathologic findings in nine patients. *American Journal of Respiratory and Critical Care Medicine* 155(1):296-302.

Teixeira MJ, Teixeira CR, Andrade BB, Barral-Netto M, Barral A. 2006. Chemokines in host-parasite interactions in leishmaniasis. *Trends in Parasitology* 22(1):32-40.

Watanabe K, Fujimura M, Kasahara K, Yasui M, Myou S, Kita T, Watanabe A, Nakao S. 2002. Acute eosinophilic pneumonia following cigarette smoking: A case report including cigarette-smoking challenge test. *Internal Medicine* 41(11):1016-1020.

Wessely S. 2004. The long aftermath of the 1991 Gulf War. *Annals of Internal Medicine* 141(2):155-156.

Zapor MJ, Moran KA. 2005. Infectious diseases during wartime. *Current Opinion in Infectious Diseases* 18(5):395-399.

Zilinskas RA. 1997. Iraq's biological weapons. The past as future? *Journal of the American Medical Association* 278(5):418-424.

APPENDIX

BIOGRAPHICAL SKETCHES FOR MEMBERS OF THE COMMITTEE

Robert E. Black, MD, MPH (Chair), is Edgar Berman Professor and chair of the Department of International Health at Johns Hopkins University Bloomberg School of Public Health. Dr. Black serves on a number of advisory boards related to international health and is chairman of both the Child Health and Nutrition Research Initiative for the Global Forum for Health Research and the Child Health Epidemiology Reference Group for the World Health Organization and United Nations Children's Fund. He received his MD from Hahnemann Medical College and his MPH from the University of California, Los Angeles. Dr. Black has served on the Board on Global Health and many National Academies committees, most recently on the Committee on the Middle East Regional Infectious Disease Research Program. He is an IOM member.

Martin J. Blaser, MD, is Frederick H. King Professor of Internal Medicine, chair of the Department of Medicine, and professor of microbiology at New York University School of Medicine. Dr. Blaser is president of the Infectious Diseases Society of America and cofounder and member of the Board of Directors of the Foundation for Gastrointestinal Mucosal Pathogens. He is a member of the editorial boards of numerous journals on infectious disease. He received his MD from New York University.

Richard D. Clover, MD, is professor and dean of the School of Public Health and Information Sciences at the University of Louisville. In addition, he is director of the Center for Deterrence of Biowarfare and Bioterrorism and associate vice president for health affairs and health informatics at the University of Louisville. Dr. Clover has been on several advisory panels and committees, including many on immunization practices for the Centers for Disease Control and Prevention. He received his MD from the University of Oklahoma.

Myron S. Cohen, MD, is J. Herbert Bate Distinguished Professor of Medicine and Microbiology, Immunology and Public Health at the University of North Carolina (UNC) School of Medicine. Dr. Cohen is the chief of the Division of Infectious Diseases and director of the UNC Center for Infectious Diseases. He has received numerous professional honors and awards and has served on committees for the Centers for Disease Control and Prevention and the International Society for Sexually Transmitted Diseases Research. He received his MD from Rush Medical College. Dr. Cohen served on the IOM Committee on HIV Prevention Strategies.

Jerrold J. Ellner, MD, is professor and chair of the New Jersey Medical School at the University of Medicine and Dentistry of New Jersey. Dr. Ellner has served on numerous advisory panels and committees for the National Institutes of Health and is a founding member and codirector of the Academic Alliance for AIDS Care and Prevention in Africa. He received his MD from Johns Hopkins University. Dr. Ellner served on the IOM Committee on the Evaluation of the Department of Veterans Affairs Uniform Case Assessment Protocol.

Jeanne Marrazzo, MD, MPH, is medical director of the Seattle STD/HIV Prevention and Training Center and associate professor in the Division of Allergy and Infectious Diseases in the

Department of Medicine at the University of Washington School of Medicine. She is a member of several national committees related to sexually transmitted infections and HIV/AIDS, including the Expert Consultants' Group for the Centers for Disease Control and Prevention's STD Treatment Guidelines and the Curriculum Committee for the Advancing HIV Prevention Initiative of the CDC. She also serves on the Institutional Review Board for the Program for Appropriate Technology in Health. Dr. Marrazzo received her MD from Jefferson Medical College and her MPH from the University of Washington.

Megan Murray MD, ScD, MPH, is assistant professor of epidemiology at the Harvard University School of Public Health and an infectious-disease physician at Massachusetts General Hospital. Her research focuses on using molecular and genomic epidemiology and mathematical modeling to understand the transmission dynamics of tuberculosis. She received her MD, ScD, and MPH from Harvard University.

Edward C. Oldfield III, MD, is professor of medicine, microbiology and molecular cell biology and director of the Division of Infectious Diseases at Eastern Virginia Medical School. Dr. Oldfield is chair of the Infection Control Committee and a hospital epidemiologist at Sentara Norfolk General Hospital. His clinical interests include tropical and travel medicine. He received his MD from the University of Virginia Medical School.

Randall R. Reves, MD, MSc, is professor of medicine in the Division of Infectious Diseases at the University of Colorado Health Sciences Center. Dr. Reves is medical director of the Denver Metro Tuberculosis Clinic of the Denver Public Health Department and is a member of the National Tuberculosis Controllers Association, of which he was president in 2003. His research experience includes participation in multicenter clinical research in the Centers for Disease Control and Prevention Tuberculosis Trials Consortium and Tuberculosis Epidemiologic Studies Consortium. He received his MD from the University of Texas Medical Branch and his MSc in Epidemiology from the London School of Hygiene and Tropical Medicine.

Edward T. Ryan, MD, is associate professor of medicine at the Harvard Medical School and director of the Tropical and Geographic Medicine Center at Massachusetts General Hospital. Dr. Ryan is an active member of two National Institute of Allergy and Infectious Diseases (NIAID) committees and has served on several other committees for NIAID, the American Society of Tropical Medicine and Hygiene, and the Centers for Disease Control and Prevention. His research focuses on enteric infections and the development of vaccines that protect against such infections. He received his MD from Harvard University.

Sten Vermund, MD, PhD, is professor of pediatrics, medicine, preventive medicine, and obstetrics and gynecology at the Vanderbilt University School of Medicine. He holds the Amos Christie Chair in Global Health and serves as director of the Vanderbilt Institute for Global Health. Dr. Vermund is an infectious-disease epidemiologist and pediatrician with substantial research and training experience overseas. From 1988 to 1994, Dr. Vermund was chief of the Vaccine Trials and Epidemiology Branch, Division of AIDS, at the National Institute of Allergy and Infectious Diseases. His work in HIV vaccine clinical-trial preparedness led to the 1994 Superior Service Award, the highest civilian honor in the Public Health Service. Dr. Vermund works on HIV prevention and care with support from the National Institutes of Health and the Centers for Disease Control and Prevention.

Dawn M. Wesson, PhD, is an associate professor in the Department of Tropical Medicine and Parasitology at Tulane School of Public Health and Tropical Medicine and director of the training program in Vector-Borne Infectious Diseases at Tulane University. Her research interests include the ecology of mosquito- and other insect-transmitted diseases and development of novel control and prevention strategies for those diseases. Dr. Wesson is past president of the Louisiana Mosquito Control Association, in which she remains a member of the Board of Directors, and past chair of the Medical and Veterinary Entomology Section of the Entomological Society of America. She received her PhD in medical entomology from the University of Notre Dame.

INDEX

A

B

D

E

F

G

H

I

K

L

M

S

T

Z